Global Clinical Trials Playbook

To my beloved wife Zewdi, my kids Winta Bairu, Dawit Bairu, my family and friends:
Over the last 25 years, Zewdi had and continue to be my steadfast and loyal supporter of my various personal and professional pursuits. There are not enough words to appropriately thank my wife's dedicated parenting of our two wonderful children, love, companionship, and our kids continuous encouragement in my various projects.

Menghis Bairu

This book is dedicated to my family, who have given me unwavering support throughout the years, and have been the source of strength and inspiration.

Richard Chin

Global Clinical Trials Playbook

Capacity and Capability Building

Edited by

Menghis Bairu

Elan Biopharmaceuticals, San Francisco, California, USA

and

Richard Chin

UCSF School of Medicine,
San Francisco, California, USA

Amsterdam • Boston • Heidelberg • London
New York • Oxford • Paris • San Diego
San Francisco • Singapore • Sydney • Tokyo
Academic Press is an imprint of Elsevier

Academic Press is an imprint of Elsevier
32 Jamestown Road, London NW1 7BY, UK
225 Wyman Street, Waltham, MA 02451, USA
525 B Street, Suite 1800, San Diego, CA 92101-4495, USA

First edition 2012

Notice
No responsibility is assumed by the publisher for any injury and/or damage to persons or property as a matter of products liability, negligence or otherwise, or from any use or operation of any methods, products, instructions or ideas contained in the material herein. Because of rapid advances in the medical sciences, in particular, independent verification of diagnoses and drug dosages should be made

British Library Cataloguing-in-Publication Data
A catalogue record for this book is available from the British Library

Library of Congress Cataloging-in-Publication Data
A catalog record for this book is available from the Library of Congress

ISBN : 978-0-12-415787-3

For information on all Academic Press publications
visit our website at www.elsevierdirect.com

Typeset by TNQ Books and Journals

Working together to grow
libraries in developing countries

www.elsevier.com | www.bookaid.org | www.sabre.org

ELSEVIER   BOOK AID
              International   Sabre Foundation

CONTENTS

v

CAPACITY BUILDING FOR GLOBAL CLINICAL TRIALS

Edited by
Menghis Bairu & Richard Chin

Prof Saleh A. Bawazir
Vice President for Drug Affairs, Saudi Food and Drug Authority,
and Prof of Clinical Pharmacy, College of Pharmacy, King Saud University.
Riyadh Saudi Arabia

Suzanne Gagnon MD, FACP
Chief Medical Officer, NuPathe Inc.

Douglas Love Esq
Executive Vice President, Head of Tysabri, Elan Biopharmaceuticals

Michael Makanga MD, PhD
Director South-South Cooperation and Head of Africa Office,
European & Developing Countries Clinical Trials Partnership (EDCTP),
Francie van Zijl Drive, Parow, P.O. Box 19070, Tygerberg 7505,
Cape Town, South Africa

Rubin Minhas MD
Editor-in-Chief: 'Clinical Evidence', 'Best Practice' & Clinical Director,
BMJ Evidence Centre, Clinical Director, BMJ Evidence Centre, BMJ Group ,
BMA House, Tavistock Square , London WC1H 9JR

Fidela Ll. Moreno MD
Visiting Professor, Faculty of Medicine and Surgery, University of Santo Tomas and Former
Vice President, Global Clinical Site Management and Monitoring, Allergan Inc.

Prof S.D. Seth MD, FAMS, FNASc, FIPS, FCAI, FISCD
Advisor, Clinical Trials Registry - India, National Institute of Medical Statistics,
Indian Council of Medical Research, Ansari Nagar, New Delhi - 110029, India

Yaw Asare-Aboagye
United Therapeutics, Durham, NC, USA

Mehtap Asenaoktar
Kuantum CRO and Logistics, Izmir, Turkey

Serdar Asenaoktar
Kuantum CRO and Logistics, Izmir, Turkey

Menghis Bairu
Elan Biopharmaceuticals, San Francisco, California, USA

Lesley Burgess
TREAD Research, Stellenbosch University, Tygerberg Hospital, Parow, South Africa

Herng-Der Chern
Center for Drug Evaluation, Taipei, Taiwan

Havana Chikoto
Triclinium Clinical Research, Sandown, South Africa

Richard Chin
UCSF School of Medicine, San Francisco, California, USA

James (Dachao) Fan
ICON Clinical Research Pte Ltd/Asia Pacific, Singapore

Suzanne Gagnon
ICON Clinical Research, North Wales, Pennsylvania, USA

Don Hayward
Triclinium Clinical Research, Sandown, South Africa

Jakub Hort
2nd Medical Faculty, Charles University and University Hospital Motol, Prague, Czech Republic, and International Clinical Research Center, St. Anne's University Hospital Brno, Brno, Czech Republic

Ankit Joshi
ECCRO, Mumbai, India

Lynn Katsoulis
The Aurum Institute, Parktown, South Africa

Elizabeth Messersmith
R & D Operations, Balance Therapeutics, Inc USA

Bogdan O. Popescu
University Hospital, "Carol Davila" University of Medicine and Pharmacy, Bucharest, Romania

Philip Scheltens
VU University Medical Center, Amsterdam, The Netherlands

ix

Peter Schueler
ICON Clinical Research, Langen, Hessen, Germany

Victor Strugo
Triclinium Clinical Research, Sandown, South Africa

Quintin Van Wyk
ICON Clinical Research Pte Ltd, Hampshire, UK

Nermeen Varawalla
ECCRO, London, UK

Dong Wei
Janseen Alzheimer Immunotherapy R&D, LLC, South San Francisco, California, USA

Janice B. Wilson
Wilson Quality & Compliance Consulting, Antioch, California, USA

Zhijie Xia
ICU Department, Shanghai Huashan Hospital, Fudan University, Shanghai, China

Juncai (Jack) Xu
Shanghai Clinical Research Center, Shanghai, China

Jing Yin
Covance Central Laboratory Services, Singapore

Clinical Trials

CHAPTER 1

Introduction

Menghis Bairu
Elan Biopharmaceuticals, San Francisco, California, USA

Wherever in the world we stand, the majority of clinical trials are being conducted somewhere else in the world, under a different regulatory framework and in different cultural settings. However, we all rely on the same trials to make decisions; as regulators, to allow or disallow marketing authorizations, and, as patients and healthcare providers, to use or not to use a medicine.

Fergus Sweeney, Head of Inspections at the European Medicines Agency (September 2010)

Thirty years ago, the United States Food and Drug Administration (FDA) formalized a process for the inclusion of data derived from clinical trials conducted overseas that could be included in a new drug application (NDA) submitted for marketing approval by pharmaceutical sponsors. The impetus for this new FDA guideline derived from clinical trials being sponsored by US government agencies, academic research medical centers, and US pharmaceutical companies which were being conducted outside the USA. At that time, 41 foreign clinical investigators were conducting drug research under an investigational new drug application. By 1999, over 4400 foreign investigators were participating in US-sponsored research, and by 2008, more than 200,000 patients were enrolled in over 6500 research sites outside the USA for over 80 percent of the NDAs submitted to the FDA that year.

This trend in globalization of clinical trial research was by no means limited to regulatory submissions in the USA. During the years 2005–2009, registration studies submitted to the European Medicines Agency (EMA) involved more than 44,000 investigator sites in 89 countries. Only 38.8 percent of patients within the European Union or European Economic Area were enrolled in studies sponsored by local institutions. The remainder of patients were recruited offshore.

The forces that have driven the globalization of clinical trial research are multifactorial, with potential benefit for patients, sponsors, local communities, and foreign governments. Government-, non-government-, and pharmaceutical industry-sponsored research conducted in emerging nations reflects the desire to study medicines in populations with locally endemic diseases and infections which may also be found in developed countries. In addition, for pharmaceutical companies that anticipate selling in key global markets, the impetus to use overseas study sites undoubtedly reflects the potential to reduce operational costs and recruit larger numbers of drug-naïve patients over shorter periods, while establishing a research and marketing presence in these developing countries.

Nevertheless, the globalization of clinical trial research has revealed significant challenges, especially in developing countries, with regard to understanding good clinical practice, informed consent, patient safety, ethics review capacity, access to medical equipment, integrity of acquired data, and regulatory oversight. Low- and middle-income countries in which clinical trials are conducted vary substantially in the extent of their capabilities and experience with clinical trial research. Many developing countries have limited or no institutional regulatory infrastructure and ethics review boards to oversee the conduct of clinical trials at globally accepted standards. Local clinical investigators have varying degrees of skill, training, and experience requisite to supervise the conduct of a clinical trial. The extent of understanding and sophistication of patients, coupled with local cultural idiosyncrasies, affects informed consent, study participation, and overall expectations.

Recognition of these challenges over the past decade has led to a variety of publications, workshops, training programs, and guidelines in an effort to enhance the quality of the clinical trial enterprise in developing countries. Key stakeholders, including regulatory agencies in developed nations, the Word Health Organization (WHO), ministries of health, academia, the pharmaceutical industry, non-governmental organizations (NGOs), contract research organizations (CROs), and non-profit foundations, have forged a variety of partnerships to advance the quality of clinical research. For example, the Strategic Initiative for Developing Capacity in Ethical Review (SIDCER) was organized in 2001 "… to develop competent, independent, in-country decision making for promoting responsible conduct of human research and to monitor the quality and effectiveness of ethical review worldwide, with mutual understanding and respect for cultural, regional and national differences". The European and Developing Countries Clinical Trials Partnership (EDCTP) was created in 2003 "… to accelerate the development of new or improved drugs, vaccines, microbicides and diagnostics against HIV/AIDS, malaria and tuberculosis, with a focus on phase II and III clinical trials in sub-Saharan Africa". The US FDA holds ongoing training programs such as "Train the Trainer Good Clinical Practices", to enhance the regulatory oversight of clinical trials in various regions around the world. Although these examples illustrate the enormous strides that have been taken to improve the quality of clinical trials conducted in developing nations, there has yet to be the consolidation of best practices regarding the various components of the clinical research enterprise that may be resourced for establishing high-quality clinical research institutions.

This book was written to provide resources under one cover which elucidate the various elements required for the successful implementation of clinical trials in developing countries. For the first time, the reader has a practical manual for developing and enhancing the infrastructure and processes required to conduct clinical research in developing countries. This book is divided into eight sections addressing the essential aspects of how to build and enhance global clinical trials capacity in emerging markets and developing countries. In Section 1, an introduction to the subject of global clinical trials is provided, with a focus on design and planning. The African perspective of appropriate and necessary training in good clinical practice of all personnel involved in conducting clinical trials, in both urban and rural locales in African countries, is discussed. Clinical trial site capabilities and the importance of establishing adequate standard operating procedures in sub-Saharan Africa are discussed, while addressing the challenges of informed consent, clinical execution by principal investigators and staff, partnering with local pharmacy, and processing of laboratory specimens, practices that should be intended to endure from trial to trial. Building and strengthening clinical trial site capabilities and capacity in other developing/emerging markets, including India, China, Eastern Europe, Singapore, and Turkey, are covered in Section 2. Partnering with the right contract research organization is a vital component in conducting a successful clinical trial; the different perspectives of working with global and niche CROs and the options available for choosing a CRO when conducting an overseas clinical trial are presented. The final chapters of this section provide the reader with guidelines for prioritizing clinical trial research based on national interests, as well as addressing the management of resources, budgets, and personnel, with an emphasis on future planning to sustain the clinical research enterprise locally.

Section 3 provides a roadmap for local regulatory agencies to build and enhance their capacity to evaluate investigative new drug and NDA applications, with recommendations of best practices to develop the regulatory capacity for the monitoring, oversight, enforcement, and approval of clinical trials. Section 4 addresses the establishment of infrastructure, operating procedures, and personnel training for pharmacovigilance and risk management by local government agencies.

The challenges and opportunities for outsourcing of electronic data collection and data management in developing countries, with examples of best practices for minimizing data dilution, are presented in Section 5. Section 6 contains a chapter dealing with the important concept of the establishment and maintenance of highly functioning investigational review boards, with special consideration of vulnerable populations in developing nations. The critical importance of identifying local talent, optimizing recruitment and retention of staff to ensure continuity during a clinical trial and from trial to trial, and the means for ensuring the protection of intellectual property are also discussed. Section 7 addresses best practices and challenges for acquiring and managing clinical data of high quality through strategic planning, and the process and preparation for external monitoring by sponsors and regulatory agencies. Finally, in Section 8 (Appendices), samples of study protocol, a consent form, job descriptions, case report forms, and a statistical analysis plan, as well as the International Committee on Harmonisation (ICH) guidelines, are provided.

This book is the first of its kind to provide guidelines and best practices to the reader for enhancing the capacity of developing countries to participate in clinical trial research at the highest level. As a complement to the recently published *Global Clinical Trials: Effective Implementation and Management* by the same authors, this book is aimed at individuals in the WHO, ministries of health, pharmaceutical companies, clinical researchers in academia, non-profit organizations such as the Bill and Melinda Gates Foundation, the World Bank, and NGOs who are involved in clinical research around the world, and will serve as a vital reference for anyone interested in building and enhancing clinical and research capacity in developing countries.

CHAPTER 2

Global Clinical Trials: Study Design and Planning

Richard Chin
UCSF School of Medicine, San Francisco, California, USA

Material in this chapter is based on or excerpted with permission from Chin and Lee.[1]

INTRODUCTION

The design of any study has direct effects on the execution of the study and the quality of the study results. A well-designed and well-written study protocol is clear on the inclusion and exclusion criteria, and it is clear on the procedures to be followed. It does not demand unreasonable or infeasibly stringent criteria on schedules and procedures to be followed, and it takes into account the limitations that the site may face. Such a protocol facilitates a smoothly run study. A well-designed study also makes it possible to interpret the results and draw clear conclusions.

This chapter discusses the fundamentals of clinical study design and planning. This material is drawn from and is discussed in more detail in Chin and Lee.[1]

While the fundamentals of good study design are the same for studies conducted in developed and developing countries, there are several considerations that must be taken into account when conducting trials in developing countries.

First, there are clinical practice differences between countries. A patient with congestive heart failure may receive different care in different countries. Standards of care can differ significantly even within the same country depending on geography and the social and economic strata of the patients.

Second, there are genetic, dietary, and other differences in populations between different countries. Genetic or dietary differences may result in different responses to drugs, including metabolic differences. Another difference is variation in weight. Patients in developing countries who have a lower caloric intake may have smaller statures and lower rates of obesity. Rates of background diseases, including tuberculosis, can vary from country to country.

In some countries, many of the women of childbearing age may be pregnant or nursing, making it difficult to recruit young women if exclusion criteria exclude pregnant and nursing women. It is important to carefully assess the differences and to determine whether such differences may require revisions in the study design.

Third, there may be regulatory differences between countries and jurisdictions. Laws on privacy, collection of genetic material, and other issues may vary from country to country and may require changes in the study. In some jurisdictions, there is a requirement that the sponsor pay for all medical care for the patient. In some cases, the ethical considerations may require additional prudence, as discussed in Chapter 15.

Fourth, the facilities and training of the investigators and the site personnel may limit the types of studies and procedures that can be performed. For example, magnetic resonance imaging (MRI) is not widely available in many countries. Many sites may not have ready access to a nearby acute care facility for adverse events. In rural areas, reliable electricity may not be available, necessitating that diesel generators be provided. However, in developing countries, the principal investigator may be much more actively involved in the study than in developed countries, and sometimes, therefore, a more complicated study is possible. In addition, clinical diagnostic skills such as auscultation and ophthalmic examination skills may be much more sophisticated in a setting where echocardiograms and other types of diagnostic machine are not readily available.

Fifth, transportation in developing countries, especially in rural areas, can be challenging. A patient may need to walk for an entire day to reach the clinic. In such cases, studies that are normally outpatient may need to be conducted as inpatient studies. Communication can sometimes be a challenge as well, but the availability of cellphones is now almost ubiquitous and contacting sites and patients has become significantly less challenging.

Sixth, cultural and national calendars may make it difficult to conduct studies during certain periods. Just as it is difficult to recruit patients during August in France, recruiting patients during Ramadan in Muslim countries or during October in India can be a challenge.

Being aware of the potential issues and working with the local medical director, contract research organization (CRO), or investigator during the design of the study will make the study much more likely to succeed.

PRINCIPLES OF CLINICAL STUDY DESIGN

There are three key parameters in the design of a clinical trial: endpoint, dosing, and patient selection. Although there are multiple additional parameters that can be modified in a trial, these three account for nearly all of the differences between study designs that lead to success and those that do not.

Endpoint

The first critical factor, endpoint, is the clinical or surrogate item that you are assessing to determine whether the drug or intervention is effective. This item can be a disease characteristic, health state, symptom, sign, or test (e.g. laboratory, radiological) results. Regulatory agencies base drug and device approval decisions on clinical trial endpoints. Early in the development and evaluation of an intervention, endpoints are used to determine the safety and biological activity of an intervention. Later on, endpoints help investigators to decide whether a drug provides a clinical benefit.

There are several key characteristics of a good clinical endpoint. It should:

- be clinically relevant
- closely and comprehensively reflect the overall disease being treated
- be rich in information

- be responsive (sensitive and discriminating, with good distribution)
- be reliable (precise and reproducible, with low variability), even across studies
- be robust to dropouts and missing data
- not influence the treatment response or have a biological effect in and of itself
- be practical (implementable at different sites, measurable in all patients, economical, and non-invasive).

The endpoint must closely and comprehensively reflect the overall disease being treated, and it must be clinically relevant. An endpoint that only captures one aspect or component of a disease may not suffice. For example, if the disease being treated were systemic lupus erythematosus (SLE), an endpoint focusing just on skin manifestations may miss the cardiac, pulmonary, and renal manifestations of lupus. If the intention of the therapy were to improve the overall status of a patient with SLE, a skin manifestations measure would be an inappropriate endpoint. However, if the drug were only intended to improve skin manifestations, this endpoint may be acceptable.

One of the most important aspects of selecting and defining an endpoint is its clinical relevance. The most sensitive and reliable measure is of little use if the results do not have clinical meaning or cannot be extrapolated to an endpoint that has clinical meaning. Clinical relevance is dependent on several factors, including the importance of the endpoint being measured, the magnitude of the change, and functional outcome. Ultimately, though, what is clinically relevant is what matters to the patient.

The choice of clinically relevant endpoints often depends on the type of disease. What is relevant to one disease may not be relevant to another disease. Reduction in symptoms would be a better endpoint than mortality for acute, self-limited, non-fatal diseases such as seasonal allergies or colds; but mortality would be a more appropriate endpoint for potentially rapidly fatal diseases such as aneurysm ruptures or myocardial infarctions.

The endpoint should capture enough appropriate information that can be used to analyze and to draw appropriate conclusions, and it should be responsive. In general, knowing more useful information is better. For example, knowing the actual cardiac ejection fraction by percentage is usually better than just knowing whether the ejection fraction was normal or reduced.

Responsiveness (i.e. sensitivity of the measure to actual changes in a phenomenon) is a critical characteristic of a good endpoint. When there is a change in the phenomenon, the value of the endpoint should change as well.

Endpoints with good responsiveness (i.e. large changes in the endpoints when the phenomenon changes) allow smaller sample sizes and permit a better estimate of the clinical benefit. Of course, when the endpoint is too sensitive, it may detect too many small clinically insignificant changes, such as a three percent decrease in tumor size or a six-hour increase in the median survival. The key is balancing responsiveness and clinical significance.

The endpoint should be reliable. Reliability is the "consistency" or "repeatability" of the endpoint. Repeated measurements for an endpoint should produce similar values, i.e. the endpoint should be reproducible and verifiable. The measurement should not vary significantly depending on who measures it.

The endpoint should be robust to dropouts and missing data. Patients will drop out of trials. Data will be lost. So you will have to predict what measurements would have been. For example, all-cause mortality is relatively robust to a few dropouts because you may count dropouts as deaths. However, frequency of flare is not robust because you cannot predict how many flares dropouts would have had during the study.

Finally, the endpoint should not influence treatment response or have a biological effect on the patient; the endpoint should be practical from an implementation, economic, and patient comfort standpoint.

Surrogate endpoints are measures that correlate with and can replace measuring clinically important outcomes in a trial. They include:

- pharmacokinetic/pharmacodynamic measures
- in vivo biomarkers (e.g. CD4 count, viral load, glucose level, cholesterol level)
- clinical surrogates (e.g. blood pressure)
- ex vivo measures
- minimal inhibitory concentration (MIC) of an antibacterial agent
- adenosine diphosphate (ADP)-induced platelet aggregation inhibition
- non-clinical measures [e.g. forced expiratory volume in 1 second (FEV_1), radiographic findings].

Surrogate endpoints are used when it is not practical or feasible to use real clinical outcome endpoints. It may take too much time (when the outcome occurs in the distant future) or too many patients (when the outcome is relatively uncommon) to see a real clinical outcome endpoint. They are also used when it may be too costly or cause too much discomfort to measure a real clinical outcome.

Surrogate endpoints commonly guide treatment decisions in clinical practice; for example, a 95 percent stenosis in a coronary artery may lead to a percutaneous coronary intervention, high glycosylated hemoglobin levels may lead to an increase in the insulin dose, and active urine sediment may precipitate aggressive immunosuppression in a lupus patient. Therefore, many clinical trials use surrogate endpoints, and their results often can drive clinical practice.

> ### BOX 2.1 EXAMPLE OF A FAILED SURROGATE ENDPOINT: CARDIAC ARRHYTHMIA SUPPRESSION TRIAL (CAST) STUDY
>
> High rates of premature ventricular contractions (PVCs) are predictive of sudden death after myocardial infarction. Several drugs were developed with suppression of PVCs as the goal, with the ultimate goal of reducing death after myocardial infarction. The CAST study was initiated in 1987 with flecainide, moricizine, and encainide, which had been shown to be highly effective at reducing PVCs. At initiation of the trial, there was debate over whether it was ethical to randomize patients to placebo when the drugs had been demonstrated to reduce PVCs. In all, 2309 patients were randomized.
>
> The Data Safety Monitoring Board (DSMB) stopped the study early because the patients receiving antiarrhythmic therapy had an unacceptably high mortality. The relative risk (RR) of death and non-fatal events at 10 months was 4.6 in favor of placebo.
>
> As an aside, the rate of mortality seen in the antiarrhythmic group was lower than historical controls. If it had been deemed unethical to conduct a placebo-controlled trial, then we might still be using these drugs in post-myocardial infarction patients.

However, a surrogate endpoint is never as informative as the clinical endpoint, and in many instances, surrogate endpoints have turned out not to be predictive of clinical response at all. For example, antiarrhythmics that prevent premature ventricular contractions have actually increased mortality. Some drugs that lower blood pressure do not lower the risk of cardiovascular problems. Moreover, a surrogate endpoint that works for one drug may not for another drug with a different mechanism of action. As a result, regulatory authorities and many clinicians insist on clinical rather than surrogate endpoints.

Dosing

The second critical parameter in clinical study design is dosing. A dose is the amount of an intervention administered. There are several aspects to dosing: the amount of dosing can vary; the route of administration can vary (oral, intravenous, subcutaneous, etc.); the dosing interval can vary; and, for interventions that are administered over a long period, the rate and duration of administration can vary. Infusing 500 mg of a medication over 10 minutes (which may result in higher levels of medication in the blood at a given time) can be very different from infusing 500 mg over one hour (which may result in lower levels over a longer period).

The overall goal of dose selection, exploration, and characterization is not just to identify doses that are safe and effective but also to paint a comprehensive picture of:

- the relationships between dose and different efficacy, safety, and convenience parameters
- the parameters that affect these relationships
- the dosing regimens that appropriately balance efficacy and safety.

Researchers need to understand fully how different doses behave in a wide variety of situations, such as the distribution of efficacy and toxicity in the population and whether the patients experiencing adverse events are those exhibiting a response. Being able to predict (if possible) which patients will respond and which will suffer toxicity would allow clinicians to select the right doses and appropriate measures to avoid or alleviate adverse effects.

Designing appropriate dosing regimens requires close collaboration with pharmacokineticists, toxicologists, and preclinical scientists. Data from preclinical experiments such as animal, modeling, and pharmacokinetic data help to determine the dosing interval and the initial doses in early clinical development. Later on in clinical development, the clinical efficacy and safety profiles from early-phase studies play a much larger role in guiding dose selection, but understanding pharmacokinetics, toxicology, and preclinical information is still important.

When great heterogeneity in patient response or a narrow therapeutic window exists, any number of methods may have to be used to customize the dose.

- **Dosing by baseline characteristic.** Customizing doses by baseline physiological factors is the most common method. For example, if you find that drug response varies by patient weight, you may have to give heavier patients higher doses than lighter patients.
- **Titrating to an endpoint.** An alternative method is choosing a relevant clinical endpoint (i.e. outcome) and adjusting the dose for each patient until the endpoint reaches a certain value (e.g. changing the medication dose until a certain blood pressure is achieved or a certain plasma level of the drug is reached).
- **Dosing by subpopulation.** Another method is to identify subpopulations that may respond differently to the drug and giving each subpopulation a different appropriate dose (e.g. men may receive higher doses than women, African Americans may require different doses than Latinos, or patients with liver failure may only tolerate lower doses). In some cases, the drug may not be indicated or safe for certain subpopulations.

Convenience and practicability are extremely important but often underappreciated facets of choosing the right dose regimen. The optimal dose from a pure risk–benefit standpoint is not necessarily convenient or practical. For example, many oral medications would be more effective and less toxic if given intravenously, since intravenous administration delivers the drug directly to the bloodstream. However, taking oral medications is much more convenient and requires significantly less time and effort. Similarly, frequently titrating the dose to a patient's daily fluctuations in body weight, temperature, blood pressure, fluid intake, and urine output could improve the risk–benefit ratio of a medication but would be confusing and impractical for a patient.

A dose–response curve is an x–y graph that plots the dose (or the logarithm of the dose) on the x-axis and the response (which can be any measure or endpoint) on the y-axis. Figure 2.1 illustrates a typical dose–response curve. Commonly, the x-axis plots the dose (in units of intervention per unit mass of test subject) or dose function (the log of the dose) and the y-axis

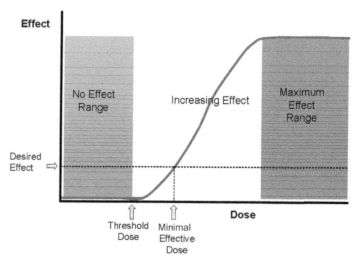

FIGURE 2.1
Dose—response curve. (Please refer to color plate section)

plots the percentage of the population that exhibits the response (e.g. desired effect or toxicity). The more powerful the intervention, the steeper the curve becomes. The clinical trial generates data points to plot the dose—response curve. In general, the trial should provide as many data points as possible to draw an accurate curve.

By plotting a dose—response curve in which response is the desired effect of the intervention, a number of important efficacy parameters can be determined. The threshold dose is the lowest dose at which there is any response. This is the point at which the vertical height of the dose—response curve first starts to rise above zero. So, if you were using a dose—response curve to demonstrate the effectiveness of a blood pressure medication, the threshold dose would be the dose at which any decrease in blood pressure in any test subject occurs. Usually slightly higher than the threshold dose is the minimal effective dose (MED), the lowest dose that will generate a specific effect. If the specific desired effect is lowering the blood pressure by 20 mmHg, then the MED will be the dose at which at least one test subject's blood pressure decreases by at least 20 mmHg. Finding an MED is especially important when toxicity is of concern (e.g. small molecule drugs that tend to have toxicities at almost all doses or completely novel drugs that must be developed quickly to fill an important unmet need). For small molecules, the MED tends to be the dose where the efficacy and safety curves diverge the most.

Patient Selection

The third critical parameter in clinical study design is patient selection. There are many ways to define patient populations and diseases. It is not always optimal to define the patient population by a previously recognized disease category, as disease categories are arbitrary intellectual constructs. Disease categories are based on a number of possible criteria, including:

- **histological changes** (e.g. Crohn's disease and ulcerative colitis alter the intestinal lining in different ways)
- **pathophysiological mechanisms** (e.g. lack of insulin secretion results in type 1 diabetes while lack of response to insulin results in type 2 diabetes)
- **causative agent** (e.g. hepatitis A is caused by the hepatitis A virus, asbestosis is caused by asbestos)
- **physical manifestations** (e.g. rheumatological conditions are defined by the joints they affect and how they affect them)

- **symptoms and signs** (e.g. stable angina is the presence of chest pain during exertion and unstable angina is the presence of chest pain at rest)
- **body part, organ, or organ system affected** (e.g. iritis is inflammation of the iris and uveitis is inflammation of the uvea)
- **predisposing, preceding, or concurrent conditions** (e.g. concussions occur after head trauma, frostbite occurs with extreme cold)
- **prognosis and natural history** (e.g. cancerous masses can spread to distant locations while benign masses do not)
- **measurement thresholds** (e.g. hypertension is defined as a systolic blood pressure above 140 mmHg and a diastolic pressure above 90 mmHg).
- **response to treatment**: two very similar conditions may have different treatments (e.g. ST and non-ST elevation myocardial infarction) or several conditions with very different mechanisms and clinical manifestations will be defined as a single disease if their treatments are the same (e.g. schizophrenia includes catatonic and paranoid schizophrenia).

Of the above, the most common way to classify disease is by response to therapy. Several distinct conditions with very different pathophysiology and clinical manifestations may be classified as the same disease if the treatment is the same (or, more commonly, if no good treatments exist for any of the conditions). For example, schizophrenia has very different possible manifestations that range from catatonic to paranoid schizophrenia. These conditions all fall under the umbrella of one disease, partly because they respond to similar therapy. Classifying diseases based on the available treatment options is often more pragmatic (e.g. distinguishing between ST elevation myocardial infarction and non-ST elevation myocardial infarction was unnecessary before thrombolytics were shown to be effective in one but not the other; since that discovery, one disease has become two).

So, it is important to think carefully about the "disease" that a clinical trial is targeting. A trial may have to be expanded beyond the normal confines of a disease (e.g. by grouping all patients with arterial atherosclerosis together, including patients requiring coronary artery bypass surgery, percutaneous coronary interventions, and stroke interventions) or limited to a subgroup of patients (e.g. classic or occult age-related macular degeneration). There are many different ways to group conditions together. For example, conditions that have:

- the same symptoms (e.g. patients with joint pain)
- any combination of signs or symptoms from a list of criteria (e.g. different lupus patients have different symptoms. but all must have a minimal number of symptoms from an established list)
- the same pathophysiological criteria (e.g. a positive blood culture for an organism)
- the same cause (e.g. patients with tuberculosis may have pulmonary or gastrointestinal manifestations)

can be grouped together.

Using etiology to group conditions can be problematic. Although assigning a single cause to diseases is common, very few diseases have just one cause. Most are the result of interaction among the environment, genes, and other factors. Here are three examples:

- *Helicobacter pylori*: *Helicobacter pylori* is present in many people. Although it causes peptic ulcers, many infected patients do not have ulcers. Other factors must be present for ulcers to result.
- **Phenylketonuria (PKU)**: PKU is often called a genetic disease. But if the "normal" human diet had very low levels of phenylalanine, even people who were homozygous for the recessive PKU gene would not demonstrate any signs of PKU. Only people with abnormally high levels of phenylalanine would exhibit PKU. Therefore, it may be said that an abnormal diet causes PKU.

- **Acquired immunodeficiency syndrome (AIDS)**: Mutant versions of CCR5 can keep the human immunodeficiency virus (HIV) in a chronic dormant state. If 99 percent of the population had these mutations then most would never develop AIDS despite being infected by HIV. Only those without the mutation would be susceptible. In such a scenario, AIDS could be called a genetic disease.

In addition, when choosing a study population, one should keep in mind that disease definitions may change over time as scientists gain a better understanding of the biological processes. Medical knowledge changes at a rapid rate. Conditions that were not considered diseases 20 years ago are defined as diseases today (e.g. the normal ranges for blood pressure and cholesterol continue to change). Continuing research may reveal that diseases and conditions currently considered separate may indeed be one unified disease process (e.g. a patient with hypertension, diabetes, and coronary artery disease may have the same disease: metabolic syndrome) and certain individual diseases may actually be conglomerates of multiple conditions. Researchers must be sure to define the study population in a manner that will be amenable to such potential changes in the future, particularly if the study intervention will generate or inspire the changes.

As mentioned above, using traditional disease definitions is not always the best way to define a study population. Many situations call for either expanding the study population beyond the normal confines of disease definitions (e.g. grouping coronary artery disease, cerebral vascular, and peripheral vascular disease patients together) or limiting the population to a subpopulation with a disease (e.g. patients with uncontrolled diabetes). In general, the study population should mirror the population that the intervention targets. Interventions do not necessarily target specific diseases (e.g. ibuprofen can be used for a number of different conditions), although they usually do. So, the study population may consist of patients who exhibit or have certain features:

- **Symptoms**: Some interventions alleviate particular symptoms (e.g. pain) rather than treat a disease; in such situations, defining the study population as patients who have that symptom (e.g. joint pain, which would include patients with osteoarthritis, rheumatoid arthritis, and traumatic injury) may be a better alternative.
- **Phenotypes or signs**: Interventions may be for certain body characteristics (e.g. breast reduction surgery for women with very large breasts).
- **Genotypes**: Sometimes interventions may be for patients with specific genetic sequences or types (e.g. BRCA mutation, Tay Sach's disease, or Down's syndrome).
- **Medical history**: When studying interventions designed to prevent diseases (i.e. prophylactic studies), researchers may use the patient's past medical history (e.g. history of transient ischemic attacks).
- **Causative agents**: If the intervention (e.g. antibiotic) targets a particular causative agent (e.g. *Streptococcus* bacteria), the study population may be patients with that causative agent (e.g. patients with streptococcal infections).
- **Values of a measure**: For interventions that alter specific measures (e.g. blood pressure), patients with certain values of that measure may be chosen (e.g. blood pressure above 140/90 mmHg).
- **Behaviors, habits, or activities**: Interventions may benefit individuals who exhibit certain behaviors (e.g. medical devices for those who snore), have certain habits (e.g. nicotine patches for smokers), or participate in specific activities (e.g. orthopedic braces for athletes playing sports).
- **Demographic characteristics**: Interventions can target certain age groups (e.g. vaccinations for newborns), genders (e.g. hot flash prophylaxis for women), ethnicities (e.g. sickle cell screening tests for African Americans), socioeconomic groups (e.g. special programs for patients who cannot pay for medications), or occupations (e.g. ventilators for miners).

Selection criteria are the characteristics and qualities that a patient should or should not have in order to participate in a clinical study. Selection criteria include inclusion criteria (the characteristics and qualities a patient must have to be included in or participate in the trial) and exclusion criteria (characteristics or qualities that prevent a patient from participating in the trial). Most inclusion criteria can be worded as exclusion criteria and vice versa (e.g. "patient is female" as an inclusion criterion is equivalent to "patient is male" as an exclusion criterion).

Selection criteria must be well defined, precise, unambiguous, and clearly established and stated before patient recruitment begins. Vague selection criteria can lead to the wrong patients being selected and cause a number of significant problems. Patients may be subject to inappropriate treatments that may cause serious harm (e.g. a patient with heart failure may receive a drug that worsens heart failure) or violate ethical or moral principles (e.g. testing a drug on children before testing on adults). Choosing the wrong study patients may invalidate results (e.g. if some study patients do not actually have a disease, the investigators may not be able to claim that their drug improves the disease).

Similarly, the repercussions of choosing different selection criteria should be borne in mind. The more stringent your selection criteria, the narrower and more homogeneous the study population will be. Greater homogeneity means less variability in the study population. Less variability allows for more precise and accurate comparisons and results. Greater homogeneity also limits the generalizability of results (e.g. results from a study population consisting of only white men in their forties cannot necessarily be applied to women, Asian—Americans, or people in their sixties). In addition, more stringent selection criteria make it more difficult and costly to find appropriate patients (e.g. it is much easier to find men between the ages of 20 and 65 than men who are between the ages of 20 and 65, weighing 150—200 pounds, and Samoan). The selection criteria may be so stringent that you cannot find enough patients to conduct the trial (e.g. how many 20—25-year old, 150—160-pound Samoan men do you expect to find if you are recruiting for patients in Iowa?)

The type of inclusion and exclusion criteria used will depend on the condition, intervention, study population, and trial. Patient characteristics (e.g. age, weight, geographical location, or cardiac function) and in turn patient trial eligibility may change during the course of recruitment and the clinical trial. So, specifying the exact date at which these criteria apply (e.g. on the date of randomization the patient must be less than 45 years old) may be important. For many criteria, specifying the duration, frequency, and degree may be relevant. The impact of diseases, medications, habits, and environmental risk factors can vary by how long, how often, and how much the patients have been exposed.

Excluding more patients from a study will generate a more homogeneous study population and reduce bias and confounding, but will also limit the generalizability of the study results. Choosing whether to exclude a certain set of patients is a balance between these two considerations. Some commonly excluded populations are described below.

HIGH-RISK PATIENTS

Researchers should consider excluding patients who have either a high probability of suffering side-effects or a possibility of experiencing catastrophic side-effects (e.g. death, permanent disability, or disfigurement). So, for example, one should avoid administering interventions that may cause bleeding (e.g. anticoagulants) to patients who are at increased risk for falling (and hitting their head, which may cause intracranial hemorrhages) or gastrointestinal bleeding (e.g. peptic ulcers). Unless necessary, interventions that may suppress the immune system must not be given to patients at high risk for serious infections (e.g. positive PPD). Investigators should beware of any conditions that the intervention may exacerbate (e.g. congestive heart failure in patients taking drugs that increase stress on the heart; patients with weak immune systems taking immunosuppressants).

PATIENTS UNABLE TO GIVE CONSENT

For ethical and legal reasons, studies should avoid including patients who cannot consent to studies out of their own free will, unless the trial is specifically for those patients. These include children who must receive permission from their parents or guardians, patients with impaired thought processes or consciousness (from psychiatric illness, substance use, medications, or other conditions), and patients who may be under duress to participate (e.g. prisoners). When trials require these populations (e.g. interventions designed for infants or patients with psychiatric illness), people must be identified who can serve as the patients' legal guardians.

PREGNANT PATIENTS

Including patients who are either pregnant or planning to conceive runs the risk of fetal harm or birth defects. Moreover, pregnancy-induced alterations in the mother's physiology may influence the intervention's effects. Therefore, most trials exclude any patients who are or may become pregnant. In fact, many trials (e.g. most Phase I trials) exclude any women of child-bearing age.

CHILDREN

Clinical trials often exclude children since many interventions may affect development, obtaining consent is more difficult, many adult diseases are uncommon in children, and interventions often act differently in children (e.g. different dosing and pharmacokinetics). Unless the intervention will be used in children, excluding children is reasonable.

ELDERLY PATIENTS

The elderly are potentially a high-risk, vulnerable population. Many have other medical conditions and are taking other medications that may confound the study results. Moreover, many people feel a duty to respect and protect the elderly. However, many medical conditions are most common in elderly people. It is sometimes prudent to exclude very elderly people unless necessary or the disease is common in the elderly.

PATIENTS WITH EXTREME BODY SIZES

Since the effects of many interventions (e.g. drug pharmacokinetics, pharmacodynamics, and side-effects) depend on patient body size, it may be necessary to exclude patients with extreme body size measurements (e.g. significantly underweight or overweight) compared with the general study population. Extreme body sizes also may cause logistical problems. Patients may exceed or fall short of the height or weight limits of trial equipment (e.g. CT tables may collapse or the patient may not be able to fit into a machine). Body size may impair (e.g. body fat can distort images such as ultrasound and make it difficult to find anatomical structures such as veins to insert catheters) or prevent (e.g. fasting in underweight patients may be dangerous) certain procedures.

PATIENTS WITH CONFOUNDING DISEASES OR CONDITIONS

Investigators must beware of diseases, conditions, or medications that may cause or alter the effects that they are trying to measure. For example, when trying to measure an intervention's effects on cancer mortality, one should consider excluding patients who are at high risk of dying from other causes (e.g. patients with severe heart failure). However, it should be kept in mind that many patients in real clinical practice will have multiple medical conditions and be on multiple medications. So, aggressively excluding patients with any other diseases or medications may limit the generalizability of the study results (e.g. it may be unrealistic to exclude patients who have been on any other breast cancer medications from a breast cancer drug trial, or to exclude diabetics from a trial involving peripheral vascular disease).

PATIENTS TAKING OTHER MEDICATIONS OR INTERVENTIONS

Ideally, patients should stop taking their other medications during the course of the trial, since other medications may interact and interfere with the intervention. The patient should not start the trial until a washout or medicine-free period has elapsed to ensure that the medications and their effects are completely eliminated from the body. Stopping other medications abruptly is not always feasible or prudent and may cause withdrawal or rebound effects. Slowly tapering the medications (i.e. decreasing the dose each day until the patient is completely off the medications) may be necessary.

Reference

1. Chin R, Lee BY. *Principles and Practice of Clinical Trial Medicine.* 1st ed. New York: Academic Press; 2008.

CHAPTER 3

Building a Healthy Mechanism for Good Clinical Practice-Compliant Global Trials: African Perspectives

Lynn Katsoulis*, Havana Chikoto[†], Don Hayward[†], Lesley Burgess**, Victor Strugo[†]
*The Aurum Institute, Parktown, South Africa
[†]Triclinium Clinical Research, Sandown, South Africa
**TREAD Research, Stellenbosch University, Tygerberg Hospital, Parow, South Africa

INTRODUCTION

The globalization of clinical trials and the growth of research in human immunodeficiency virus/acquired immunodeficiency syndrome (HIV/AIDS), tuberculosis (TB), and malaria have resulted in the emergence of clinical trial sites throughout Africa. The number of patients recruited in Africa into pivotal trials supporting marketing authorization applications has steadily increased from 0.6 percent in 2005 to 3 percent in 2009.[1] Of many therapeutic areas being investigated in the region, the vast majority remain in the above-mentioned infectious diseases.[2] Sponsors active in the region include pharmaceutical companies, public–private product development partnerships, and government-dependent institutions. South Africa has the continent's most mature clinical trial infrastructure and good clinical practice (GCP) culture. Trials date back to 1965, when legislation was implemented requiring both regulatory and ethical approval of clinical trials. The country has local GCP guidelines that closely mirror International Conference on Harmonisation (ICH) E6 guidelines, with an added emphasis on the protection of vulnerable population groups. Other African countries tend to follow ICH GCP.

STATUS OF CLINICAL TRIALS IN AFRICA

Clinical trials have been conducted in 45 of the 49 African countries,[2] but South Africa, ranked 21st, is the only African country in the world's top 50 countries according to the numbers of clinical trials conducted and active trial sites. The African continent represents only 0.9 percent of all trials conducted,[3] yet it represents about 15 percent of the world's population.[4] This disparity illustrates Africa's potential to conduct more clinical trials and that opportunities exist for developing additional clinical trial capacity throughout the continent.

Regulatory Infrastructure

Fully functional regulatory authorities with balanced permissiveness are key to the conduct of clinical trials in Africa.[5] Most African countries have some form of ethical review processes but face challenges of poor funding and inadequate standard operating procedures.[6] A survey of 31 ethics committees across sub-Saharan Africa, by the African Malaria Network (AMANET), noted a need for training on clinical trial design, determination of risks and benefits, and monitoring of research. The study further showed that 38 percent of respondents did not receive any formal training.[7] Regulatory authorities also face developmental challenges, mainly due to a lack of robust legislative frameworks.[8] Ethics committees and regulatory authorities suffer from chronic human resource shortages, mainly because reviewers are not fully employed by these institutions. That these institutions are often underdeveloped may be attributed to the more pressing health economic challenges facing government and public institutions.[6] Many sponsors counteract the potential lack of regulatory expertise by submitting protocols for parallel review by at least one internationally recognized authority (such as the United States Food and Drug Administration or the Medicines Control Council in South Africa) and/or an accredited institutional review board in the sponsor's country of origin.

Types of Clinical Trial Site

There are three main types of clinical trial sites throughout Africa: not-for-profit organizations, institution-associated sites (typically affiliated to a public hospital or an academic center), and privately owned sites. Proportions vary across countries but, in general, privately owned sites form the majority in South Africa, whereas academic sites predominate elsewhere.

Not-for-profit sites have proliferated since 1995. These are generally large, established with donor support to conduct studies on diseases prevalent among the poor. They can typically enroll 150–1000 subjects per study and are often associated with one or more trial site networks established to expedite the implementation of donor-funded trials. They typically employ 50–450 staff members to conduct large-scale trials predominantly on HIV/AIDS, TB, and malaria treatment and prophylaxis. Most existing sites were established or expanded through support from donor-funded trial networks such as AMANET, the Aids Clinical Trials Group (ACTG), the HIV Vaccine Trial Network (HVTN), the International Clinical Epidemiology Network (INCLEN), and several others. The establishment of these networks and the building of clinical research capacity throughout Africa were made possible through funding agencies such as the Bill and Melinda Gates Foundation (BMGF), the European and Developing Countries Clinical Trials Partnership (EDCTP), the World Health Organization (WHO),

Tropical Disease Research (TDR), the Swedish International Development Agency (SIDA), the Department for Research Cooperation (SAREC), Fogarty International Centre, National Institutes of Health (NIH), and the Wellcome Trust.

Most academic sites are managed by a senior clinician with a strong research interest. They vary in enrollment potential depending on their medical speciality and internal capacity.

Participants are typically recruited from large clinics at affiliated public healthcare facilities. Trial teams may be underresourced when staff members balance trial activities with heavy clinical workloads. Many of these sites channel revenue from conducting clinical trials into a central research fund to supplement institution-derived income. The most efficient academic trial sites are departments that reinvest trial funds into employing dedicated research staff.

Privately owned sites (usually investigator owned) are generally smaller and usually focus on diseases prevalent in the developed world, typically enrolling 10–50 subjects per trial. They are often attached to a private hospital. A site typically employs or has access to subinvestigators, trial support staff, GCP-compliant facilities, and a patient referral network. Sponsors usually execute research contracts directly with the investigator.

Therapeutic Area Experience

South Africa's clinical research infrastructure was predominantly built on funds from pharmaceutical company-sponsored trials for global drug development. This resulted in resident expertise in most therapeutic areas of interest to developed countries. The more recent severe tandem HIV and TB pandemics, coupled with the pre-existence of investigator and GCP competence, has seen South Africa take a leading role in conducting trials in HIV/AIDS and TB. Owing to its lower incidence, contributions to malaria research are mainly laboratory based.

Other sub-Saharan countries have also seen increasing involvement in all these indications. Malaria trials have been placed in 13 African countries, including Burkina Faso, Zambia, and Uganda, with Tanzania playing a leading role.[9,10]

An almost exponential growth in the number of clinical trial sites has occurred throughout Africa since 1995. Most of this growth was supported through the conduct of donor-funded trials on HIV, TB, or malaria. Consequently, most studies conducted in Africa are on these three infectious diseases. Even though the most prevalent diseases on the continent are HIV, TB, and malaria, the WHO estimates that the incidence of lifestyle diseases in Africa (cardiovascular conditions, diabetes, etc.) is reaching double or treble that of developed countries,[11] predominantly among poor communities in urban settings.[12] Moreover, in poorer countries with limited healthcare funding, trial participation may often be the best medical option available to patients.[13] As developed countries increasingly struggle to enroll participants owing to competing trials and commercially available treatments, it is expected that over the next decade or two, more trials will seek to accelerate enrollment by involving African countries in research across a broader range of therapeutic indications. Rapid site development under prevailing economic circumstances will, in turn, require an intensification of capacity-building activity, involving skills transfer, mentorship, and training by more established collaborative sites (e.g. in Europe, North America, and South Africa) and expedited monitoring support through the use of modern technologies such as telemedicine.

Location of Clinical Trial Sites and Associated Challenges

Most clinical trial sites in Africa are located near major economic centers with commercial airports for practical reasons, such as the greater ability to attract and retain experienced investigators; to establish training for support staff around academic institutions; to access densely populated pools of potential participants; and for access to adequate road and communication infrastructure that facilitate logistics and site accessibility for monitors, technicians, and suppliers.

Because most clinical research units are affiliated to tertiary academic institutions or hospitals, the availability of clinicians and health scientists interested in conducting clinical research is not a serious limiting factor in urban areas. In less developed countries, expatriate specialist health scientists have been employed to conduct trials and engage in capacity building of site-based personnel. Semi-skilled workers, generally from less affluent backgrounds, may require training in basic skills ranging from computer literacy to driving motor vehicles as well as research-specific skills. Interestingly, in African countries, high-quality training has been seen as a double-edged sword in that retention of trained and skilled workers becomes a challenge as new trial sites open and start to recruit staff.[14]

These staffing considerations apply equally when setting up on-site laboratories, which face the additional challenge of ensuring efficient supply lines and technical support. Technicians must often travel from South Africa or overseas to repair or calibrate laboratory equipment. Nevertheless, the general absence of proximal back-ups makes laboratory self-sufficiency a critical need, particularly for specialized tests that require extemporaneous processing shortly after drawing blood (e.g. peripheral blood mononuclear cells). Moreover, as few African countries possess national accreditation systems, many clinical trial laboratories currently subscribe to the South African National Accreditation System (SANAS) or one of the accrediting boards in Europe or North America.

The above factors are not insurmountable, but should be considered when choosing locations for new sites or when assessing the cost-effectiveness of choosing sites for new trials. However, enrollment potential and the ensuing healthcare and social benefits provided to research-naïve communities have spurred the creation of unexpected pockets of research excellence in several remote locations.

Clinical Research Skill and Human Capability Availability in Africa

The growth of clinical research in South Africa's public health sector has been limited by "inadequate human resource capacity and planning, and poor stewardship, leadership and management".[15] This problem has been exacerbated by medical emigration, increasing the resource gap between public and private healthcare systems and causing a staffing crisis in the public health service, especially at district and community levels.[15]

The development of careers in clinical research on the African continent has historically been hampered by the paucity of clinical trial centers capable of training African clinicians, health scientists, and technical staff,[14,16] and of specialist training that focuses on clinical research.[17] The resulting scarcity of skilled research personnel, compounded by emigration of African clinicians and health scientists seeking more stable opportunities elsewhere,[14] breaks the vital chain of knowledge transfer, especially in less developed countries. Moreover, it is accepted that academic structures in Africa have difficulty in stimulating creative thought and problem-solving abilities in young students of considerable potential. This results in impaired ability to interpret results, recognize inconsistencies, and find potential solutions.[18]

The persistence of adequate funding and supervision from the international community can build adequate and self-sustaining research sites and infrastructures, staffed and managed by resident nationals. This process will be critical to meet future demand for functioning trial sites on the African continent.

SITE MANAGEMENT STRUCTURES

Clinical trials are intricately detailed and complex projects that need to be completed according to stringent global regulations and standards, so effective sites require multiple skill sets that harmonize under strong hands-on management. The greatest challenge of establishing new sites in emerging regions is finding experienced research managers and investigators who fulfill the requirements of ICH E6: "investigator(s) should be qualified by education, training, and experience to assume responsibility for the proper conduct of the trial". To overcome the management challenge, sponsors and site networks have used various models such as employing remotely situated leaders (in a first world country) and seconding experienced trialists to reside in developing sites. Whatever model is used, basic project management principles must be applied. According to Jim Collins' evidence-based assessment of the key principles to success,[19] each site needs a credible leader who is humble, acts in the site's best interests, and is strongly driven to produce sustained results. Site staff must be disciplined in thought and action, and able to cooperate in developing and maintaining systems that lead to successful implementation of clinical trials. Staff selection is therefore critical, followed by intensive and ongoing training geared to producing high-quality data.

The data trail principle of clinical trials prohibits erasing errors, which remain in project files for scrutiny by monitors and auditors. Corrective actions often require much more work than correct initial performance. Staff must thus be primed to perform tasks accurately the first time, so the presence of hands-on managers is self-evident. Remotely managed sites run the risk that delayed detection of small errors can translate into large problems.

CURRENT FUNDING MODELS AND IMPACT ON IMPLEMENTATION OF STUDIES

Grant-funded and privately funded clinical trials tend to follow different models for funding the implementation of the trial. The classic private funding model is participant based, ascribing a finite value to each completed case, calculated according to protocol-specific procedures (clinical, dispensing, diagnostic, etc.) carried out at each clinic visit and for supporting activities such as staff training, equipment leases, and patient advertising. Payments are usually made periodically, after monitoring confirms what protocol-compliant work has been completed to date, what recruiting milestones have been reached, and so on. These budgets may sometimes be incentivized, motivating investigators to meet enrollment targets, timelines, and quality standards. Such budgets are well received by experienced sites with already trained staff that conduct multiple studies with high cumulative enrollment, and are able to negotiate a fair value to the time required (and consequent monetary value) to execute all functions itemized in the budget.

In contrast, most not-for-profit and academic sites built around public healthcare facilities have tended to be funded by grants that are based on salaries of staff members required to conduct a given trial, facility construction, leasing, and equipment and related overheads, which may include computers, mobile phones, and sometimes motor vehicles to ensure high protocol compliance and retention by shuttling low-earning participants to and from scheduled clinic visits.

Budgets calculated according to staff salaries may lack incentives for teams to meet targets, but they typically cover hidden costs such as recruitment of participants and staff training. Incentivized participant-based budgets inherently motivate investigators to reach targets. They need careful compilation to avoid overlooking hidden costs.

Both approaches thus have their pros and cons. When proposing a funding model, sponsors should seek to optimize site benefits in the most cost-efficient manner. It is essential that sites are consulted early in the budget negotiation process so that fees and grants are realistically structured to maximize the performance of quality research within the shortest achievable timelines while also contributing to achieving site stability and longevity. Sponsors should also be aware that with academic sites there is often a mandatory levy payable to their governing institutions. Prospective clarification should be sought if this is already built into the budget or will be surcharged.

In time, an optimized hybrid model (between grant and private funding) is likely to develop, capitalizing on the advantages of both.

BUILDING ADDITIONAL CAPACITY

Ongoing Need for Capacity Building

Capacity building is an ongoing global initiative. Sites must continually adjust processes and capacity in accordance with changing regulatory requirements, sponsor needs, and scientific developments.

Between 2006 and 2008, the Global Alliance for Tuberculosis Drug Development assessed 84 clinical trial sites and associated mycobacteriology laboratories in 39 countries for readiness to conduct TB treatment studies. Many sites with trial experience were identified, yet significant capacity-building efforts to impart the requisite skills for conducting GCP-quality trials were required.[20] It is expected that as sites become more diverse and sustainable they will require fewer external donor resources to be capacitated for changing demands.

Furthermore, training increases the mobility of clinical research staff, so it must be realized (by both local and foreign donors and sponsors) that investment in skills training and capacity building is a continuing process. This investment applies not only to liquid assets, but also to the availability of specialists and support staff to facilitate ongoing education and skills training.

Need for Additional Sites

Until now, the development of clinical trial capacity in tropical and equatorial Africa has kept pace with the capacity needs for numerous Phase II developments, but when several antimalarials, microbicides, and TB vaccines enter Phase III trials, the required capacity will augment substantially. A Malaria Clinical Trial Alliance (MCTA) case study found that few clinical facilities in Africa are geared toward conducting either early- or late-phase trials.[16] They further observed benefits in developing a new site around one particular trial, with consolidated training. Once experience grows, sites need to maintain a degree of autonomy to ensure sustainability by engaging with multiple sponsors.

Furthermore, if the large patient numbers required for efficacy trials and public health implementation strategies are to be found and enrolled, it is important to educate the general public about research and develop a culture of adherence to treatment regimens.[21]

Enhancing Skills and Internationally Acceptable Best Practices

Skills shortages in Africa can be addressed by investing in infrastructure that would facilitate the training of greater numbers of qualified health scientists who specialize in more than one disease or condition. In turn, this would lead to the creation of more stable and longer term career opportunities wherein African health scientists could be retained and motivated to reach career goals by performance-driven excellence over a longer period. It has been suggested that this may be achieved through first building on existing and operational facilities and then founding satellite facilities staffed from the parent facility in other areas. The major obstacle that confounds this plan is that sponsor companies seldom have the budget to invest in support, maintenance, and training of sites and staff. Attracting new investments from sponsor companies for trials is dependent on the operational state of the site. In South Africa, it was observed that even clinical research units associated with tertiary institutions situated ex campus are expected to be self-reliant and self-financing, with only minor input from the tertiary institution.

In South Africa, mandatory GCP training is required for all research staff, including investigators, study coordinators, pharmacists, and support staff. There are, however, currently no accreditation and/or standardization guidelines for such training, and this has resulted in a plethora of GCP training courses being offered by various institutions and organizations, often at substantial cost. These courses typically run over two or three days, with shorter refresher courses offered for the mandatory three-yearly update. The lack of accreditation is further compounded, in some cases, by the qualifications and/or the expertise of providers and trainers being questioned.[22] In addition, GCP training has been compared to learning the rules of the road but not being taught to drive the car.[23]

Investigator Training

When investigators sign the FDA 1572 form (Statement of the Investigator), they are certifying that they are qualified to conduct all aspects of the clinical trial. However, there is currently no standard method of assessing such competence. Despite recent growth in the clinical trial industry and the acknowledgment that trials are becoming increasingly more complex, clinical research is not recognized as a speciality with formalized training, other than GCP.[22,24] Specialized training would serve not only to improve investor and patient confidence, but also to promote the generation of quality data.[25] However, such training is neither easily defined nor easily accessible. Internationally, a masters in public health is regarded as the traditional degree for clinicians interested in research. There are also international associations offering investigator certification programs, including the Association of Clinical Research Professionals (ACRP), the Society of Clinical Research Associates (SoCRA), and the Drug Information Association (DIA), but few researchers obtain such certification.[23,26]

Recently, several universities (e.g. those of Montpellier, France; and Liverpool, UK) have established master's degrees in clinical research, and new specialized courses are emerging.

Training for Support Staff

25

Study coordinators are typically registered nurses, auxiliary health workers (including paramedics, biokineticists, and pharmacists), or graduates in a health-related science. Study coordinators have been described as "the glue that holds studies together", yet a recent survey conducted in Australia and New Zealand demonstrated that 75 percent of all study coordinators had no formal grounding in clinical trial methodology training prior to starting in their current positions. Current training reported generally consists of on-the-job training with (38.8%) or without (17.3%) a mentor.[27] No such information is available from Africa, although it is likely that the situation is similar. Formal training programs and certification courses are beginning to emerge in the study coordination area.

Other support staff, including pharmacists dispensing for clinical trials and core laboratory personnel, should at least attend GCP basic and refresher courses so as to understand how their technical responsibilities apply in the research setting. In addition, with an ever-increasing volume of international transport of clinical trial supplies to sites and biological specimens to laboratories, site managers should ensure that key site personnel are trained in national regulations and International Air Transport Association procedures. Such courses are now available in South Africa.[25]

ESTABLISHING NEW SITES

The greatest challenges in new sites are ensuring that inexperienced staff understand the complexities of clinical trials and establishing robust systems that safeguard data quality and regulatory compliance. Classroom-style teaching of broad research principles is most effective when supplemented by tutored job experience. Internal audits are also very instructive in conveying the interrelated complexity of trials and develop the habit of identifying potential problems before they occur.

A very effective way of activating a new site is to seed the team with highly experienced key staff members, or at least to have new staff visit well-established facilities, to observe and learn the dynamics and systems of effective sites. A more advanced form of training, although time consuming, can be to conduct a dummy trial, to help staff understand how processes should function and go wrong if not tightly managed in real time.

Another option, employed by several Product Development Partnerships (PDPs), is for a new site to run epidemiological, non-interventional or Phase IV trials to help the establishment of systems before progressing to more rigorous and challenging preregistration trials. Effective training continues during trial execution, through monitoring visits or audits when errors are detected, and is most effective when corrective action is coupled with targeted training.

Notwithstanding the technical and training challenges, like any enterprise a clinical trial site needs to be rooted in sound management principles and be managed by strong leaders who inspire staff and ensure efficient running of the site.

References

1. European Medicines Agency. *Clinical trials submitted in marketing authorization applications to the EMA: overview of patient recruitment and the geographical location of investigator sites*; 2010. EMA/INS/GCP/154352/2010. Compliance and Inspection.

2. Clinicaltrials.gov. Map of All Studies in Clinicaltrials.gov. United States National Institute of Health. http://clinicaltrials.gov/ct2/search/map/click?map.x=417&map.y=233 [accessed 11.05.11].

3. Thiers FA, Sinskey AJ, Berndt ER. Trends in the globalization of clinical trials. *Nature Reviews Drug Discovery* 2008;**7**:13–4.

4. United Nations. *World Population Prospects, the 2010 Revision*. http://esa.un.org/unpd/wpp/Analytical-Figures/htm/fig_2.htm; 2010 [accessed 4.5.11].

5. Maiga D, Akanmori BD, Chocarro L. Regulatory oversight of clinical trials in Africa: progress over the past 5 years. *Vaccine* 2009;**27**:7249–52.

6. Noor RA. Health research oversight in Africa. *Acta Tropica* 2009;**112**(1):S63–70.

7. Nyika A, Kilama WR, Chilengi R, Tangwa G, Tindana P, Ndebele P, Ikingura J. Composition, training needs and independence of ethics review committees across Africa: are the gate-keepers rising to the emerging challenges? *Journal of Medical Ethics* 2009;**35**:189–93.

8. Whitworth JAG, Kokwaro G, Kinyanjui S, Snewin VA, Tanner M, Walport M, Sewankambo N. Strengthening capacity for health research in Africa. *Lancet* 2008;**372**:1590–3.

9. Kilama WL, Chilengi R, Wanga CL. Towards an African-driven malaria vaccine development program: history and activities of the African Malaria Network Trust (AMANET). *American Journal of Tropical Medicine and Hygiene* 2007;**77**:282–8.

10. AMANET. *AMANET Annual Report*. http://amanet-trust.org/ext/reports/annual/2009/AmanetAR2009.pdf; 2009 [accessed 4.5.11].

11. Househam KC. Africa's burden of disease: the University of Cape Town Sub-Saharan Africa Centre for Chronic Disease. *South African Medical Journal* 2010;**100**:94–5.

12. Mayosi BM, Flisher AJ, Lalloo UG, Sitas F, Tollman SM, Bradshaw D. The burden of non-communicable diseases in South Africa. *Lancet* 2009;**374**:934–47.

13. Petryna A. *When Experiments Travel: Clinical Trials and the Global Search for Human Subjects*. Princeton, NJ: Princeton University Press; 2009. p. 3.

14. Stilwell B, Khassoum D, Zurn P, Vujicic M, Adams O, Dal Paz M. Migration of healthcare workers from developing countries: strategic approaches to its management. *Bulletin of the World Health Organization* 2004;**82**:595–600.

15. Coovadia H, Jewkes R, Barron P, Sanders D, McIntyre D. The health and health system of South Africa: historical roots of current public health challenges. *Lancet* 2009;**374**:817–34.

16. Ogutu BR, Baiden R, Diallo D, Smith PG, Binka FN. Sustainable development of a GCP-compliant clinical trials platform in Africa: the Malaria Clinical Trials Alliance perspective. *Malaria Journal* 2010;**9**:103.

17. Siegfried N, Volmink J, Dhansay A. Does South Africa need a national clinical trials support unit? *South African Medical Journal* 2010;**100**:521–4.

18. Kimanani E. Good clinical practice in East Africa: a review. *East African Medical Journal* 2001;**78**:550–4.

19. Collins JC. *Good to Great: Why Some Companies Make the Leap … and Others Don't*. New York: HarperCollins; 2001.

20. van Niekerk C, Ginsberg A. Assessment of global capacity to conduct tuberculosis drug development trials: do we have what it takes? *International Journal of Tuberculosis and Lung Disease* 2009;**13**:1367—72.

21. Lingappa JR, Lambdin B, Bukusi E, Ngure K, Kavuma L, Inambao M, Kanweka W, Allen S, Kiarie JN, Makhema J, Were E, Manongi R, Coetzee D, De Bruyn G, Delany-Moretlwe S, Magaret A, Mugo N, Mujugira A, Ndase P, Celum C, for the Partners in Prevention HSV-2/HIV Transmission Study Group. Regional differences in prevalence of HIV-1 discordance in Africa and enrollment of HIV-1 discordant couples into an HIV-1 prevention trial. *PLoS ONE* 2008;**3**(1):e1411.

22. Burgess LJ, Sulzer NU. GCP accreditation — a worthwhile investment? *South African Medical Journal* 2006;**96**:161—2.

23. Hartnett T. Investigator certification: a pivotal role in assuring trial quality. *Clinical Researcher* 2003;**3**:11—6.

24. Getz K. Rising clinical trial complexity continues to vex drug developers. *ACRP Wire*. May 13, 2010. www.acrpnet.org; 2010 [accessed 9.6.10].

25. Burgess LJ, Sulzer NU. Clinical trials in South Africa: need for capacity building and training. *South African Medical Journal* 2010;**100**:402.

26. Arrant T, Soo B, Boepple P, Halloran L, Parmentier JL, Sauer A, Koski G. Advancing your clinical research career through educational opportunities. *Monitor* 2007;19—23.

27. Duane CG, Granda SE, Munz DC, Cannon JC. Study coordinators' perceptions of their work experience. *Monitor* 2007;39—42.

CHAPTER 4

Clinical Trial Sites Capabilities: Standard Operating Procedure Implementation in Effective African Models

Lesley Burgess*, Havana Chikoto[†], Don Hayward[†], Lynn Katsoulis**, Victor Strugo[†]
*TREAD Research, Stellenbosch University, Tygerberg Hospital, 7505 Parow, South Africa
[†]Triclinium Clinical Research, 135 West Street, 2196 Sandown, South Africa
**The Aurum Institute, 29 Queens Road, 2193 Parktown, South Africa

INTRODUCTION

The implementation of good clinical practice (GCP) guidelines has undoubtedly had a beneficial effect on the quality of clinical research. According to these standards, trial sites conducting Phase I–IV clinical trials must use documented systems of quality control and quality assurance and ensure adherence to written, detailed standard operating procedures (SOPs) in order to obtain accurate, reproducible results.

The concept of standardizing procedures was first developed in the manufacturing sector to ensure that products conform to specifications and standards and to eliminate interbatch variability; it was later adopted by most industries. SOPs are particularly relevant to research as they minimize extraneous variances in data by standardizing data collection methods, thereby increasing the probability of obtaining accurate and reproducible results.

SOPs, according to International Conference on Harmonisation (ICH)-GCP Guideline 1.55,[1] are defined as "detailed, written instructions to achieve uniformity of the performance of a specific function". They are mentioned repeatedly in these guidelines, e.g. ICH-GCP Guideline 2.13 states that "systems with procedures that assure the quality of every aspect of the trial should be implemented".[1] SOPs have therefore become mandatory in all clinical research settings, including pharmaceutical companies and other sponsors, contract research organizations, regulatory authorities, ethics committees, investigative sites, laboratories, pharmacies, and couriers. In this chapter, the term "research organization" has been used generically to refer to functional groups throughout which procedures should be standardized, ranging from a small research site comprising an investigator and a trial coordinator to large multifunctional institutes employing numerous people to fulfill a diverse spectrum of clinical and support functions.

One of the most frequent findings in regulatory audits is failure to adhere to SOPs. Significant deviations noted by the US Food and Drug Administration (FDA) in recent FDA Forms 483 or Warning Letters illustrate the range of activities that may be targeted for failure to meet written SOP guidelines, including:

- "Failure to establish and follow appropriate written procedures designed to prevent microbial contamination of drug products purporting to be sterile"
- "Failure to establish written procedures applicable to the function of the quality control unit"
- "Failure to develop written procedures for surveillance, receipt, evaluation, and reporting of postmarketing adverse drug reactions".[2]

Despite the importance of SOPs, neither the FDA nor the European Union regulations specifically prescribe them for clinical trial conduct. However, there are guidelines and regulations that infer responsibility.[3,4] For instance, 21CFR 312.53 states that investigators will "ensure that all associates, colleagues and employees assisting in the conduct of the trial(s) are informed of their obligations in meeting the above commitments".[5] One of the best ways to ensure that research staff are knowledgeable about obligations and commitments is by having SOPs that cover clinical trial procedures and assign responsibility. It is interesting to note that SOPs are mentioned explicitly in the manufacturing phases of the drug development process, e.g. 21 CFR 211.100, which states that "There should be written procedures for production and process control designed to assure that the drug products have the identity, strength, quality and purity they purport or are represented to possess. Such procedures shall include all requirements in this subpart. These written procedures, including any changes, shall be drafted, reviewed, and approved by the appropriate organizational units and reviewed and approved by the quality control unit".[5]

ROLE OF STANDARD OPERATING PROCEDURES IN CLINICAL RESEARCH

The primary purpose of an SOP is to document and standardize the working procedures for all functions (including the initiation, conduct, and reporting of clinical trials) implemented throughout the specific research unit organization in order to ensure accurate and reliable data. As such, SOPs reflect a research organization's attitude to GCP and quality data.

SOPs thus have a beneficial role in an organization:

- First and foremost, an SOP documents the way in which a process that may be followed by several individuals should be carried out in a research organization, to ensure consistent implementation. Such standardization and reproducibility of a process increase the credibility of results and ensure uniformity between successive trials.

- SOPs assign responsibility to components of a process, thereby assisting in the identification of weaknesses and training requirements in the research organization.
- SOPs act as step-by-step instructions for the training of new and temporary staff, thereby reducing supervisory time and effort.
- The existence of SOPs in a research organization provides a written record of quality control and quality assurance processes. They ensure that important procedures are organized, applied, and documented consistently, while concurrently maintaining the high standards of GCP. By having and maintaining SOPs, the organization builds quality into trials from their outset and assures the rights and welfare of participants.

STANDARD OPERATING PROCEDURES, POLICIES, GUIDELINES, AND STUDY-SPECIFIC PROCEDURES

It is important that research staff understand the differences among SOPs, policies, guidelines, and study-specific procedures (SSPs). According to Majchrzak,[3] SOPs provide general instruction and guidance for all widely applicable processes. They should be generated for application during any research. It is thus important to write SOPs in a sufficiently broad way that is site/institution specific and not trial specific, assigning primary and back-up responsibilities to staff positions. SOPs should thus be regarded as strictly controlled documents, synonymous with the laws of an organization. Each step in each SOP has to be adhered to by all its members, who should understand that any accidental or necessary deviance from an SOP must be transparently disclosed, documented, and explained.

Policies document the attitudes, norms, and expectations of an organization towards specific concepts, such as behavior in the workplace, dress code and work-related travel. Policies do not include procedures and do not necessarily assign responsibilities to specific positions.

Guidelines are significantly more detailed than SOPs and are less stringently controlled. They are synonymous with regulations in a legal framework. Guidelines should contain wisdom that advises, in situations where prescribing is too restrictive. An organization cannot be cited in an audit for not adhering to each element within a guideline. Guidelines typically include details that improve quality but are not essential to meet regulatory requirements. They may require to be changed and/or updated as a result of organizational and/or equipment changes more frequently than SOP revision.

SSPs are procedural manuals supporting the implementation of a specific trial protocol. SSPs contain the details of steps to be implemented in a trial. SSPs can include plans or manuals for functions such as dispensing, laboratory processing, and monitoring, usually formulated before the start of a specific trial. SSPs are not regulated, so modifications do not require regulatory or ethics committee approval before implementation. Strict version control by the management team is important, though, to ensure that the same version is implemented by all teams participating in the study (Figure 4.1).

SUGGESTED LIST OF STANDARD OPERATING PROCEDURES

There is no single definitive list of SOPs that should be implemented for all research organizations. Each organization should identify the full range of their deliverables by reviewing its own functions and processes, and consequently decide what SOPs need to be written. The following SOPs are suggested as fundamental needs for a site that conducts clinical trials:

- Preparation, approval and revision of SOPs (i.e. an "SOP on SOPs" that sets standards for writing).
- Review and validation of protocols and protocol amendments.

31

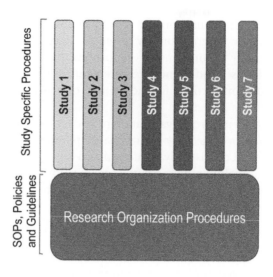

FIGURE 4.1
Standard operating procedures (SOPs), policies, and guidelines are applicable throughout an organization, whereas study-specific procedures provide additional detail to support the implementation of a specific protocol to standardize procedures throughout all the organizations involved in implementing the study. (Please refer to color plate section)

- Informed consent process: This is a mandatory and critical SOP. Flaws in the consenting process are among the most commonly cited FDA audit findings.[5] The consent process must not only conform to GCP, national laws, and institutional guidelines, but also be tailored to the site's activities. Thus, a site conducting pediatric trials would need to have an SOP that covers consenting by the parent/legal guardian and assenting by the minor; a site dealing with psychiatric trials would need an SOP dealing with consenting of patients with impaired capacity for reasoning, including provisions as to when a legal guardian is required.
- Case report form (CRF) completion, including completion of electronic CRFs and query resolution.
- Adverse event and serious adverse event reporting: This SOP should comprehensively cover investigator obligations to local authorities and sponsors; it should be general enough to harmonize with sponsor-specific pharmacovigilance processes, which may vary among trial protocols.
- Recruitment and screening of trial participants.
- Retention of trial participants and steps that should be taken to trace or follow-up defaulters.
- Pharmacy issues, including receipt, storage, dispensing, accountability, and destruction/removal of investigational product. Local pharmacy laws and procedures must here be harmonized with GCP. Protocol-specific requirements should be addressed in an SSP.
- Clinical procedures that must be systematically standardized, e.g. blood sample collection and processing, measuring blood pressure (BP), performing electrocardiography (ECG). This SOP must be customized to the site's current circumstances (e.g. the location of processing laboratory or ECG department), equipment (e.g. manual or automated sphygmomanometer), and specialities (e.g. lung function tests in pulmonology units, psychometric testing for psychiatric trials).
- Setting up and maintaining the site's required trial files.
- Medical records and source documents.
- Staff training, including training on SOPs.
- Preparation and hosting of monitoring visits.
- Preparation and hosting of sponsor or regulatory audits/inspections.
- Trial termination.

- Archiving of records.
- Back-up power supply (to ensure patency of storage facilities for refrigerated medicines or frozen laboratory specimens).
- Managing "needle-prick injuries" (especially relevant in countries with a high HIV prevalence).

LOGISTICS ASSOCIATED WITH STANDARD OPERATING PROCEDURE IMPLEMENTATION

SOPs can only fulfill their function in a clinical trial site if they are read and followed by all staff members. It is thus essential that the writing, as well as the subsequent implementation and training thereof, is done systematically.

Writing, Approval, and Implementation of Standard Operating Procedures

SOPs generally follow a characteristic format, as shown in Figure 4.2. Consistent formatting is essential when writing SOPs, so that instructions and general information do not become muddled. In addition, the following writing guidelines are advised:

- Try to keep SOPs concise.
- Use simple words and terms.
- Use short sentences with instructional style in the active (e.g. "dispense the medication"), not passive ("the medication should be dispensed") voice.
- List the instructions in sequential order (like a recipe).
- Limit the content to essential elements of procedures.

When writing SOPs, it is imperative to consult ICH-GCP, regulatory, and other applicable guidelines and related reading matter for specific guidance on implementing the correct procedure. If necessary, also consult the ethics committee, regulatory body and/or sponsor or contract research organization (CRO) companies for additional insight. It is also always advisable to consult the core staff members who will carry out a particular procedure, to ensure that processes are described in a familiar and practically feasible way, such that user compliance is maximized. Unclear writing and theoretical, over-detailed style are common reasons for non-compliance with SOPs.

The writing of SOPs can be a particularly time-consuming and laborious task, and many sites opt to make use of templates designed for this purpose.[6–8] Although there are numerous templates available both on the Internet and in published books and journals, it is essential that these templates are customized for the specific research site.

The most challenging aspect of writing SOPs is achieving a balance between including sufficient information for standardization of procedures throughout an organization and keeping text sufficiently generic to cover all projects conducted within the organization. This becomes increasingly difficult as organizational activities diversify. Because auditors will seek evidence that SOPs have been followed, procedural steps should be written in such a manner that execution will construct an audit trail. For example, if an SOP states that regulatory letters must be checked for completeness before being filed, the responsible reviewer should sign and date the document when doing so, and mark deficiencies as evidence of the checking. If there is no way of leaving an audit trail, or if a step is not essential, the writing team should consider excluding it from the SOP.

Once completed, an SOP needs to be reviewed by the staff representing those who will be implementing the SOP, the most senior person responsible for the content of the SOP, and the organization's quality representative. For a research site, this could translate to the trial team, the principal investigator, and the person responsible for quality and training. Once satisfied,

33

Distribution	Doc. No.	Version	Effective Date	Page
		DD/MM/YYYY	DD/MM/YYYY	1 of 2

STANDARD OPERATING PROCEDURE

Title: [Short and Instructive]

Approval

Author	Name	Signature	Date
	Role		
Reviewer 1	Name	Signature	Date
	Role		
Reviewer 2	Name	Signature	Date
	Role		
Reviewer 3	Name	Signature	Date
	Role		

1. Purpose
[Describe the aim of this procedure.]

2. Scope
[Describe the extent of the area or subject matter dealt with and to whom it is relevant.]

3. Abbreviations
[List all abbreviations used in the text. List abbreviations in alphabetical order followed by the definition. Remember all abbreviations must be expanded the first time they are used in the text.]
For example:

ABB   Abbreviation

4. Definitions
[Define all unique or important terms used in this document.]

5. Responsibility
[List by job title a summary of the responsibilities of each person involved in the implementation of this SOP.]

Distribution	Doc. No.	Version	Effective Date	Page
		DD/MM/YYYY	DD/MM/YYYY	2 of 2

6. Procedures
[Detailed step-by-step instructions for completing the task. The instructions must be detailed enough so someone with no knowledge of the task can pick up this procedure, follow it, and successfully complete the task. The instructions should document who is responsible for the steps. Other tips: Include a list of equipment needed, problem-solving steps, and escalation pathways. Use clear language. If any steps are optional, clearly label as such.]

7. Related Procedures
[List all related policy, SOP, WPGs, or clinical guidelines. As a minimum, all procedures referred to in the text must be listed here. The aim is to reduce duplication of instructions; if the instructions for a particular process are contained in another procedure document, simply refer readers to that procedure in the text, do not replicate the content in your SOP.]

8. References
[List all legislation, regulations, guidelines, industry standards, or other reference material that informed the content of the SOP.]

9. Attachments
[List all form templates, checklists, flowcharts, or other documents attached to this form. Do not attach references. Only attach form templates for critical documents that will not be changed. If an attachment is changed the SOP must be revised as a new version. It may be better to simply refer to required documentation, e.g. the current leave form.]

10. Revision History

Version	Approval Date	Next Review Date	Significant Changes
1	DD/MM/YYYY	MM/YYYY	N/A – First authorized version
2	DD/MM/YYYY	MM/YYYY	Replaces XXXXXXX List all significant changes

Standard Operating Procedure Template V 0.0

FIGURE 4.2

Suggested standard operating procedure format.

the responsible staff (typically three tiers of responsibility) stipulated in the "SOP on SOPs" must add authorizing signatures and dates before the SOP is released, distributed, and implemented. Distribution should be done in a timely manner, ensuring that each employee documents training or reading of the SOP.[2] To optimize learning, it is also advisable to introduce SOPs in a gradual way, prioritizing the most important SOPs.

The following simple list is useful as a final check before releasing an SOP:

- Does it answer the basic "who, what, when, where, why, and how?" questions for execution?
- Are the steps listed in logical order of execution?
- Are controlling and back-up persons identified?
- Does it conform to GCP and local regulations?
- Will execution be coupled with an audit trail of procedural steps?
- Is there an audit trail of set-up and revision of the SOP itself (i.e. a "history" section)?

Filing of Standard Operating Procedures

The descriptive title and subsequent filing of an SOP are imperative in the long-term adherence thereof. An inability to locate an SOP within a collection of SOPs invariably leads to non-compliance.[9] Several different filing systems for a research site have been suggested. Kolman et al.[6] make use of a simplified method using four basic sections, namely (1) General Study SOPs, (2) Prestudy SOPs, (3) During the Study SOPs, and (4) End of Study SOPs. This method is adequate for new and smaller sites. Larger sites with larger numbers of staff and more specialized functions may prefer the system advocated by Shefran et al.,[7] namely: (1) General Administration, (2) Study Start-up, (3) Study Management, (4) Participant Management, (5) Data Management, (6) Quality Assurance, (7) Privacy Practices, and (8) Miscellaneous. For larger or more diverse organizations, it is suggested that SOPs are categorized by functional area.

It is essential that all staff have ready access to the current versions of all SOPs. Convenience and efficiency can be maximized using an intranet, according staff read-only and printing access but not downloading rights, to reduce the risk of staff storing and referring to outdated versions. If an electronic system is not available, paper copies of current versions should be accessible to all staff for reference in dedicated master files. Whatever system is used, the responsible person must ensure that all files are kept current and complete at all times.

Control of Standard Operating Procedures

All procedural documents should be numbered and version controlled, using a system that simplifies identification. For example, the first two characters could indicate the functional area, the next two digits for the SOP number within the functional area, and the last two digits reserved for the version of the SOP. Moreover, the number could be preceded by the letters S, P, or G, indicating whether the document is an SOP, a Policy, or a Guideline. Thus, the document codes S-QC-01.02 and G-EQ-03.01 could be used to identify, respectively, the second version of the first Quality Control SOP and the first version of the third Equipment Maintenance guideline.

External Standard Operating Procedures

Several sponsors and international trial networks provide SOPs and insist that all sites, CROs, and other partner research organizations implement a single set of SOPs. This can be very convenient for fledgling organizations; however, maintaining several sets of SOPs in parallel becomes problematic when an organization starts to grow and work with several sponsors or networks. It is essential that each organization develops its own internal centrally filed set of

SOPs, while external SOPs are filed in applicable trial or project files with a note to file stipulating which set of SOPs will be used for each project.

Training on Standard Operating Procedures

Robust SOPs are necessary, but do not automatically result in good quality data; their "inefficient existence" can also lull research staff and management into a false sense of security.[9] It is imperative that research staff know and understand the contents of all applicable SOPs. Training on the implementation of SOPs is thus crucial for any site and should be conducted in such a way that the trainer explains GCP and other guidelines within the context of the site's SOPs. Such training should be carried out with all existing and new staff, and documented in the site and/or project training records.

Periodic Review of Standard Operating Procedures

Changes in regulations and/or staff turnover can highlight weaknesses in an SOP, which may become outdated without staff being aware of this. At the same time, during an audit or inspection, the site's work will be audited against SOPs that were applicable during work execution (possibly more than one version). It is thus essential to review SOPs a few months after they are written, and thereafter on a regular basis. Most auditors advocate updating SOPs every one to two years. This activity should preferably be a "team task" that involves experienced implementers of the procedures.

SOPs regarded as inadequate should generally be revised as soon as possible. Between revisions, it is very useful for the responsible person to maintain a detailed log of identified problems, deviations, and corrective actions that can inform the next review. Maintaining and discussing such a log will also raise awareness of new SOPs that need to be created.

Whenever a new version is released, it is of paramount importance to remove from circulation the outdated and superseded versions. One official set of all older documents must then be centrally archived for general site and auditor reference.

CONCLUSION

SOPs are critical to a research organization's achieving efficient operations, quality control, and regulatory compliance.[2] When properly designed and implemented, they provide research staff with a practical reference tool that promotes efficient, accurate job performance. When properly managed and reviewed, they provide site managers with an overview of existing deficiencies and identify knowledge gaps requiring additional training. They can also be used as a tool for an organization to achieve compliance after being cited for non-compliance in an audit or inspection.

References

1. International Conference on Harmonisation. *Guideline for Good Clinical Practice*; 1997. E6.

2. Peterson DC. *Assuring the effective use of standard operating procedures (SOPs) in today's workforce. BioPharm International*, September 2. http://biopharminternational.findpharma.com/biopharm/Article/Assuring-the-Effective-Use-of-Standard-Operating-P/ArticleStandard/Article/detail/371024; 2006 [accessed 11.03.11].

3. Majchrzak K. Presentation entitled "A blueprint for clinical research: standard operating procedures". http://www.mc.vanderbilt/edu/root/ppt/rss/Blueprint_for_clinicalresearch_sops_FINAL.ppt [accessed 13.03.11].

4. Sajdak R, Thomas K. Presentation entitled "The importance of standard operating procedures (SOPs) in clinical trials". http://www.wrsnm.org/presentations_v2/oct21/Rebecca%20Sajdak%20CNMT.pdf [accessed 13.03.11].

5. US Food and Drug Administration. Code of Federal Regulations Title 21. Website last updated January 4, 2010. http://www.accessdata.fda.gov/scripts/cdrh/cfdocs/cfcfr/cfrsearch.cfm?cfrpart=312 [accessed 13.03.11].

6. Kolman J, Meng P, Scott G, editors. *Good Clinical Practice: Standard Operating Procedures for Clinical Researchers.* New York: Wiley and Sons; 1998.

7. Shefrin A, Saunders C, Rusnak E, DeMarinis AJ. *Standard Operating Procedures for Good Clinical Practice at the Investigative Site.* Center for Clinical Research Practice: Wellesley, MA; 1998.

8. Clinical Trial Magnifier. http://www.clinicaltrialmagnifier.com/ [accessed 13.03.11].

9. Farmovs/Parexel. Presentation on "Standard operating procedures", Corporate GCP course. Presented March 14, 2002. UCT Lung Institute, Cape Town.

CHAPTER 5

How to Select and Oversee Contract Research Organizations

Elizabeth Messersmith
R&D Operations, Balance Therapeutics, Inc, USA

INTRODUCTION

Pharmaceutical and biotechnology companies all face the same challenge of managing operational costs and execution associated with bringing a drug to market. Of the US $130 billion spent on research and development (R&D) in 2008,[1] approximately 70 percent was spent on clinical stage activities.[2,3] Knowing that the return on investment (ROI) must be greater than the dollars spent in the R&D product development cycle, operational strategies

Global Clinical Trials Playbook. DOI: 10.1016/B978-0-12-415787-3.00005-9

must be in place to achieve cost control for a positive ROI. The billion-dollar R&D market drives various choices in the types of contract research organization (CRO) available to support R&D outsourcing.

Focus on outsourcing to support clinical trial execution from planning, through recruitment, to program close-out is essential to control timelines and costs. Slow enrollment or difficult patient recruitment is typical for most trials, with 7 percent of clinical trials beginning on time and 70 percent of sites failing to meet recruitment targets.[4] The faster a trial completes, the faster the approval and the shorter the development time to market. The development cost can be reduced by approximately two-thirds when the development time is reduced by 50 percent. It also provides a longer post-approval patent term in which to recoup ROI.[5] The right choice for clinical trial outsourcing can facilitate the ease of clinical trial execution and decrease the timeline to completion. These deliberate choices can lead to overall reduced costs and an increase in ROI.

It has become more commonplace for emerging markets to be incorporated in clinical trials. Emerging markets, defined as those outside the USA and Central Europe, have outsourcing and vendor choices that cover the regulatory planning stages, clinical trial maintenance activities, program close-out, and report writing. Clinical trial experience has risen in emerging markets, with the number of Food and Drug Association (FDA)-regulated investigators increasing by 15.9 percent in Central and Eastern Europe, 12.1 percent in Latin America, and 10.2 percent in the Asia Pacific region between 2004 and 2007.[6] Emerging markets have demonstrated past clinical trial successes through their ability to tap patient populations, increase patient enrollment rate, and even achieve early trial completion timelines. Vendors in these emerging markets have gained valuable experience and successes, as well as mis-steps, which better prepared them for successful trial execution. This chapter examines the many alternatives and variables to consider when selecting and overseeing a CRO to support a global clinical trial.

PERSPECTIVE OF WORKING WITH GLOBAL AND NICHE CONTRACT RESEARCH ORGANIZATIONS

The combined CRO market in 2009 was estimated at $23.7 billion, with a projected growth to $33.7 billion by 2012.[7] This growth is a reflection that the percentage of outsourced R&D expenditure is expected to outpace the total in-house pharmaceutical growth. This means that more CRO choices will exist when deciding on an outsourcing strategy. The most commonly outsourced services in a clinical trial are clinical site management, monitoring, drug supply management, medical writing, data management, and statistical analysis. These can be found across global CROs and individually within niche CROs.

The choice of services to outsource is solely dependent upon the sponsor's ability to support an internal function/department and the sensitivity of the sponsor to maintain direct hands-on control of its regulatory "sponsor" responsibility, i.e. liability for ensuring quality execution of a clinical trial. For example, clinical site management and monitoring as well as drug supply management are often outsourced, with the sponsor auditing the services of the CRO throughout the study. In this instance, the sponsor ensures its oversight, without directly managing the day-to-day operations. A shared responsibility for program management is often duplicated across the sponsor and CRO, where the sponsor manages its internal development program team and the CRO manages its operational team. Third-party vendor management could occur at either sponsor or CRO. For competitive value, data management, statistical analysis, and regulatory strategy are also often kept in-house, especially in cases where the trial design, endpoint analysis, and registration approval path is less defined. Where a registration path is more defined, outsourcing is feasible. Once a sponsor has built its business model for in-house competencies, CRO choices can be made. When faced with multiple CRO choices, one approach is to consider the services offered between the two broad CRO categories, i.e. global CROs versus niche CROs. In 2005, the top five global CROs by market share laid claim to 36 percent of total industry revenue for outsourcing.[8] These dominant CROs offer a full range of services, developed over years of experience in all aspects of clinical trial execution. The niche CROs comprise the remainder. The definition of a global and niche CRO can be based on the reach of services offered, namely full service and/or functional service, regional depth, technology breadth, and investigator access.

What is a Global Contract Research Organization?

A global CRO typically offers a comprehensive spectrum of full service departments which operationally integrate across the organization. They can support a global clinical trial program managed by country-specific locations, which are all integrated with respect to the systems and processes. They typically have experience in the entire spectrum of clinical development phases (I–IV) for multiple therapeutic areas. These organizations offer services across a large geographical area, and have considerable technology breadth, numerous and broad access to experienced investigators, patient centers, and well-defined controls supported by standardized processes. For the sponsor, positioning a single CRO to execute a global clinical trial can be favorable from a sponsor management perspective, as the dollar value for the program means that the CRO can build the best team to service the trial. If, however, the trial does not require global execution, the full service offering can also be segmented into functional service offerings at the sponsor's request. This approach can be important for companies to bridge their internal functional expertise with outsourcing. For a global CRO, the day-to-day interactions of conducting a global clinical study encompass:

- country-specific amendments to protocol and informed consent that are aligned with a global protocol and informed consent
- responsiveness of query handling for protocol and operational execution
- staff training and qualification, both within the CRO and at the investigator's site
- emphasis on all aspects of study monitoring and quality
- integration of technology systems or processes to efficiently streamline workflow to effectively handle data input and output
- transparency and clarity in reporting.

A global CRO, with its set systems and standards implemented across its organization, can effectively manage a global clinical program. In this framework, a global CRO's success will be measured as the total output of its organization. For a sponsor who chooses not to utilize the full service option, but limit outsourcing to a few functional service options, issues within program integration can arise quickly. As an example, take the integration of a third party monitoring service to verify site activities or data verification of the global CRO that has been awarded study execution. The systems and standards that allow the global CRO to integrate well across its organization immediately become an obstacle for the third party vendor to conduct monitoring or verify data. The sponsor and global CRO then have to define an integrated solution. The set of systems and standards that is the strength of the global CRO can become the source of inflexibility in which new solutions for program integration across the sponsor, CRO, or third party vendors have to be defined.

What is a Niche Contract Research Organization?

A niche CRO typically specializes in a therapeutic area or technology-based service, or builds infrastructure to access specific patient populations in narrow geographical locations. The narrow geographical markets are defined as second or third tier city centers (based on population) in emerging markets, where there is less global CRO competition. Key to providing the sponsor access is the niche CRO's location. Maintenance of local office(s) in the second and third tier city centers facilitates the niche CRO's access to the local network of regulatory processes, local language, and cultural integration.[6] These CROs can offer many types of service but are geographically limited to local areas; alternatively, they may offer single technology operational services, for example, monitoring, electronic data capture (EDC) to data entry, electronic patient recorded outcomes (ePROs) and investigator meeting planning, across multiple second and third tier cities. In contrast to global CROs, niche CROs have greater flexibility in operational and innovative procedures, primarily because their internal systems and standards are meant to integrate with other third party providers. Niche CROs will often propose alliance or partner companies to the sponsor for services that they do not offer, since the niche CRO has past integration project experience on which to build. In addition, niche CROs have a strong understanding of cultural influences and considerable experience with local regulatory authorities. Local regulatory approval is a key step to entry within an emerging market. Niche CROs typically have a smaller customer base and thus are often more responsive to the needs of a sponsor, but they are also targets for mergers and acquisitions. There are numerous choices available when identifying a niche CRO to service a particular area of a clinical trial. Niche CROs can be netted together to cover most clinical trials needs, but it is up to the sponsor to provide and manage integration.

How to Leverage the Menu of Services Offered by a Global or Niche Contract Research Organization

Each type of CRO has a menu of services to offer through a variety of financial models with different incentives. Five different financial classifications are used to describe these models: time and materials, fixed unit, fee for service, outcomes based, and risk milestone sharing (Table 5.1).

Most of these pricing models can be used to engage the CRO in their range of services. Typically, global CROs can offer incentives for functional sourcing for multiple programs or full service modalities to support a single program. They can also offer à la carte services for a price premium to the sponsor if there is an immediate need to fill a functional or capacity gap within the sponsor organization. In contrast, niche CROs specializing as functional service providers typically cannot support all the needs of an entire drug development program but rather have developed considerable depth in a technology, speciality laboratory, or procedure that can be leveraged to fill expertise, process, or capacity gaps in the organization. The financial incentive for the niche provider is typically seen in the unit pricing, where cost reflects not only their optimization in technology, but also less infrastructure and lower management overheads. As an example, consider the past emergence of niche data management CROs in India, where unit pricing was substantially lower owing to reduced labor market infrastructure costs. Economic changes and competition can rapidly change, affecting labor costs; therefore, the validation of these assumptions should be questioned before making outsourcing decisions.

Although not utilized to a great extent, financial incentives and penalties can be negotiated into most financial models. Financial incentives, reported to occur in about 11 percent of contracts, incorporate performance incentives recognized as financial bonuses to the project team and company.[9] These performance incentives have typically been defined as high-level milestones for a program: meeting timelines early, meeting or beating patient enrollment goals, coming in on or below budget, quality of deliverables, and low project team turnover. Financial penalties have been reported to occur in slightly more cases, 17 percent, and are expressed in terms of withdrawal of future business, delay or decrease in payments due to missed timelines, poor deliverable quality, study delays, not meeting patient enrollment goals, or being over budget.[9] It is not clear whether defined incentives or penalties improve pricing or really affect communication between the sponsor and CRO to achieve the common goal of study completion with quality.

TABLE 5.1 Financial Models	
Pricing model	**Comment**
Time and materials: Estimates cost-based hours required to complete the task; charged for hours worked to complete task **Time and materials with a cap**: Places a cap on the charges for both materials and work	Time and materials (with or without cap) works well for services typically in the scope where the deliverable is technology or speciality expertise based. Examples include chemistry-based deliverables, packaging, and labeling for clinical trial materials.
Fixed unit: Charge is based on a projected dollar cost to deliver a specific, well-defined task or deliverable; charged fixed price is less or more work than projections required to complete tasks **Fixed fee/fixed price**: Also includes charges for pass-through costs, as well as personnel costs	CRO typically needs to leverage an integrated technology platform to gain maximum cost reductions and efficiencies. Both sides must recognize that is it difficult to introduce change into this system platform without incurring additional costing changes to both sponsor and CRO. Both CRO and sponsor benefit by spending less time tracking invoice rates and negotiating pricing. **Sponsor perspective**: If budgeted appropriately, there are fewer scope changes to negotiate and better control of funding demands over time. **CRO perspective**: There is better planning of resources to support in-house efficiency gains in accounting, program tracking, more accurate accounts payable/receivable, and the opportunity to build long-term performance-based relationships.
Unitized: Based on defined activity units, such as time interval or frequency of repetition **Fee for service**: Dollar cost is charged for time spent for a specific individual's actual work time provided to the sponsor	Typically this is a single isolated functional service, charged by the unit. It is very flexible for the sponsor to achieve the best product. The final cost is driven by a number of factors: (1) professional level/qualifications of the individual providing the service; (2) clarity in the expectations delivered at initiation of the project, where a changing work scope will alter production fees; and (3) differing incentives to control billable hours between CRO and sponsor.
Outcomes based: Focused on deliverable where rates are dependent on a prespecified delivery date requirement for a well-defined task	Predicated on a clear definition of feasibility and scope. The operational scope typically shifts over completely to the CRO. A CRO can apply this model to support multiple programs within a single CRO and gain synergy for the volume of work. The sponsor gains cost efficiencies in the preferred pricing. Both CRO and sponsor gain efficiencies by centralized management for the proposed work scope. The milestones are incentives/penalties for both sponsor and CRO.
Risk sharing: Cost is preset to achieve major milestones within a program. Either reduced hourly or fixed units can underlie the cost estimates, but in addition there are milestone payments for meeting the timelines of key program deliverables	The cost of services is typically discounted with milestone-based incentives acting as the reward or penalty for service delivered. This model places great emphasis on the

Continued

43

TABLE 5.1 Financial Models—continued	
Pricing model	**Comment**
	sponsor having a fully vetted and finalized clinical development plan, and the CRO accurately estimating costs and resources, managing profit margins, and assessing the overall operational success of the clinical development plan.
	Both sponsor and CRO have a financial interest in efficient execution, so there needs to be an additional level of transparency and communication across the organizations to enable active collaboration to address and resolve issues quickly.

CRO: contract research organization.

Advantages of Working with a Global Versus a Niche Contract Research Organization and Vice Versa

A global CRO advertises that it provides CRO personnel training and maintains a depth in personnel background and experience which can be used to accommodate the resourcing challenges in a large-scale global clinical trial. This quality of meeting resourcing demands has been identified as one of the top reasons for working with a global CRO.[9] Another advantage of working with a global CRO is that typically a past working relationship with either the company or individual exists which can be leveraged to set expectations or proactively address CRO inadequacies. The third most cited working advantage lies with knowledge of past pricing and leverage to preferred pricing.

A niche CRO also leverages the advantages of prior experience, personnel training, and background. Although personnel is of a similar standard to a global CRO, there is less depth in the ability to resource. Therapeutic experience or technological advantage is one of the key factors identified as preferred in the selection of niche over global CROs.[10] Niche CROs are also recognized as being easier to incorporate into a sponsor's program from a strategic and cultural perspective.

Whether one chooses global, niche, or a combination of CROs, it should be kept in mind that there is no standard solution to outsourcing, as the successful mix of clinical trial outsourcing is most dependent on the business needs and strategic direction of the sponsor organization and the program goals.

UNDERSTANDING YOUR OPTIONS WHEN OUTSOURCING AN OVERSEAS TRIAL

The first step in defining a successful outsourcing plan for an overseas trial is to have a clear understanding of the clinical trial design, role, and responsibilities of the sponsor and CRO. A sponsor organization can either take complete ownership to define all the details and workflow within a clinical trial design or start with a study concept that is outsourced to a CRO to complete both the final clinical study design protocol and execution. While health authorities will hold the sponsor liable for study oversight in either case, the approach chosen is up to the sponsor. In the former example, the sponsor maintains and drives the clinical science focus of the design and dictates operational execution, while often overlooking the operational feasibility and associated cost of the design. This outsourcing strategy can lead to cost inefficiencies as well as missed program deliverables if the sponsor requires the CRO to work outside its processes. While the latter strategy leverages the operational feasibility, it may lack integration of the particular specific therapeutic being evaluated, especially if the product goal focuses on more exploratory endpoints, biomarkers, and study population segmentation. A balanced approach, where the sponsor's therapeutic and drug target expertise is merged with the CRO's operational expertise and feasibility assessment, can be used to leverage the best of sponsor and CRO organizations. This is especially the case where the sponsor has great depth in the therapeutic area and trial design but is less familiar with the operational caveats in regions outside its own geography. The decision to leverage the CRO's expertise in these regions and utilize their functionality to support the trial is a key point of consideration in completing the outsourcing strategy for an overseas clinical trial. The driving factors should consider both the CRO's versus the sponsor's expertise, and the sponsor's ability to provide effective staffing for the trial capacity.

Defining the Scope of Work: Aligning the Outsourcing Strategy to Meet the Organizational Capacity

Understanding the type of service to be outsourced is the result of the sponsor's completing a gap analysis in a number of areas: therapeutic depth and experience, site management and scale capability, integrated tracking of the project, defined standards and repeatable processes, infrastructure capacity in application expertise in core laboratories, data management, and speciality services such as imaging, analytical assays, specialized medical assessments, or technology/medical devices to capture patient data. The State of the Clinical Trials Industry (2009) surveyed the top reason for outsourcing cited by sponsors; the lack of internal resources or capacity to support a clinical trial was identified.[11] Staffing up and down to meet the demands of a single trial can readily tax other infrastructure parts of an organization, so the decision to use a CRO to meet this delta in demand is recognized. Nearly equal in responses were reasons regarding portfolio fit of the program within the organization, i.e. the program was considered a non-core competency to the organization or a single indication opportunity for the company. This speaks to aligning the outsourcing strategy with the organization's product development goals.

Defining the Scope of Work: Aligning the Outsourcing Strategy to Meet the Product Development Goals

A clear goal for the product is required to effectively align the appropriate operational strategy. The level of operational investment is dependent on the sponsor's intent: launch of a product, or defining the therapeutic potential to support licensing of the product. The key strategic question around country selection not only sets the path to support initial product launch but begins to define the operational and outsourcing boundaries. For example, if the organization's goal is ultimately to sell off the asset during the early phase of drug development but before initiation of a registration clinical study, an initial clinical trial entry targeted in emerging countries can gain product experience along with decreases in time to study enrollment/completion. The follow-on choice of outsourcing to complete the clinical trial then becomes focused on time to execution and operational efficiencies looking to leverage the integration services within that central geography. At the other extreme, if the sponsor clearly has functional capability to support the trial and the sponsor organization is trying to establish itself as an innovative leader in a particular therapeutic area, then operational execution and clinical strategy become a key element of focus. This latter choice often comes with a timeline and cost increase, as the sponsor gains experience, both strategic and operational, which is then applied to the coordination, integration, and analysis of data. One of the most challenging time factors remains time to complete patient recruitment. Even in this extreme scenario, there is the option to include emerging countries and CROs to bolster patient enrollment.

A practical step in aligning the scope of work is to ensure that the transfer of obligations between sponsor and CRO is clearly documented. While the decision on what to transfer to a CRO is made by the sponsor, the delegation of these responsibilities must be detailed and appropriately documented to demonstrate that the investigational new drug studies conducted (regardless of geographical location) must follow GCP guidelines to be accepted by the larger regulatory authority (FDA or EMEA).

The International Conference on Harmonisation Good Clinical Practice (ICH-GCP) E6 Guidelines[12] note:

5.2.1 A sponsor may transfer any or all of the sponsor's trial-related duties and functions to a CRO, but the ultimate responsibility for the quality and integrity of the trial data always resides with the sponsor. The CRO should implement quality assurance and quality control.

5.2.2 Any trial-related duty and function that is transferred to and assumed by a CRO should be specified in writing.

5.2.3 Any trial-related duties and functions not specifically transferred to and assumed by a CRO are retained by the sponsor.

Even in the light of transfer of work responsibilities, the sponsor retains the responsibility for providing oversight of the CRO. Table 5.2 shows a list of scope activities to consider when defining the transfer of obligations matrix. The list is ICH- and FDA-centric, and it cites the supporting regulatory guidance and a generic description of the responsibility. When progressing into emerging markets, the selected CRO within the region, along with the sponsor, should update the transfer of obligations with specific requirements for the region according to the appropriate regulatory body.

Defining Top-Line Criteria to Successfully Evaluate Contract Research Organization Choices

The setting of criteria to meet and measure quality, financial goals, and timeline progress should be completed before CRO selection to ensure successful management of any outsourced service. Recognizing that the sponsor is ultimately responsible for the quality, investment, and time to service completion of the product, the choice of CRO is critical in successfully supporting that responsibility.

The most common criteria utilized to select a CRO are staffing to fill a capacity or expertise gap; experience of the CRO in terms of quality, experience, and retention of staff; preferred ranking of the CRO, directly with the sponsor or with individuals now employed with the sponsor; and therapeutic expertise of the CRO in type, number, size, and geographical footprint of the trial experience. These common criteria are good to rely on when country selection of the past trials is being implemented, but may hold little value when country selection includes emerging or naïve markets. The perspective that sites bring to evaluating past performance is underestimated when the outsourcing strategy involves emerging or naïve markets.

Site evaluation of CRO performance is typically not a criterion for CRO selection for countries where clinical sites and GCP have been in place for a number of years. However, a sponsor can gain insight over the site's perspective of its CRO working relationship and the sponsor may apply these factors in evaluating a CRO's working relationship in emerging markets. Center-Watch surveys of CRO responsiveness to site service have been conducted over a number of years (2001–2007)[11] and provide a set of attributes that can be applied to CROs offering services in emerging countries. In general, these attributes have steadily improved across the USA and Europe, resulting in higher site satisfaction over the years: organization and preparedness of CRO staff, setting of realistic timelines and patient enrollment goals, responsiveness to protocol enquiries, usability of case report forms (CRFs), realistic grant payment schedule, prompt payment of services and the CRO's role in effective liaison with the sponsor. Setting criteria and

TABLE 5.2 Scope Activities

Guidance		Description of responsibility to consider transferring by line item
Preparation and document submission	21 CFR §312.23	• Document preparation • Document submission • Regulatory approval
Maintain effective filing with respect to the investigation	21 CFR §312.50, 312.30, 312.31	• Main filing amendments, as required • Protocol amendments (new protocols, changes in protocols and adding new investigators) • Information amendments: chemistry, manufacturing, and controls; pharmacology/toxicology; clinical
Select investigators and monitors	ICH GCP E6, 2.8, 4.1, 5.18, 5.61 21 CFR §312.50, 312.53a–d, 312.55	• Select qualified investigators • Verify that proposed investigators are not debarred/disqualified • Disseminate appropriate information to investigators to conduct the investigation properly • Control distribution of study drug • Obtain from each investigator: completed and signed form FDA-1572, curriculum vitae, clinical protocol, and financial disclosure • Inform investigators • Select qualified monitors to monitor the progress of the investigation
Monitor the investigation	ICH GCP E6, 5.18 21 CFR §312.56a–d, 312.59	• Monitor the progress of clinical investigations being conducted under the submission • Secure compliance or discontinue investigator participation • If investigator participation discontinued, ensure return and disposition of study drug per 21 CFR §312.59 • If investigator participation discontinued, notify agency of discontinuation of investigator

Continued

47

TABLE 5.2 Scope Activities—continued

Guidance		Description of responsibility to consider transferring by line item
		• Review and evaluate evidence relating to safety and effectiveness of the drug as it is obtained and report to regulatory board, as appropriate • Discontinue investigation when appropriate and notify regulatory agency, all IRBs, and all investigators
Investigator records and reports	ICH GCP E6, 5.18 21 CFR §312.62, 312.64, 312.66	• Monitor that investigators are maintaining proper records and making proper reports

Sponsor records and reports	ICH GCP E6, 5.5
	21 CFR §312.57 a, c, 312.32, 312.33
		• Prepare and submit as appropriate:
		  – records of shipment and disposition of drug
		  – retention of all records and reports required
		  – safety reports
		  – investigational drug annual reports

IRB records	ICH GCP E6 5.11 21 CFR §312.66	• Verify that IRB review and approval of investigation are obtained prior to study drug shipment
Regulatory request for records and reports	21 CFR §312.58a	• Provide records or reports upon regulatory request
Disposition of unused supply of study drug	ICH GCP E6, 5.14.4 21 CFR §312.59	• Return and disposition of unused study drug
Apply for approval to export study drug	21 CFR §312.110	• Apply for regulatory approval to export study drug
Sample retention for bioavailability and bioequivalence studies	21 CFR §312.57 c, d, 320.38	• Retain reserve samples of study drug and reference standard

CFR: Code of Federal Regulations; ICH-GCP: International Conference on Harmonisation Good Clinical Practice; IRB: institutional review board.

ranking responsiveness to these qualities could be helpful in separating out experienced and naïve CROs bidding for work in trials being conducted in emerging markets.

COMPARING THE CAPABILITIES OF GLOBAL AND NICHE CONTRACT RESEARCH ORGANIZATIONS TO SUPPORT CLINICAL TRIALS

Capability comparisons when considering CRO clinical trial operations rest on the CRO's ability to demonstrate past success in a number of areas: GCP training and compliance, quality of professionals, interface experience with health and ethics committees, experience in training investigators and maintaining quality data and documentation at clinical sites, experience and familiarity in working for approval to conduct a trial, knowledge of local restrictions, and ability to access patient populations in an efficient manner. CROs, both global and niche, relatively new to the clinical trial industry in the countries of Central and Eastern Europe, have over the past five years begun to demonstrate a presence in successful participation in global clinical trials. Global CROs can easily access and address this past performance through their existing processes and systems infrastructure. Niche CROs, lacking this infrastructure base, will have to augment their data with plans to actively build and manage these capabilities through qualified personnel and key relationships with sponsors.

Key Performance and Relationship Attributes

Performance attributes for both global and niche CROs can be evaluated before CRO selection by rating staff qualifications in terms of years of experience, training, and staff turnover, and evaluation of key standard operating procedures to understand the incorporation of good clinical practice attributes into procedures such as site qualification, patient informed consent, data management, drug shipment/accountability, and site monitoring. Once a CRO has been selected, ongoing metric reports to evaluate adherence to study execution milestones and clinical management objectives can be evaluated at preagreed intervals. Relationship attributes can be evaluated and managed by review and specialization of the quality oversight and clinical risk management plans, which address issue escalation, tracking, and resolution. Successful management of these key attributes supports successful trial completion regardless of the type of CRO chosen for study execution.

Top Emerging Markets for Clinical Trials

Local CROs in top emerging clinical trial markets outside North America and Western Europe include those in the countries of Eastern Europe such as Poland, Hungary, the Czech Republic, Romania, and Bulgaria; Russia and Ukraine; Asian countries, especially India and China; and Latin America, particularly Brazil and Argentina, and Mexico. These countries have demonstrated growth in participation in clinical trials, where foreign-based sites have continued to increase steadily from 16.3 percent in 2001 to 33.5 percent in 2007.[16] Given that clinical trial globalization comprises over one-third of clinical investigator experience, the practice of conducting trials and the ease of trial execution will continue to enhance a CRO's ability to support current trials while they continue to improve upon their capabilities for future trials.

In addition, the portfolio of drug development will continue to play a central role in determining which countries will comprise future emerging clinical trial markets. As the operational procedures to tap into these new markets become more established, the access to patients with a particular disease or condition becomes less of a barrier. Therefore, the scope of clinical research may change in response to knowing that drug development opportunities may now exist where patient opportunities and regional disease or therapeutic indications were viewed as inaccessible in the past.

Special Considerations when Using Contract Research Organizations in Emerging Markets

The primary issue at stake when considering clinical trial conduct in emerging markets rests with the sponsor to ensure data accuracy, compliance with respect to world standards, and trial conduct without bias. Operational aspects can then focus on a review of the emerging market's genetic diversity and/or limitations, predicted enrollment rates, standard of medical care for the particular indication, cost of procedures, cultural acceptance of patients to comply for the duration of the clinical trial, and qualifications of investigators. Additional regulatory and government barriers to execution of a clinical trial in a relatively new geography can include the role of the country in supporting registration, the potential for bureaucracy and excessive procedures, vague legislation, lack of implementation of regulatory standards, costs and logistics to ship drug or biological samples, unplanned taxes, negative attitudes in the media, and lack of cooperation within trial centers. If not managed appropriately, all these can negatively affect the ability to enroll patients in a timely manner and increase the time and costs of the clinical trial.

To successfully address these special considerations, selecting a CRO that understands geographical differences in patient centers, differences in medical practice diagnosis, and standard of care, is key in emerging markets. For example, in some countries acupuncture and herbal medicine are often part of standard practice and their use can complicate clinical trial results. Clear acceptance criteria for use during the trial need to be defined within the clinical protocol and included and monitored as part of the investigator training.

While management of these special considerations may seem daunting, often the management can be centrally located from either a global or a local CRO because the large patient pools that exist in Russia, South America, China, and India have the advantage of being located in large urban areas with central medical facilities. In addition, these centers can act as central points of operational management hubs to increase patient accessibility and decrease burden costs for extensive travel, as required by patients from smaller communities or rural regions.

Special strategic considerations for evaluating a specific drug product profile can exist in emerging markets, which have larger naïve patient populations. These regions can support trials of a potential product as first- or second-line therapy with more rapid enrollment rates. They can also support the need for a placebo-based trial versus a comparative trial. The key to successful implementation of either strategy lies within the regulatory approval process for trial initiation, which can be levered through a knowledgeable CRO, assuming that the sponsor lacks such expertise.

Incremental Criteria for Contract Research Organization Selection

The main driver for outsourcing in clinical markets outside North America and Western Europe is time to enrollment. There are some advantages where unit pricing can be lower owing to labor cost differences or procedure pricing, but these drivers are second to patient availability and the impact on overall clinical trial timelines. An additional five criteria are presented below as topics to discuss in more detail with potential CROs during the bidding and contracting process.

- **Resource flexibility during the different stages in a clinical study**: The ability of a CRO to proactively manage the resource differences that occur between study start-up, maintenance, database lock and close-out of a clinical study should be clearly presented in the request for proposal (RFP) during the bid solicitation process. For example, clear application of resources during site start-up ensures timely execution to bring online the majority of clinical sites and is essential for setting and validating the initial rate of enrollment. If site activation lags, then time lost in realizing that the predicted enrollment rate is lower than the target can rarely be recovered. Resource differences should be documented through functional assessments of the proposed work to ensure that costly charge orders are not required to accommodate the ramping-up of activity during study start-up and database lock.
- **Accessibility to import/export drug and biological samples from clinical trial sites or geographical regions without hindering customs and operational shipping delays**: Queries on country-specific requirements, potential hurdles and examples of risk mitigation to regional specific issues should be addressed during the bid defense. The handling of biological samples, as well as informed consent requirements detailing how the patient samples will be used, can have country-specific limitations. A niche, geographically specific CRO can typically be leveraged to resolve these issues.

- **Monitoring plan and frequency**: Site monitoring is one of the higher cost items in a clinical trial. A change in the frequency of monitoring will have a large budget impact on a clinical study. Many factors control the expected time spent on monitoring and drive the expected costs. A complex study with complicated CRFs and EDC will require more time on site and probably more monitoring time throughout the study. Operational assessment of these complex parameters can help to align the expected CRF review time and EDC query resolution. EDC allows greater visibility and more frequent checks for data field completeness and can be a cost-efficient use of monitoring time. Use of EDC checks can better prepare monitors for on-site areas of focus, yet should not be viewed as a replacement, but rather as means to supplement, on-site monitoring visits. This is especially important when considering monitoring frequency in emerging markets with less overall clinical trial experience. During the bidding process, a CRO should actively present the cost drivers for monitoring, experience level of their monitoring staff, expectations for activities to be completed during monitoring, and separate out the cost drivers for focus on site compliance and documentation, as well as defining trends in operational challenges and protocol design issues.
- **Clinical project meetings and reports**: Aligning the expectations of cross-functional meetings and reporting metrics should be addressed during the RFP process. Depending on the type of relationship between sponsor and CRO meeting, participation could be set to ensure that essential personnel are in attendance as defined by the meeting agenda, or a broader approach could be taken in which the CRO team personnel attend all meetings to maintain program awareness. This working style should be set by the sponsor and billed accordingly.
- **Pass-through costs**: During the RFP review, process funds are allocated into the pass-through cost category. This category tends to be poorly defined and often grows unexpectedly. Setting a definition of items captured within this category as well as setting an agreement not to exceed limits can help to set awareness triggers for unexpected costs incurred during a clinical study.

51

ASSESSING THE BENEFITS OF INTERNATIONAL REACH VERSUS LOCAL KNOWLEDGE

Benefits of international reach compared with local knowledge can be grouped into three main areas: regulatory reach versus local knowledge, staffing of a clinical trial, and the appropriate use of the patient population. The selection of the outsourcing plan needs to take into account how the choice of a CRO can affect each of these benefits.

Government forces can have an impact on the regulatory and trial review process and thus the time to clinical trial initiation. Knowing how the country-specific regulatory standards align with harmonized regulatory standards is critical. The effects of government forces vary from making it more demanding for the regulatory and trial review process to receive approval to a more collaborative process of working through regulations and facilitation of protocol reviews. If the sponsor lacks the internal expertise to navigate the regulatory process, then outsourcing to a CRO in which that expertise can be validated may guard against lost time in study initiation, as well as time later in meeting that country's specific expectations of a qualified and properly conducted clinical study. The level of awareness of these issues will depend on the breadth of the CRO's international reach and depth of local knowledge. It may be necessary to balance the choice of CRO with the sponsor's internal capability or to identify the gaps in either to successfully navigate the regulatory and trial review process.

In emerging markets, staffing for a clinical trial can be under scrutiny by government forces or regulatory granting agencies that support protocol review. Where medical markets are under rapid development, the expertise in conducting trials is relatively new and limited. Health agencies within these countries have an interest in ensuring that patients and medical professionals are offered access to medical care and trained appropriately to develop GCP, and that the experience and expertise stay within the country to support access to subsequent clinical trials and advances in the healthcare offered. Choosing a local CRO, where knowledge is preserved within the country, addresses this concern, whereas a global CRO, with its international reach, will need to demonstrate how they support knowledge transfer to a local level.

At the completion of a trial, the granting agency conducts an evaluation to assess whether the clinical population used in the trial represents the proposed target population for treatment. If the patient pool varies too widely by geographical region, there may be underlying differences in pharmacokinetic and pharmacodynamic profiles in the outcome data, as well as variations with respect to the interpretation of clinical inclusion or exclusion criteria, in medical diagnosis or acceptable treatment. The inclusion of too many countries may lead to local regulatory authorities requiring additional clinical bridging studies in order for the trial to be accepted. Similar rules of acceptance apply to international trials conducted in the USA and European Union, in that data must be relevant and apply to the population, with a preference for including patients from the country granting approval. These conditions are in addition to verifiable data, and involve qualified and competent clinical investigators.[17]

Addressing Cultural Barriers

Cultural standards regarding disclosure, informed consent, data ownership, and investigator rights to publish should be evaluated with care, as the standards within Western clinical trials should not be assumed to be universally adopted. For example, disclosure of the patient's diagnosis upon entry into trial can be culturally filtered. The informed consent process can often be viewed as being the decision of the physician, rather than that of the patient. The decision to participate in a trial can also extend to other people, as reported in a clinical study in India in which 30 percent of patients chose to involve other people before providing trial consent, compared with the practice followed by US patients.[18] This can also be true with respect to ownership of data and publication rights. The sponsor has a responsibility to endorse the standards of informed consent and practice of the informed consent process. It is important to address local knowledge of these challenges with a CRO and proactive management may be required in some emerging clinical markets.

Importance of Translation

Language must be used correctly and documents associated with a clinical trial should be translated accurately. Local translators who are qualified to translate clinical study documents, such as clinical protocol summaries, informed consent, and patient-oriented information, can offer translations into a native language. Ensuring that translations are completed with accuracy can bridge culture gaps and protect against trial delays, increased costs, and potential litigation. It is critically important to address the need for translation in countries with multiple dialects. CROs with local knowledge of the country or region are likely to be most suited to addressing translation appropriately, especially when local dialects are of concern.

Awareness of Work Styles

The benefits of international reach and local knowledge can be evaluated through the top factors reported for delays in clinical trials. The factors resulting in clinical trial delays typically focus on patient enrollment, investigator selection, contract/budget approval, and protocol amendments. The last three of these involve a great deal of process and documentation. Reports from trials sites in North America found that 70 percent of delays were typically one month or longer, whereas in Europe and Canada this figure was 56 percent, and only 41 percent in Asia Pacific and Latin America.[11] Although North America and Canada would be expected to have equivalent knowledge and experience through their substantial years of experience, the trial delay discrepancy is probably due to working style, in that Canadian sites

TABLE 5.3 Items to Consider when Designing Key Performance Indicators

Key performance indicator	Threshold (set limits for meets/exceeds/ does not exceed)	Target	Results (average) (measured output)	Subcategories/comment
Site recruitment				Threshold and target can be based on time allotted per study enrollment feasibility
Trip reports	10 days	10 days	7.2 days	Site management and pharmacy management
Site issue resolution	> 85%	> 90%	100%	All issues and data queries addressed immediately or resolved within a window
Site visits	> 90%	> 95%	100%	Per scheduled frequency for initiation and monitoring visits
Utilization for site management	Days on site per x personnel	Days on site per x personnel	Days on site	
Query rate				No. of eCRF; no./100 data field: < 5/eCRF pages for a typical 40 page uncomplicated clinical design
Time from query to query resolution				Set day threshold and target to clean database which can be changed as the study progresses, e.g. longer allowable time at study start, down to 24 hours before last patient's last visit
Last patient, last visit to database lock	100%	100%	100%	
Training	> 95%	100%	100%	CRO training metrics to support study, as well as CRO SOPs
Turnover	15%	10%	0%	CRO study staff departures or promotions
Time to fill positions	85%	90%	100%	CRO study staff time to fill turnover

eCRF: electronic case report form; CRO: contract research organization; SOP: standard operating procedure.

are more efficient than US sites. The drivers for this discrepancy are likely to be process related. While emerging markets may lack standardization of processes, too much process can also be a hindrance. Finding the right CRO with knowledge of the working style and expectations regarding regulatory and shipping processes can help to prevent these types of trial delay.

EXAMINING QUALITY AND RELATIONSHIP MANAGEMENT TO FINALIZE CONTRACT RESEARCH ORGANIZATION SELECTION

At the conclusion of a trial, the performance standards and lessons to be incorporated in future work should be identified. However, waiting until trial conclusion will be too late to ensure that current trial performance meets expectations. The performance standards used by a CRO must be identified at the beginning of CRO selection and measured throughout a trial. Key to CRO selection is ensuring that high performance standards in the areas of service, quality, compliance, effectiveness, and finance can be validated by a repeatable and measurable methodology. Key performance indicators (KPIs) of operational related key outcomes can be assessed regularly. In general, these metrics are measures of cycles, quality, productivity, and efficiency. The metric is typically tracked for items that are performed repeatedly over the course of the study. By tracking on a regular basis, one can implement corrective actions and improve performance. For each metric, it is important to define the precise start and end points used for measurement; for example, time increments for site recruitment, document approvals, institutional review board approvals, database development, completion of edit check writing and programming, monitoring cycle, and drug receipt by the first subject at each site. Measures of contract and finance performance may include time for contract approval, on-time/on-budget enrollment, financial reporting, invoice compliance, and contractual compliance to ensure clear financial transparency. Lastly, evaluating processes for relationship management between the sponsor and CRO is essential to setting up effective in communication, issue resolution, and overall project success. Some items to consider when designing KPIs are listed in Table 5.3. To gain sponsor oversight of the CRO and visibility of the CRO's management of a clinical program, performing an ongoing evaluation of KPIs at monthly, or at a minimum of quarterly intervals, will provide additional sponsor oversight. This approach will assist in the merging of the sponsor's and CRO's working style into one common goal of product development.

References

1. Space S. *Competition challenges US site profitability.* CenterWatch Monthly (November); 2007.
2. Pfizer: Research and Development Clinical Trials,www.pfizer.com/research/clinical_trials/clinical_trials.jsp; May 22, 2009.
3. PhRMA. *Pharmaceutical Industry Profile: 2009.* Washington, DC: PhRMA; 2009.
4. Clinical Research Report. *Pharmaceutical Industry Competitive Task Force.* UK Department of Health; 2002.
5. DiMasi JA. The value of improving the productivity of the drug development process — faster times and better decisions. *PharmacoEconomics* 2002;**20**(Suppl. 3):1–10.
6. Gambrill S. *Central and Eastern Europe triples global trial participation.* Center Watch Monthly (August); 2008.
7. Hoang T, et al. *Contract Research Helps Keep Drug Pipelines Flowing.* Sector Focus Report. Berwyn, PA: Turner Capital Investment; 2008.
8. Tufts Center for the Study of Drug Development. *Outlook 2007.* Boston, MA: Tufts CSDD; 2007.
9. CenterWatch. Volume 12, Issue 10. Boston, MA: CenterWatch; 2005.
10. Thomson CenterWatch. *State of the Clinical Trials Industry.* Boston, MA: Thomson Healthcare; 2005.
11. Lamberti MJ, editor. *State of the Clinical Trials Industry: A Sourcebook of Charts and Statistics.* Boston, MA: CenterWatch; 2009.
12. ICH Topic E6 Guideline for Good Clinical Practice, Consolidated Guideline 17 January 1997 (CPMP/ICH/135/95) Section 5.2, Contract Research Organization (CRO); 5.7, Allocation of Duties and Functions; 8.0 Essential Documents for the Conduct of a Clinical Trial.

13. FDA. *Guidance for industry — acceptance of foreign clinical studies*, www.fda.gov/RegulatoryInformation/ Guidances; 2009.

14. International Conference on Harmonisation. Technical requirements for registration of pharmaceuticals for human use. Ethnic factors in the acceptability of foreign clinical data. E5(R1); 1998.

15. CFR §312.52, Investigational New Drug Application, Subpart D: Responsibilities of sponsors and investigators: transfer of obligations to a contract research organization.

16. Getz KA, Zuckerman R. Today's global site landscape. *Applied Clinical Trials (June)*:34–8, http:// appliedclinicaltrialsonline.findpharma.com; 2010.

17. US 21 CFR §314.106. The acceptance of foreign data in a new drug application.

18. Berman-Gorvine M. Understanding patient culture key to recruitment in India. *Clinical Trials Advisor (June 11)*; 2009.

CHAPTER 6

The How-To of Global Clinical Trial Forecasting, Budgeting, and Project Management

Dong Wei

Janssen Alzheimer Immunotherapy R&D, LLC, South San Francisco, California, USA

RECENT TRENDS IN CLINICAL TRIALS

Global Rising Costs of Clinical Trials

The cost of drug development has risen steadily during the past few decades, from approximately US $300 million in 1987 to about $800 million in 2000[1] and $1.3 billion in 2005.[2] A significant driver for escalating costs is declining productivity in the clinical trial phase of development. Indeed, a recent study showed that from 1995 to 2002, the average Phase III development cost increased from $131 million to $200 million, while the probability of registration approval fell from 73 to 59 percent.[3] It now takes, on average, 37 separate Phase I to Phase III clinical trials to gain one new drug approval.[4] In addition, clinical trials often require more complex procedures, more subjects, and longer duration than in the past.

Rise in Clinical Trial Complexity

Clinical trials have become increasingly complicated with more endpoints to observe and test, driven by advances in scientific and medical knowledge, shifting the focus to chronic and more complex diseases, and higher demand for safety, efficacy, and outcome by patients, physicians, and regulatory authorities. From 1999 to 2005, the total procedures per trial protocol increased by 65 percent, with unique procedures per trial protocol increasing by 46 percent.[5] Consequently, in order to reach valid study conclusions, i.e. by achieving statistical significance, larger sample sizes and longer treatment durations are often needed. An investigation of 300 clinical studies reported in major medical journals in 1995 and 2005 found that the median patient population required has increased from 215 to 661[6] and the length of trials has increased from 460 to 780 days.[7]

Stagnant Volunteer Participation

Meanwhile, participation and enrollment rates of clinical trial volunteer subjects have been stagnant. In the USA, only about 2 percent of the population is involved in clinical trials sponsored by academic institutions and biopharmaceutical companies. Even among people who suffer from severe and chronic diseases, the participation rate is only 6 percent.[8] Competition for these subjects has intensified as the number of compounds in clinical development has increased: in the USA alone in 2009, approximately 2950 compounds were in clinical trials or waiting for approval, compared with about 2000 in 2000.[5] Consequently, only 6 percent of clinical trials are completed on time, while 80 percent of total trials are delayed by at least one month because of enrollment challenges.[9] According to a report by Cutting Edge Information,[10] clinical trials last 42 percent longer than expected in Phase I, 31 percent longer in Phase II, and 30 percent beyond planned deadlines in Phase III, all because of recruitment delays. On average, such delays result in approximately 4.6 months being lost per trial.

Heavier Work Burden for Investigators

The workload for investigators and site study staff has increased significantly, posing additional challenges for clinical trial execution. Regulations governing clinical research activities have become more complex, increasing the work burden on investigators in terms of additional needs for compliance, documentation, and training. A recent study showed that the work burden for clinical researchers increased by 67 percent from 1999 to 2005.[7] Furthermore, investigators have to adapt to a consolidating pharmaceutical industry landscape and continuous evolving relationship between the sponsor companies and the contract clinical research organizations (CROs). As indicated in a survey of US sites, "contract & budget negotiation & approval" was cited as the number one cause of study initiation delays, ahead of "patient recruitment & enrollment".[11]

Increasing Globalization for Efficiency

Facing unprecedented challenges from increased competition, patent expiration, higher demand from regulatory authorities and cost pressure from payers, the biopharmaceutical companies have been focusing on driving efficiency and controlling cost in key operations including clinical trials. A broad range of operation models has been developed and implemented, from strategic outsourcing partnership with CROs to moving more clinical trials into developing countries. A recent study of industry-sponsored Phase III clinical trials showed that approximately one-third of the trials (157 of 509) are being conducted solely outside the USA and that a majority of study sites (13,521 of 24,206) are outside the USA.[6] Since 2002, the number of active US Food and Drug Administration (FDA)-regulated investigators based outside the USA has grown by 15 percent annually, whereas the number of US-based investigators has declined by 5.5 percent.[12] Compared to the USA, developing countries in Asia, Eastern Europe, and Latin America offer attractive alternatives with considerably lower study conduct costs, well-trained professionals, and established clinical trial centers. The expansion of global CROs and rapid growth of local CROs in these countries are bridging the critical gaps in conducting global clinical trials with high quality. In addition, developing countries can provide the large, genetically diverse patient pools willing to participate in clinical trials, potentially easing the recruitment challenge.

Progressive Improvement by Regulatory Authorities in Developing Countries

The regulatory environment in developing countries remains challenging, with problems such as inconsistent standards, inadequate enforcement, and complex processes. To take advantage of the globalization trend in clinical research, regulatory authorities in developing countries have been improving the national infrastructure and regulatory environment, including adoption of the International Conference on Harmonisation of Technical Requirements for Registration of Pharmaceuticals for Human Use Good Clinical Practice (ICH-GCP) guidelines and stronger intellectual property protections. In recent years, they have significantly increased collaboration with the US FDA, and have been improving the organizational structure and the regulatory process to make them simpler, more comprehensible, and faster. For example, India is establishing a new regulatory body, the Central Drugs Authority of India, modeled on the US FDA. In China, the State Food and Drug Administration has been increasing enforcement of good manufacturing practice (GMP) standards, has passed new regulations to facilitate clinical research, and is establishing clinical practice centers to train investigators and staff.[13] The Korean FDA has adopted clinical trial standards to comply with international standards, and streamlined the clinical trial authorization process. Furthermore, to encourage the domestic drug development industry, which is better at making incremental improvements than developing new molecular entities, the Korean FDA has recognized a new class of products called incrementally modified drugs, granting this group of drugs expedited review and favorable pricing regulation.[14]

CLINICAL TRIAL FORECASTING

Despite the myriad challenges associated with successfully executing clinical studies, all is not lost. Sound clinical trial forecasting and execution practices can meaningfully reduce trial costs while enhancing productivity. At the clinical study planning stage, forecasting is a critical activity to translate the strategic objectives of the clinical trial into operational elements and project the cost and resources, while aligning the clinical trial design and execution with the overall product development strategy. Usually, this exercise is conducted by the cross-functional project team, with members from related functions such as clinicians, clinical operations, regulatory affairs, project leaders, and project management.

The forecasting exercise starts with the study concept. Each clinical study is designed to achieve specific study objectives, and approaches vary accordingly, from a dose-escalating design to placebo-controlled, double-blinded parallel arms. The subject population is defined, and specific inclusion/exclusion criteria are designed to further refine the target population. Tiered endpoints are designed to achieve the desired safety, efficacy, pharmacokinetics, and pharmacodynamics objectives in the appropriate hierarchy. The testing regimen is designed according to the drug's mechanism of action and preliminary profile, and the study size is determined based on statistical calculations and key assumptions such as treatment effect and variability.

With the critical elements of the study defined in the study concept, the project team can develop the study timeline with key milestones, based on historical benchmarks of clinical trials of similar design and key assumptions such as subject enrollment rates and number of study sites. As shown in Table 6.1, the timeline is then integrated with other cost drivers, including strategic design elements, subject population, countries and sites, and study conduct, to forecast the cost and resource needs. Each cost driver has its unique characteristics and complex interdependencies may exist among different cost drivers. For example, a challenging screening procedure not only will increase the study conduct costs, but also will increase the screen failure rate and may lead to a longer recruitment timeline and the need for additional sites or countries. By varying key assumptions around those elements, the project team can evaluate multiple scenarios and, by incorporating operational considerations, develop the cost forecast model. Forecasting software, such as ClearTrial (ClearTrial LLC, Westmont, IL, USA), is often used in combination with internal and external benchmarks to facilitate the exercise.

TABLE 6.1 Summary of Key Cost Drivers for Forecasting

Category	Key Cost Drivers
Strategic design elements	Therapeutic area
	Phase of the study
	Study design
Timeline	Initiation of start-up activities, including site activation
	First subject screened and first subject randomized/treated
	Last patient randomized/treated
	Treatment period and follow-up period
	Close-out period
Subject population	Total number of subjects
	Screen failure rate
	Subject attrition rate
	Expected number of serious adverse events per subject
Countries and sites	Countries (including sites per country, subjects per country)
	Total number of sites, including number of sites using local IRB/EC
Study conduct	Screening visit(s): schedule, procedures performed and analysis required
	Pretreatment visit(s): schedule, procedures performed and analysis required
	Treatment visit(s): schedule, procedures performed and analysis required
	Follow-up visit(s): schedule, procedures performed and analysis required
	Monitoring frequency
Clinical supply management	Drug supply labeling/packaging
	Drug depot management
Data management	Number of expected CRF screens or pages per patient including number of unique screens
	Number of queries expected for each patient CRF record
Quality assurance	Target number of sites to be audited
	Target number of audit visits
Patient recruitment and retention	Specific services needed, in addition to the site recruitment campaign
Training	Investigator meeting
	Investigative site training; CRO training

IRB: institutional review board; EC: ethics committee; CRF: case report form; CRO: contract research organization.

Conducting a clinical trial requires resources from a pool of shared functions, including clinicians, clinical pharmacology, clinical operation, biostatistics, regulatory affairs, pharmacovigilance, clinical supply management, bioanalytical, contract management, legal, and project management. Depending on the specific study, the skill sets and workload demand for each type of resources can vary. With the increasing outsourcing trend, such resources can come from either internal functions or external partners, leading to further demand for efficient resource planning. It is important to schedule the right resources to establish the clinical study team with appropriate oversight at the beginning, given the dynamic nature of the clinical trials portfolio for companies, and the criticality of continuity to minimize delay in clinical trials. For key personnel in pivotal trials, back-up resources may be identified and personnel trained in parallel to minimize ramping-up time and avoid trial delays in case of need.

In the current cost-conscious and timeline-driven business environment, the forecasting exercise often goes through an iterative process, with rigorous re-evaluation and disciplined rebalancing among the strategic and operational elements of the clinical study. A successful forecasting exercise not only provides the forum for the cross-functional project team and senior management to align on key assumptions for the clinical trial and business constraints, but also delivers a robust forecast model to be integrated as an important part of the clinical trial plan and the product development plan. Increasingly, globalization strategy, study design optimization, technology enablement, and operation efficiency have become the focus of assessment and planning at this stage.

Globalization Strategy

For studies such as clinical pharmacology studies in healthy volunteers, a single site may be desirable to achieve best consistency and efficiency, with site selection mainly driven by cost advantage for study conduct and simplified regulatory processes. For proof-of-concept studies and pivotal studies requiring a sizable number of subjects of target diseases, a multinational setting provides significant advantages of access to larger patient pools and quality investigative sites, as well as potentially lower operational costs, especially in developing countries. By reviewing multinational epidemiology studies on the target population, as well as competitive intelligence on ongoing studies of similar products and historical performances, strategic scenarios can be developed with a different mix of sites and countries for comparative evaluation. It is important to consider all implications from such mixes and optimize the plan in the context of the overall study outcome and objectives. For example, if projected subject enrollment rates vary widely across the countries, country specific enrollment targets may need to be preset to ensure that the data from the final patient population support the overall product registration strategy.

Study Design Optimization

Refinement and optimization of the study design should take into consideration patient demographics, language, clinical practices, and anticipated feedback from the regulatory authorities across selected regions or countries. The final design should satisfy the study objective, while ensuring robust interpretability of final data from such a population mix, general applicability of potential study conclusion, and acceptability by the regulatory authorities. At this stage of planning, patient population (including inclusion and exclusion criteria) and safety and efficacy endpoints are often the most important drivers for cost and timeline.

- **Patient Population** The definition of the patient population has a direct impact on the final label, as well as the operational costs and timeline. In a world of dynamic progress in scientific and medical fields, it is important to balance what data are desired with what can be achieved practically under the cost and timeline constraints. For example, including an invasive diagnostic procedure during screening may help to stratify and enrich the right patient population, but it may impede patient recruitment owing to safety risks (real or perceived by investigators and patients) and additional scrutiny by regulatory authorities and institutional review boards (IRBs) or ethics committees (ECs), leading to a longer regulatory review, higher screen failure rates, and longer recruitment timeline. Extensive planning and negotiation among key stakeholders, including clinicians, clinical operation, and regulatory affairs functions, are often needed in order to reach the final alignment.

- **Endpoints** Clinical trials, especially proof-of-concept and pivotal studies, are designed and conducted to gain critical scientific insight to complete the drug profile in the target populations. Besides the essential safety and efficacy endpoints, it may also be desirable to include data elements that may serve as context-setting variables in anticipation of less likely findings, or help to identify new product opportunities. Collecting all these data not only increases the costs of conducting additional procedures, but also can limit options regarding site selection, increasing the site burden and lowering patient retention. Vigorous reviews are needed to justify each data element needed against the incremental budget amount and operational burden that must be incurred to obtain those data. In the end, such reviews help to minimize the collection of unnecessary data, and streamline the protocol design, containing costs and reducing demands on sites and patients.[15]

Information Technology Enablement

Information technology (IT) in the management of clinical trials has evolved significantly in the past few years. Suites of software systems, such as project and resource management software, clinical trials management systems (CTMS), electronic data capture (EDC), and document management systems,[16] enable more efficient and effective management of important study tasks, from study design and data entry to resource scheduling and invoice tracking. The wide availability of Internet-based interfaces enables the broad adoption of technology at investigative sites across different countries, while minimizing the IT infrastructure investment and staff training burden. Depending on the study and business circumstances, these systems can be adopted in different modular fashions and integrated with other third party vendors to accommodate the local technology standards and practices across countries. Business processes have to be modified according to the technology required and differences in the local country setting, in order to maximize the returns from these enabling technologies and minimize risk in data quality.

Operational Efficiency

Multinational clinical trials bring in operational complexities, such as differences in regulatory requirements and review time, variability in local clinical practices, and requirements from local IRBs and ECs, as well as data quality concerns. As biopharmaceutical companies focus more and more on their drug development expertise, global and regional CROs play an increasingly important role in efficient study planning and execution.[17] By partnering with CROs instead of going it alone, the companies can leverage CROs' deep understanding of industry-leading practices, broad geographical operational footprint, and local knowledge and relationships in specific countries to maximize operational efficiencies.

CLINICAL TRIAL BUDGETING

The budgeting process is triggered by the investment decision, and is built on the foundation of the forecast model and the finalized clinical protocol. The final budget consists of the internal resources allocated through advance scheduling and negotiation with key internal functions, and external costs through contract negotiations with CROs, third party vendors, and investigative sites. As shown in Table 6.2, a typical clinical trial can be allocated into multiple stages, within which a number of different tasks with different scopes and processes are conducted by various functions according to their respective function plans. Consequently, the budgeting process is often carried out by collaboration among the cross-function project team, the clinical study team, and the individual functions. As drug development companies are increasingly turning to CROs for their operational expertise and capability to manage a clinical study, often at this stage, a CRO partner is engaged to work with internal functions and teams to further define the function tasks and scope, and in some cases hold contracts with third party vendors and investigator sites. Projections for costs and resource needs are developed and finalized in the form of contractual agreements with various service providers, according to the expectation and specification of key deliverables and the agreed timeline.

As shown in Table 6.3, key cost categories includes the costs of site activities, third party vendors, study execution and management, data management, and recruitment and training. For a Phase I study, the costs of site activities and third party vendors can represent the majority of the total study budget; yet for a multicenter Phase III study, such costs may represent less than 50 percent of the total study costs. As the complexity of the study increases, the study execution and management cost represents a bigger proportion of the total cost and becomes a major focus for cost efficiency planning.

TABLE 6.2 Summary of Key Activities and Function Plans across the Clinical Trial

Stage	Key Activities	Selected Plans
Design and planning	Assemble the project team Design and review the study protocol, informed consent and investigator brochure Prepare regulatory document Prepare the drug supply	Study plan Clinical supply plan Risk management plan Communication and issue escalation plan Country and site selection plan
Start up	Select target countries and sites Negotiate and finalize CRO and vendor contracts Initiate and activate sites Design and build eCRF and database Set up data collection	Vendor management plan Document management plan Data management plan Quality plan Medical and safety management plan Site management plan
Study conduct	Recruit, screen, and treat eligible patients Perform medical and safety assessment Manage investigator sites Manage drug supply Enter and clean data	Site monitoring plan Site auditing plan Data management plan Statistical analysis plan Study close-out plan For key studies, also include the topline data communication plan and publication plan
Data analysis and reporting	Verify and reconcile data Lock database Conduct statistical analysis Write the study report Finalize the trial master file Close out sites	

CRO: contract research organization; eCRF: electronic case report form.

63

TABLE 6.3 Summary of Key Budget Categories

Budget Category	Key Budget Components
Site activity	Site start-up, e.g. site initiation activity, initial site training
	Study procedures performed and supporting activities for screening, treatment, and follow-up visits
	Time and expense for investigator and study supporting staff
	IRB/EC submission and review
Third party vendors	Centralized service providers (e.g. central lab, central ECG reading, central IRB, IVR)
	Speciality vendors (e.g. specific imaging techniques, genomic assays)
	Translation service providers
	Bioanalytical service vendors (e.g. pharmacokinetics and biomarker analysis)
	Supply chain vendors (e.g. drug depot, labeling/packaging vendor)
Study execution and management	Project planning/project management
	Study start up (e.g. protocol/informed consent form development, vendor and site contract negotiation, site qualification)
	Regulatory package preparation and submission
	Medical monitoring and pharmacovigilance
	Clinical operation (e.g. site monitoring and management, site close-out)
	Site audit and corrective action implementation
Data management	Biostatistics support for study design and statistical analysis
	Electronic data capture design and implementation
	Database design, build, and management
	Data clean and reconciliation
	Medical writing and final reporting
Recruitment and training	Patient recruitment service
	Patient retention service
	Training service

IRB: institutional review board; EC: ethics committee; ECG: electrocardiogram; IVR: interactive voice response.

For multinational clinical trials, a key input to finalize the budget comprises data from the global feasibility study, conducted in the selected regions and countries. Usually, the clinical study protocol, important background information about the candidate drug, and a detailed questionnaire are sent to a number of investigators in the selected countries for feedback. In addition, similar input is obtained from experts on the subject matter within the sponsor and the CRO partner companies. Key elements of the output are summarized in Table 6.4. These data further guide the final selection of the countries and sites, refinement of key enrollment assumptions, and optimization of key deliverables scope and timeline, especially on the following four aspects of a region- or country-specific operations budget.

Local Patient Population

A global and country-level overview of the prevalent patient population (including total, diagnosed, treated), derived from epidemiological data from governmental or commercial sources, can provide important insights into the country selection strategy. A global feasibility study will provide detailed country-specific findings, including demographics, willingness and

TABLE 6.4 Key Elements of Feasibility Study Outcome

Category	Key Elements
Patient population	Demographics
	Standard of care
	Insurance coverage
Recruitment considerations	Target patient population
	Historical recruitment experience
	Impact of inclusion and exclusion criteria
	Impact of the study procedures
	Patient recruitment and retention techniques
Investigator	Patient population treated by the investigators
	Reported enrollment projections
	Investigator interest
	Key motivation
Site selection	Site environment
	Site experience
	Competitive studies
	Optimal site profile
Regulatory considerations	Considerations from regulatory authorities
	Potential responses from IRB/EC reviews

IRB: institutional review board; EC: ethics committee.

motivation to participate in clinical trials, accessibility to primary and secondary care, and cultural perspectives for the disease and the testing treatment. Target countries and enrollment goals can then be determined, taking into consideration subject recruitment and retention rates. Accordingly, the scope of potential recruitment and retention strategies can be determined. Throughout the planning and execution, the population mix must be calibrated against the study objectives to ensure that the data from the final population continue to support the registration strategy.

Investigators and Treatment Patterns

Feedback from the investigators and key opinion leaders (KOLs) in specific countries provides important information on the treatment-seeking pattern of patients and the specific clinical environment to guide the contract negotiation with the sites and selection of appropriate global or regional vendors. It is important to include all types of practitioner in the survey (e.g. primary care physicians and specialists) to provide an adequate overview of their motivation. Meanwhile, interest in the candidate drug by the investigators and site experience of conducting similar clinical trials, in combination with ongoing competitive clinical trials in their centers, will provide another level of input. Suitability and practical challenges of inclusion and exclusion criteria and diagnostic/treatment procedures included in the specific protocol also help to guide the selection of countries as well as to assess the need to modify certain procedures. In addition, logistical factors such as the availability of transport to investigative sites and facilities need to be considered, as these may affect the quality and timeliness of a clinical trial.

Regulatory Authorities

The budgeting exercise needs to take into consideration the regulatory and IRC/EC requirements in target countries, in anticipation of potential challenges to the current protocol and informed consent form (ICF). In multinational trials, because of differences in regulatory requirements, approval processes, and timelines, it is highly desirable to minimize the number of regulatory submissions and languages, and to avoid any country- or site-specific amendments. Considering the nature of the regulatory process and timeline in different countries, additional time and costs may be budgeted as contingencies in anticipation of regulatory feedback from certain countries.

Language and Cultural Barriers

In multinational trials, especially in developing countries, cultural and linguistic differences may become a significant challenge. The project team should anticipate and prepare for language-related misunderstandings during the course of the study. Repeated feedback to correct errors in translating administrative and research documents could delay the timeline and increase the costs. Therefore, it may be necessary to have contracts ready for experienced translation agencies in specific countries, and local resources to manage the study conduct and relationship. Such services should not only cover the translation of key documents, but also address language challenges in data input and query resolution, as well as developing appropriate training materials for the sites and staff in different countries.

After the clinical trial has started, key budgeting assumptions may change and, as a result, the budget may need to be modified through the change order process. For significant changes in budgeting assumptions, it is important to adjust the budget to reflect all relevant cost components, including one-time costs (e.g. site start-up fees), duration-driven costs (e.g. vendor project management fees), and unit-driven costs (e.g. costs of study procedures performed). While it is important to manage the study conduct within the budget, it is also important to assess the budget implication in the context of the overall product development plan; for example, for a candidate drug with blockbuster potential, incremental costs to accelerate or avoid delay of the clinical trial may be well justified by potential gains in future revenues, making such a budget variance an attractive investment with a positive net present value.

CLINICAL TRIAL PROJECT MANAGEMENT

The planning and execution of clinical trials involve numerous activities with unique attributes and interdependencies, across different stages of the lengthy timeline, conducted by stakeholders in different organizations, and which are affected by a broad range of factors associated with the study, including the regulatory environment and competitive landscape. The project manager plays a critical role in this process, by planning, coordinating, and tracking key tasks associated with the study, as well as managing communication among key stakeholders. In different organizations, parts of these responsibilities may be carried out by personnel from internal functions other than project management, such as clinical operation and resource planning or external CROs, but the demand for the project management responsibilities remains the same. With the increasing complexity in clinical trial design and execution, the project manager needs to possess a deep understanding of the clinical trial itself and business needs, as well as skills in relationship management and communication, in order to serve as the effective interface between multiple internal and external teams while managing the clinical trial with discipline and efficiency.

Working closely with the project team and owners of the key function plans for the study, the project manager focuses on the following elements of study execution: timeline, budget, performance metrics, communication, and risk and contingency planning.

Timeline

Stakeholders, including the project team, CRO and vendors, agree on major milestones from initial kick-off to completion of the final report and trial master file. Then, a detailed timeline with schedules for all tasks and interdependencies is developed, and the overall project critical path activities will be monitored closely. Key timeline assumptions (e.g. screen failure rate, enrollment rate) need to be calibrated in real time to ensure the accuracy of the projection. In each stage (see Table 6.2), it is also important to focus on critical path activities for that particular stage. For example, during the start-up stage, contract negotiation with vendors and investigative sites is likely to be on the critical path, and needs to be monitored closely to ensure timely initiation of the study. Meanwhile, submission to the regulatory authorities and IRBs/ECs in different countries and regions need to be coordinated to accommodate difference in the review cycle, with flexibility built in to accommodate anticipated feedback. These tasks will, in turn, drive the site activation rate and subsequently patient enrollment in each country.

Budget

Typically, the budget is set against the base-case timeline with key execution assumptions and the agreed milestones. The adoption of enabling technologies such as CTMS allows the project team to enhance business process and capture the productivity gains through real-time study status monitoring and efficient cashflow management. Changes in execution assumptions, such as slower enrollment rate or unexpected regulatory feedback, may have direct budgetary consequences. Depending on the specific study, it is helpful to set up a contingency budget to address such uncertainties to a certain extent without additional administrative burden. For material changes that will result in significant budget revision, appropriate triggers can be set up to initiate a change order in advance to minimize any trial disruption. Bonuses and/or penalties may be built in to motivate enhanced performance for the team or a specific stakeholder. These need to be prudently balanced with potential compromises in quality and other subjective characteristics of deliverables, as well as implications for the relationship from strenuous arguments regarding who has responsibility for missed targets. When such a clause is used, it is essential to agree upfront on the roles and responsibilities of parties involved, execution assumptions, and specific metrics covering the quality of the deliverables.

Performance Metrics

Metrics need to be set up between the project team and clinical service providers such as the CRO and vendors, in order to measure their performance. Such metrics should reflect the true performance of providers, the quality of deliverables, timing, and quantity. Examples include country regulatory submission targets, site activation targets (e.g. dates for 25, 50, 75, and 100 percent sites activated), patient recruitment targets (e.g. enrollment rates, global or by country or by site), and data management targets (e.g. eCRF backlog, threshold for aging query, data query rate by discrepancy type or by country or site). The project manager needs to monitor progress against these metrics, ensure that information is shared effectively, and escalate through proper channels if there is significant deviation from the target.

Communication

The project manager is responsible for managing communication paths among all stakeholders involved in the study. These stakeholders include the project team and management as well as the CRO and vendors and, to a lesser extent, the investigators and site study staff. The communication plan covers team rosters and relative contact information, all scheduled meetings and frequency of meetings, and communication venues, with secure IT links set up to ensure confidentiality. A key communication tool is the study status report, which the project manager is responsible for defining, developing, and maintaining throughout the study. As shown in Table 6.5, the report contains status updates ranging from site contract negotiation to key milestones, and is an important tool for study management by the project team and for communication with senior management.

In a multinational trial, communication planning should take into consideration any language and cultural differences. Language-related misunderstandings in multinational

TABLE 6.5 Key Elements of the Study Status Report

Category	Key Elements
Timeline update	Updated projection of key milestones
	Risk status for key milestones
Country status	Regulatory submission and approval status
	Drug supply readiness status
Site status	Legal contract negotiation status
	IRB/EC status
	Site initiation and activation status
	Amendment submission status
Subjects' enrollment status	Number of subjects screened, randomized, or dosed
	Number of subjects having completed the trial, or having completed the follow-up phase
	Number of subjects failed during screening or patients terminated prior to completion
Data management status	Data cleaning metrics
	Site monitoring status
	Site auditing and correction action status
Budgetary status	Contract and change order status
	Contract budget versus invoiced expenses
	Aging payment status

IRB: institutional review board; EC: ethics committee.

clinical trials should be anticipated and prepared for. To overcome this barrier, it is important to have resources located strategically across the trial locations, with expertise in regional and country-specific regulatory requirements, and relationships with local regulatory authorities and sites.

Risk and Contingency Planning

At the inception of the study, key risks within the study plan need to be mapped out across the key tasks by the responsible stakeholders. Such risks can then be prioritized according to probability, timing, and impact on the success of the clinical trial, and appropriate contingency plans can be developed. Inevitably, issues will arise and it is important to establish the issue escalation path to triage the issues quickly, communicate to the appropriate stakeholders effectively, and ensure timely resolution of the issues before any significant disruption to the study occurs. For example, minor issues with the sites, such as small deviations from the protocol, may be passed upwards to principal investigators and study coordinators, and resolution requested with an established timeline. Major issues, such as those requiring modification of the protocol and ICF, may need to be passed to the project team on the day of discovery, with the issue tracked and resolution implemented globally.

For key risks with a high probability of serious negative impact, specialized vendors can be engaged in the planning stage to develop a proactive risk management plan and integrate seamlessly into the study conduct plan. For example, in the current competitive environment with evolving scientific understanding and increasing regulatory demands, risks in subject recruitment and retention have become more prominent in multinational clinical trials. If not managed effectively, these risks may lead to significant consequences: delays in patient recruitment will have a direct impact on the study cost and timeline, as subjects have to be fully enrolled for the study to have sufficient power to deliver valid conclusions; lower than expected subject retention may affect the data integrity and validity of the study conclusion, as well as the product profile. Both risks can be driven by product-specific attributes, such as tolerability and safety profile, as well as operational and communicational complexities.

TABLE 6.6 Examples of Subject Recruitment and Retention Risk Mitigation Activities

Recruitment Risk Mitigation

Segment the investigators based on the fit of their patient pools with the protocol and historical record of meeting the enrollment target, and assign recruitment target and support accordingly[18]

Optimize the advertisement campaign to develop the message best fit for the patient motivation and deliver the message via the most effective venue and collaboration with appropriate advocacy organizations according to the profile of the target patient population

Set up financial incentives for quick turnaround of essential regulatory packages and reaching specific patient enrollment target

Qualify additional investigative sites as back-up; these sites can be activated immediately if needed to replace non-performing sites

Enhance communication

  Hold investigator meeting

  Implement site motivation strategies, such as deploying knowledgeable, well-trained clinical team for site visits, providing tools for easy study reference, and allowing easy access to project team for rapid resolution of questions

  Set up teleconference and newsletters to encourage site collaboration and friendly competition

Retention Risk Mitigation

Modify the study design; for example, modifying visit schedules or eliminating procedures for non-critical data points may help to lower the burden for patients and caregivers

Implement support packages for patients and caregivers to ease the logistical and emotional burdens for visits

Implement the open-label extension study, to encourage retention of patients looking for longer term potential treatment benefit

Deploy knowledgeable, well-trained clinical team and training programs to communicate with investigators and study staff, addressing key concerns related to early termination

Enhance communication to patients/caregivers and site staff regarding the study progress and background information (e.g. a study-specific web portal)

Third party vendors with expertise in subject recruitment and retention in the target countries and target patient population are often engaged to develop robust multitier plans (examples of activities are shown in Table 6.6), with timing of the activities and scale of investment adjusted up or down depending on preset thresholds for subject enrollment and retention.

References

1. DiMasi JA, Hansen RW, Grabouski HG. The price of innovation: new estimates of drug development cost. *Journal of Health Economics* 2003;**22**:151–85.

2. DiMasi JA, Grabouski HG. The cost of biopharmaceutical R&D: is biotech different? *Managerial and Decision Economics* 2007;**28**:469–79.

3. Gilbert J, Henske P, Singh A. Rebuilding big pharma's business model. *In Vivo* 2003;**21**(10).

4. DiMasi JA, Paquette C. The economics of following drug research and development: trends in entry rates and the timing of development. *Pharmacoeconomics* 2004;**22**:1–14.

5. PhRMA. *Profile of Pharmaceutical Industry.* PhRMA Report; 2010, http://www.phrma.org/research/publications.

6. Glickman SW, McHutchison JG, Peterson ED, Cairns CB, Harrington RA, Califf RM, Schulman KA. Ethical and scientific implications of globalization. *New England Journal of Medicine* 2009;**360**:816–23.

7. Tufts Center for the Study of Drug Development. http://csdd.tufts.edu/reports/description/impact_reports. *Growing Protocol Design Complexity Stresses Investigators;* 2009. Volunteers. Tufts CSDD Impact Report, 10.1.

8. Getz K. *The Gift of Participation: A Guide to Make Informed Decisions About Volunteering for a Clinical Trial.* Bar Harbor, ME: Jerian Publishing; 2007.

9. CenterWatch. *State of the Clinical Trials Industry.* Boston, MA: CenterWatch; 2008.

10. Cutting Edge Information. *Accelerating Clinical Trials: Budgets*; 2004. Patient Recruitment and Productivity (May), http://www.cuttingedgeinfo.com/reports/

11. CenterWatch. *CenterWatch Sourcebook*. Boston, MA: CenterWatch; 2009.

12. Getz KA. Global clinical trials activities in the details. *Applied Clinical Trials*; 2007 (September 1).

13. Bailey W, Cruickshank C, Sharma N. *Make Your Move: Taking Clinical Trials to the Best Location*; 2006. AT Kearney Report, http://www.atkearney.com

14. Bernstein Research. *Global Pharmaceuticals: Emerging Markets Should Infuse Badly Needed Revenues for Years to Come*; 2009. Bernstein Research Report (October), https://www.bernsteinresearch.com/brweb/Public/Login.aspx?ReturnUrl=%2fbrweb%2fHome.aspx

15. Getz K. With clinical data, less is more. *Applied Clinical Trials*; 2010 (January 1), 28–30.

16. Marwalia S, Patil S, Singh N. *Use IT to speed up clinical trials*. Spring: McKinsey on IT; 2007.

17. Goldman Sachs. *Goldman Sachs Report*. US Pharmaceutical Services; 2004 (August 24), http://www2.goldmansachs.com/?cid=PS_01_05_06_99_01_01

18. Rowe JC, Elling ME, Hazlewood JG, Zakhary R. *A cure for clinical trials*. McKinsey Quarterly; 2002 (June).

Strengthening and Building Clinical Trial Site Capabilities and Capacity in Developing and Emerging Markets

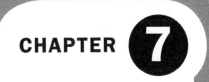
Lessons Learned in India

Nermeen Varawalla*, Ankit Joshi[†]
*ECCRO, London, UK
[†]ECCRO, Mumbai, India

73

INTRODUCTION

India offers the international clinical trial sponsor access to healthcare institutions and facilities with the potential to be among the most productive clinical trial sites in the world. India's primary healthcare system is relatively undeveloped; hence, patients attend hospitals for treatments that are elsewhere delivered in the primary care setting. This practice of patients attending centralized, urban, general and specialist hospitals for their healthcare makes India well suited for hospital-based clinical trials. Hospitals in India's cities and large towns, be they state managed, single-speciality units, or part of corporate healthcare groups, have the required patient attendance, qualified physicians, and equipment to serve as high-performing clinical trial sites. As yet, there is no process for site recognition, accreditation, or licensing. It remains a challenge to effectively utilize India's hospitals and clinics to contribute clinical trial data at international quality standards. The reasons for this are an under-resourced healthcare system, India's nascent but high-growth clinical trials sector, and little investment in building clinical trial site capability. There is an urgent imperative to correct this situation and this chapter describes the approach adopted by ECCRO, a specialist India-focused contract research organization (CRO).

INDIA'S HEALTHCARE SYSTEM

Although healthcare is one of India's largest and rapidly growing sectors, in terms of revenue and employment, with a total value of more than US $34 billion per year, this translates to a mere $34 per capita and represents only about 6 percent of gross domestic product (GDP). A mixture of private and state subsidized healthcare exists in India; however, the private sector accounts for more than 80 percent of total healthcare spending,[1] an extremely high proportion by international standards. After years of underfunding, the number of public health facilities is inadequate, with most providing only basic care and, with a few exceptions, public health facilities are inadequately managed and ill equipped. Private firms provide about 60 percent of all outpatient care in India and as much as 40 percent of all inpatient care. Private and corporate hospitals often provide subsidized and charitable treatment to patients who are poor. However, the majority of their patients are private paying patients. Only 11 percent of the population has any form of health insurance coverage; this is swiftly increasing but has a long way to go. Only 25 percent of the Indian population has access to Western medicine, which is practiced mainly in urban areas, where two-thirds of India's hospitals and health centers are located. The number of hospital beds per individual remains low, at 0.9 beds per 1000 individuals, with the number of physicians per individual being still lower at 0.6 physicians per 1000 individuals. Not surprisingly, morbidity and mortality in India remain unacceptably high compared to countries within the same economic standard. This is due to a weak healthcare infrastructure, in particular in the primary healthcare setting, along with high levels of poverty and illiteracy, which contribute to patients presenting late for diagnosis and treatment. Modest improvements have been made, such that life expectancy in India has increased by approximately 9 percent over a period of six years, from 63.62 years in 2003 to 69.89 years in 2009.[2]

Therefore, it must be recognized that at any healthcare set-up, be it primary, secondary, or tertiary, situated in either rural or urban India, healthcare is provided with limited resources to a large volume of patients presenting with illnesses across a varied spectrum of diseases.

INDIA'S CLINICAL TRIALS SECTOR

India's participation in international clinical trials is a relatively recent occurrence, with the first international trials being conducted about a decade ago. Traditionally, India's pharmaceutical industry has been a generic one, with less focus on the research and development of innovative drugs. Multinational pharmaceutical companies have viewed their India offices as primarily marketing offices with limited clinical trial capabilities. This began to change in 2005, triggered by the signing of the Trade Related Aspects of Intellectual Property Rights (TRIPS) treaty. India's commitment to follow international intellectual property rights laws, the global pharmaceutical industry's need for cost-effective patient access, and India's growing reputation as a outsourcing destination have all contributed to the brisk growth of India's clinical trial industry, which has grown at approximately 15—20 percent per year since then. Access to clinical trial subjects from India's large pool of patients with diseases of both the tropical and industrialized worlds remains the key driver for the growth of the Indian clinical trials sector. The huge unmet medical need that exists in India incentivizes patients and physicians to participate in international clinical trials, particularly those that offer an opportunity to access state-of-the-art healthcare.

The Indian clinical trials sector has enjoyed and is enjoying brisk, even exponential growth, albeit from a low baseline. The number of international clinical trials conducted in India has increased by 30 percent per annum for the past three years. Global clinical trials that include India increased from 1366 to 1533, an increase of 11 percent, in the six-month period ending 15 February 2011.[3] More than half of these were Phase III trials. Oncology, infectious disease, diabetes, and cardiorespiratory disease are the most common therapeutic areas being trialed in India. At the time of writing, only 1.5 percent of the world's ongoing clinical trials include India, compared to 52 percent that include the USA.

Clinical Research Training

Over the past decade there have been numerous successful training initiatives and programs. Clinical research training to investigators, site staff, and professionals is being delivered in a number of ways. Study start-up activities include good clinical practice (GCP) training of investigators and site personnel. This is provided by sponsors and CROs, many of whom understand that this is a good way to build a pool of trained Indian investigators with whom they may continue to work. CROs are cognizant of the importance of trained clinical operation staff and continue to make substantial investment is this area. Global CROs utilize their global training resources and expertise to deliver both face-to-face and online training to their staff in India.

Training institutes have been set up that provide training, including degree courses and diplomas, to biomedical graduates seeking to develop a career in clinical research. Several of these training institutes have collaborations with Indian and foreign universities, government, and industry. Examples include the Academy for Clinical Excellence, the Indian Clinical Research Institute (ICRI) in association with the University of Cranfield, the Clinical Research Education and Management Academy (CREMA) and Catalyst clinical services. These organizations and others have helped to meet the evolving training needs of participants in India's clinical research sector, be they from industry, government, regulators, or academia. Furthermore, they have facilitated interaction between senior members of stakeholder organizations, leading to collaborative improvements in this evolving sector.[4] Apart from formal and on-the-job training, there is much conference and seminar activity which highlights best practices and current trends. The Drug Information Association (DIA) has had an office in Mumbai since 2007 and holds regular conferences in India. As a result of these activities, there is awareness among the Indian clinical research community of worldwide developments in global clinical research, an interest among biomedical students to pursue a career in clinical research, and improving capabilities and quality standards.

Players within India's Clinical Trial Sector

The players within the Indian clinical development sector are local affiliates of multinational pharmaceutical companies, Indian pharmaceutical companies, Indian affiliates of global CROs, local CROs, and support service providers.

Traditionally, the Indian subsidiaries of multinational pharmaceutical companies have been sales and marketing units, with their involvement in clinical development restricted to the conduct of local postmarketing studies. This has changed greatly; today, Indian affiliates of multinational pharmaceutical companies have substantial clinical development capabilities and contribute increasing amounts of Indian Phase II and III clinical trial data for their global clinical development programs. They do this by using in-house resources as well as engaging with CROs. The forerunners have included Pfizer, Lilly, and Sanofi-Aventis, who have substantially contributed to the early development of the sector by training investigators, ethics committee members, and clinical research professionals. As a consequence of clinical research studies placed at various hospitals, investments have been made in upgrading the research infrastructure in India. Indian pharmaceutical companies such as Glenmark, Biocon, Ranbaxy, Dr Reddy's, and Sun Pharma who are moving beyond their generic business have begun to establish clinical development capabilities to meet the needs of their own innovative new molecules. However, their contribution to site development has been minimal to date.

In 2006, the Indian CRO market was estimated to be valued at $265 million, a fraction of the total global CRO market of $14.3 billion. By 2012, this market is expected to be worth $600 million. Most global CROs have a presence in India; the market leader is Quintiles, which was founded in India in 1997. Global CROs have contributed to the training of clinical research personnel in India; however, their contributions to site development and support have been limited. An important reason for this is that they are committed to follow their global standard operating procedures (SOPs), which have been designed for the clinical trial environments of the USA and Western Europe. Although their Indian staff recognize the limitations of these global SOPs at the site level in India, they have been unable to adapt their practices to provide the site-level investment and activities that are so essential in India.

Motivated by the relatively low barriers to entry and commercial hype, over 50 local CROs have set up operations. For the majority of local CROs the provision of bioequivalence studies to domestic generic pharmaceutical companies forms a major part of their business; however, almost all have aspirations to develop their global clinical trials business. The niche nature of their business and limited international perspective have prevented local CROs investing in site development.

When assessing potential CROs, sponsors focus on their experience, systems, processes, and pricing, paying limited attention to the site relationships that they offer. Furthermore, the CRO's relationship with sites is typically short lived, transactional, and related to specific trials. The CRO is focused on persuading the site to swiftly enroll patients, within a negotiated budget, with little attention paid to developing processes or expertise at the site. In the absence of any investment or long-term relationship with the site, site selection and feasibility assessment also become ad hoc, transactional processes with little strategic or long-term intent. Hence, the contribution of CROs to site development has been limited.

Site management organizations (SMOs) have responded to the need for site support by providing site staff for the duration of trials. Their responsibilities include contract negotiations, ethics committee submissions, patient counseling, patient recruitment, patient follow-up, maintenance of trial-related documents, serious adverse event reporting, and ensuring protocol compliance. Although SMOs have invested in training their staff, there has been little attention paid to staff development and career progression, hence there is brisk staff turnover with little continuity. These resources are typically recent biomedical graduates who view this role as the first step in their clinical research career, and are keen to move on after 12–18 months. Furthermore, because they are contracted by the sponsor or CRO to provide site-based resources for specific studies, they make almost no contribution to site selection and have little opportunity to engage strategically with the site. Communication among the SMO, CRO, sponsor, and site becomes convoluted, which is another practical flaw in this approach. Notwithstanding these issues, trained resources provided by SMOs have been able to reduce site start-up timelines and support patient identification, subject recruitment, and retention. Moreover, the flexible and nationwide staffing provided by SMOs has enabled the increasing utilization of clinical trial sites in second and third tier cities of India. The larger SMOs in India have introduced sites to their site management systems and processes, and hence contributed to site development. In spite of these contributions, the roles and responsibilities of SMOs have not yet been defined in any regulatory guidelines. In addition, SMOs are not usually signatories in the clinical trial agreements, causing further ambiguity about their role, responsibilities, and accountabilities. SMOs struggle to move beyond a resourcing business to a site development one for a number of reasons. Their ability to make a more tangible difference at the site level has been hindered by the fact that SMOs are dependent on the investigators with little authority of their own, and less experienced investigators fail to recognize the importance of site support and infrastructure, thereby undermining the potential contribution that SMOs could make. Furthermore, the low margin SMO business model limits the scope for investment in developing sites. There is little space for exclusivity with sites; this deters sponsors, CROs, or SMOs from investing in site capabilities as they fear that the return on their investment will not be exclusive to them. Sponsors are loathe to pay equally high fees to both CROs and SMOs; therefore, to protect their high-value standing, CROs seek to offer site management and patient recruitment services, thereby placing the SMOs at the risk of being bypassed.

Hospital staff, usually resident medical officers, nurses, or research fellows, may take up the role of clinical research coordinator for certain sites. In contrast to their counterparts in other countries, relatively few Indian nurses take on the role of study nurse or site coordinator. Such an arrangement is not ideal since, at busy hospitals, site staff are burdened with healthcare delivery, so their focus and dedication to research activities may be compromised. International Conference on Harmonisation (ICH)-GCP training for these staff is conducted by sponsors or CROs. However, they need to follow their own career paths, resulting in high attrition. Often there are no defined SOPs, leading to much inter-individual and inter-site variability. Large medical institutions and hospital networks have set up their own in-house SMOs with varying degrees of success. Some of them also offer study monitoring and project management services; however, there remains ambiguity about the demarcation between roles and responsibilities.

Deficient Clinical Trial Site Capabilities

Numerous hospitals and medical institutions in India which have the potential to be high-performing clinical trial sites lack the required infrastructure, expertise, and trained staff. The reasons for this are the heavy burden of routine clinical work, high levels of bureaucracy, and non-availability of relatively modest financial investment. Although there are 500—600 investigative sites in India that have participated in clinical trials and have GCP trained staff, only a very small proportion of these are truly capable of achieving their potential as high-performing clinical trial sites.

There is a shortage of adequately trained investigators in India. At present, India has around 750 GCP-trained investigators; a small fraction of the total number of trained physicians. Clinical research does not feature prominently in the medical curricula in India and training in this area is typically obtained by interested physicians as they become involved in international clinical trial participation. The investigator at a typical Indian clinical trial site faces a number of challenges, namely balancing resources between patient care and clinical research; ensuring that relatively low levels of patient education, literacy, and financial status do not compromise the principles of GCP; and guarding against allowing the sponsor's requirements for rapid patient enrollment to compromise quality standards.[5]

Thus, the level of experience and expertise of investigators and clinical research personnel in India is limited and needs to be further developed, in terms of numbers, regional distribution, and the depth of expertise within centers of excellence. Important unmet needs in India's clinical research sector are clinical trial infrastructure, training for physicians and clinical site staff on regulatory, ethical, and GCP requirements, and an appreciation of the importance of maintaining quality source documentation. Efforts and investment are required to ensure that sites have the support needed to perform at their full potential.[6]

Unequal utilization of sites in India has also become an issue, with increasing numbers of trials being placed at the more experienced hospitals, typically located in India's large metropolitan cities. These sites are becoming increasingly busy with participation in numerous trials, and some are experiencing capacity constraints and finding that they are unable to meet sponsor expectations with respect to subject enrollment and data quality. The resulting competitor trial activity at these better known sites has had a detrimental effect on their data quality and productivity. Thus, it is important both to strengthen capabilities at relatively experienced sites and to invest in developing capabilities at less experienced or even "research-naïve" sites.

There are two reasons for the imperative to address these deficient clinical trial site capabilities in India. First, a failure to do so jeopardizes the ongoing international clinical trial activity in India. Second, if clinical trial site capabilities in India are not built there is a risk that the region will fail to fulfill its potential as one of the world's most attractive clinical trial geographies.

Deficiencies at the clinical trial site level expose clinical trial subjects to the risk of inadequate protection. Most clinical institutions and hospitals have ethics committees that comply with the ICH-GCP guidelines. The minority of sites without their own ethics committee utilize the services of independent ethics committees. India does not have a central ethics committee. Therefore, approvals are granted by individual ethics committees who approve all study protocols before study commencement. The investigator submits the documents for ethics committee approval and may need to make a presentation on the study to the committee prior to its decision. Ethics committees customarily meet once a month and grant approvals in four to eight weeks. India presents clinical trial subject populations with unmet medical need, reverence for physicians who remain authority figures, and linguistic and cultural barriers for subjects to understand fully the implications of trial participation. Ensuring ethical integrity and ICH compliance of the clinical trial process in such an environment presents a challenge, and ethics committees must play an important role in meeting this challenge. Recognizing this, the Indian Council for Medical Research has set up initiatives to audit the functioning of ethics committees, introduce a national ethics committee accreditation system, and offer training via the Independent Forum for Ethics Review Committees. However, these initiatives are yet to be fully implemented. If ethics committees are not functioning in compliance with ICH standards, there remain concerns about the robustness of the informed consent process, complete and timely adverse event reporting, and provisions for post-trial access. Furthermore, in the absence of well-developed site capabilities, there are concerns about data quality and the maintenance of source documentation which may compromise the ethical integrity and clinical data quality of ongoing clinical trials. In addition, poorly developed sites may struggle to meet their subject enrollment targets, in spite of the many opportunities for patient access.

One of the most compelling attractions of including India in international clinical trials is elimination of the inefficiencies and wastefulness in clinical trial conduct that have become so prevalent in the USA and Western Europe. In these regions, clinical trial sites enroll as few as 0.5 subjects per month, with many sites failing to contribute even one subject. These poorly performing sites require resource allocation for site set-up, monitoring, and site management, which is wasted if the sites are unable to deliver their promised subject enrollment. Without developed site capabilities, Indian sites too would be inefficient and unable to fulfill their recruitment potential, thereby failing on their promise to be some of the world's most productive clinical trial sites. As a result, India's clinical trial sector may fail to grow further, to the detriment of the many stakeholders in India's healthcare delivery systems. The inclusion of India in international clinical trials brings important benefits for Indian patients. Trial participants have the opportunity to access cutting-edge biomedical innovation which could be life saving. Indian hospitals receive cash, equipment, and additional staff for participating in clinical trials, which benefit all patients served by that hospital. Exposure of the Indian healthcare system to the discipline of international clinical research enhances the practice of evidence-based medicine, thorough record-keeping, and better patient communication. Stakeholders in the sector realize this and are trying to make the necessary investment so that clinical research in India may flourish.

The global pharmaceutical industry acknowledges that up to 40 percent cost and up to 70 percent time savings can be achieved by conducting Phase II–III clinical trials in emerging countries such as India. This, coupled with the need to make the most of every research and development dollar, has heightened the interest of sponsors in placing their clinical trials in India. In addition, the drive to commercialize new products and capture market share in the fast growing pharmaceutical markets of countries such as China, India, and Brazil is becoming stronger. The conduct of Phase II–IV clinical trials in a country facilitates the introduction, adoption, and commercialization of a new product in that market; hence, pharmaceutical companies seeking to build market share in these high-growth emerging countries must consider including them in clinical trials. All of this presents tremendous opportunities for India's clinical trial sector; but poor site capabilities remain a weak link and there is an urgent imperative to address this issue.

There is limited competitor trial activity in India; however, this is rapidly changing at "first tier" sites that have developed experience and a proven track record. Selected second and third tier Indian cities, still large by most standards, with populations of around one to two million, have motivated investigators keen to participate in international clinical trials based at well-developed healthcare facilities that also serve populations from surrounding rural and semi-rural areas. Hospitals in these cities are well suited to clinical trial participation, more so as they do not have the same cost and resourcing pressures that have begun to surface in India's large, metropolitan cities. Initiatives to train potential investigators based in these places, the allocation of funds to build infrastructure and resources at these sites, and the commitment to grow the network of investigative sites will contribute to the development of necessary capabilities at the site level. In order to ensure that there will be sufficient capacity within India's healthcare system to accommodate the increasing numbers of clinical trials being earmarked for India, it is essential for second tier clinical sites to develop capabilities as well.

ECCRO'S APPROACH TO SITE DEVELOPMENT AND SUPPORT IN INDIA

Against this background, ECCRO (www.eccro.com) was established as a specialist CRO focused on providing Phase II–IV clinical trial services for international sponsors in India. The inclusion of emerging countries able to contribute high-recruiting clinical trial sites is essential for the effective conduct of Phase II–III clinical trials. The choice of CRO able to offer access to these productive sites is more critical than the choice of emerging country. ECCRO offers access to some of the world's most productive clinical trial sites, which happen to be located in India. The choice of India is based on the compelling opportunities for cost-effective patient access via productive clinical trial sites and ECCRO's local expertise and relationships. Based on an understanding of the requirements of international regulators and sponsors, and an appreciation of the weaknesses within India's clinical trial environment, ECCRO recognizes that it is critical to build clinical trial site capabilities in India in order to deliver site productivity, data quality, and ethical integrity.

ECCRO's partner clinical trial site program achieves this by careful site selection, development, and management, so as to reach ECCRO's site productivity and data quality standards. Following careful selection, every ECCRO partner clinical trial site enters into a Master Services Agreement and has an ECCRO site manager placed at the site to facilitate the conduct of all ECCRO trials taking place there.

Partner Clinical Trial Site Selection

The large number of potential sites and the substantial variation in their capabilities make careful site selection very important. Local knowledge is valuable to judiciously select clinical trial sites and investigators that will be capable of delivering quality clinical data. ECCRO's SOP for partner site selection incorporates cross-industry best practices to make the process objective, transparent, and robust. The most important of ECCRO's criteria for site selection is a motivated physician who is committed to clinical research. Expertise in therapeutic areas of interest to sponsors and adequate diagnostic and therapeutic facilities for patient care are also sought. It is not essential for sites to have sophisticated imaging or laboratory facilities on site, as long as they have ready access to these facilities at nearby accredited centers. It is important that they have access to a large pool of patients; this pool needs to be a combination of new attendances and follow-up patients, ideally supplemented by a wide referral base including satellite clinics, general practices, community clinics, and other hospitals. A functioning on-site ethics committee or access to an independent ethics committee is also an important selection criterion. Recognizing the importance of well-functioning ethics committees and that this continues to be a weakness for many sites, ECCRO carefully reviews the composition and working practices of the ethics committees at partner clinical trial sites. Although ECCRO can offer guidance and assistance with ethics committee set-up and functioning, there are limitations to the extent to which a CRO can affect this process.

The investigator's and site's experience of participating in international clinical trials, although desirable, is not essential for site selection. Indeed, ECCRO has selected research-naïve centers that meet other selection criteria, with a view to developing these sites.

Recognizing the opportunities for cost-effective clinical trial conduct in India's second and third tier cities and the value in developing sites in these cities, ECCRO has chosen to focus on these cities. Given the vastness of India and this decision to focus on relatively few select sites, the second and third tier cities that ECCRO has elected to work in are near Mumbai, the location of ECCRO's office, with good transport links to Mumbai. This facilitates the training and management of site managers. ECCRO intends to have 10−15 partner clinical trial sites in each of the key therapeutic areas.

Profiles of ECCRO Partner Sites

ECCRO's partner sites represent the full range of clinical trial site options available in India, namely, select departments within teaching hospitals, multispeciality private hospitals, single-speciality, typically oncology or cardiology or diabetes community clinics, and corporate hospital networks.

Government or state hospitals have large patient numbers and are staffed by academic physicians and their trainee doctors who are keen on clinical research. For example, KEM Hospital in Mumbai is one of India's leading academic medical institutions, founded in 1926, admitting 180 undergraduate students each year, with 1.4 million patients attending outpatient clinics each year, 1400 inpatient beds, and 60,000 major operations being carried out each year. The institute has an annual budget of US $20 million, 400 academic staff, and 600 resident postgraduate doctors. However, hospitals such as this are disadvantaged by limited site support resources, rudimentary medical records, poor equipment, and a patient population that includes members of India's lowest socioeconomic groups; hence, it can be challenging to follow-up and retain clinical trial subjects enrolled here.

To meet the healthcare needs of India's 300 million-strong, increasingly affluent middle class, corporate hospital groups are developing national, regional, and local hospitals. These relatively new, well-equipped hospitals are keen to attract international clinical trials. To do so, they are investing in setting up clinical research secretariats to address the administrative and contractual requirements, including a single point of contracting across the hospital network, as well as hotel-style beds to lodge clinical trial subjects and their families during their follow-up visits. Their motivations for this are not only grants and additional resources but also the associated kudos that will, in turn, attract more sought-after physicians to be associated with these institutions. Although these hospitals serve fewer patients than the state-subsidized hospitals, their state-of-the-art equipment and more privileged patients make them particularly attractive for the conduct of international clinical trials.

Single-speciality hospitals attract referrals from large population bases, and so could be suitable for complex protocols that seek patient subsets that are ordinarily difficult to access.

Conducting clinical trials in the primary care setting in India is relatively challenging in the absence of a well-organized state healthcare service. However, it would be possible to recruit physicians working in the private sector. Indeed, privately owned and managed community clinics and hospitals are increasingly demonstrating the interest and potential to be quality clinical trial sites. Typically, these facilities are owned or controlled by physicians with an interest in participating in international clinical trials, who are keen to learn best practices; with support, they are capable of being high-performing sites.

In rural areas, healthcare camps, mobile health delivery units with trained staff and appropriate equipment that visit villages at regular intervals, have been used effectively to conduct prophylactic and preventive infectious disease clinical trials.

Working with Sites

All ECCRO partner clinical trial sites are staffed with an ECCRO site manager, whose role is to facilitate all ongoing and planned trials ECCRO trials at the site. There is a Master Services Agreement in place between ECCRO and its partner sites. The key aspects of this agreement are that the site accepts the placement of the ECCRO site manager and agrees to let him or her work according to ECCRO's SOPs to facilitate all ECCRO clinical trials at the site. In the author's experience, the wholehearted acceptance of this is a great indicator of the investigator's keenness to develop their clinical research experience and their commitment to conducting quality international clinical trials.

The roles, responsibilities, authority, and accountability of the ECCRO site manager, investigator and the site staff are clearly delineated.

According to ECCRO's SOPs, all of its trials will be supported by a site manager, who will facilitate and supervise the conduct of ECCRO trials at the site so as to ensure site productivity, data quality, GCP compliance, and subject protection on an ongoing basis. The site manager is the focal point of contact for communication between the investigator, site personnel working on the study, the ECCRO study team, sponsor, and partner vendors including the electronic data capture (EDC) provider, central laboratory, and clinical trial supplies management services. At the start of each trial, the site manager reviews the protocol with the investigator and site staff to ensure that everyone is conversant with it and understands their roles and responsibilities. The key responsibilities for the site manager are timely and correct subject recruitment, with regular progress feedback to the rest of the study team enabling a prompt call for action should expected recruitment fail to occur. The site manager supports study conduct by promptly addressing issues related to inclusion/exclusion criteria, scales/questionnaires, the informed consent process, subject visit scheduling and coordination, liaison with central laboratories and/or imaging centers, clinical trial supplies, and adverse event reporting. They also respond to monitoring queries, prepare for monitoring visits, support electronic data entry, facilitate the timely compilation of site-related regulatory documents, address contractual issues, and schedule additional study-related training on a needs basis.

ECCRO's site support services are integrated with its other CRO services, with supporting operating practices and systems. ECCRO's operating practices represent industry best practices customized for the Indian clinical trial environment, including the complete adoption of EDC and hybrid monitoring. All team members, be they site or office based, work on a robust online electronic document management system. ECCRO's SOPs demarcate site support services and monitoring, so that study monitoring, both remote and onsite, remains unbiased. Indeed, one of the key advantages of this approach is that monitors are fully focused on ensuring data quality and scientific and ethical integrity, as they are not distracted by the requirement to coordinate study conduct.

Site development activities are conducted on a medium- to long-term basis; that is, beyond the timeframe of a single trial. An important component of these activities is clinical research and GCP training for investigators and site staff, including ongoing training programs on site, notably for new staff members. ECCRO sets up the processes, systems, and tools to support effective clinical trial conduct based on its own SOPs, and offers advice on investing in additional equipment. Partner sites participate in a regular audit and quality assurance cycle. ECCRO supports the compilation of patient databases and building relationships with clinics and hospitals able to refer patients for ongoing and planned clinical trials.

81

Furthermore, the ECCRO site manager facilitates a thoughtful protocol feasibility assessment with accurate subject enrollment estimates for new trials, thus playing a key role in attracting new clinical trials to the site. The site manager is well placed to collate the investigator's recommendations and advice on trial design, with benefits for the sponsor and much satisfaction for the investigator. The site manager also facilitates a streamlined budget negotiation process and the agreement of study-specific site contracts. Having relationships to promptly address contractual issues expedites the study start-up process. A good working relationship with a partner site also enables ECCRO to identify and develop relationships with potential investigators engaged in other therapeutic areas that would be of interest to ECCRO's customer base.

The benefits of engaging with only partner clinical trial sites are reduced study start-up timelines, and improved data quality and site productivity, as measured by the number of evaluable subjects enrolled per month. ECCRO's partner clinical trial sites are typically able to contribute five or six evaluable patients per month for the key therapeutic areas; well above the industry average. In addition, there are numerous long-term advantages related to building strategic relationships with sites and helping them to develop their capabilities. This is a non-exclusive arrangement; ECCRO expects to recover its investment by being able to achieve its site productivity targets, thereby being able to deliver customer satisfaction, win business, and improve profitability. It is expected, but not guaranteed, that because sites will find working on ECCRO studies less tedious and more efficient, and hence fulfilling, they will develop a preference for ECCRO studies.

Success Story

The following case study describes the value of ECCRO's differentiated approach to site support in the Indian clinical trial setting. A European sponsor engaged one of the industry's leading global, full-service CROs to conduct its multi-country Phase III study in a cardiovascular indication. A total of 600 subjects were to be enrolled from eight European countries, but 10 months before the targeted deadline to complete enrollment it became apparent to the sponsor that the timelines would not be met and a decision was made to include India as a rescue country. Furthermore, it was decided to provide sites with additional support so as to facilitate patient identification, pre-screening, and finally enrollment for the challenging study protocol. ECCRO was engaged to provide site support and recruitment consultancy for India.

Following assessment of the 30 selected sites in India, ECCRO elected to focus on only eight sites. The decision regarding which sites to focus on was based on investigator motivation, recruitment potential, access to a wide referral base, and the availability of good-quality patient records. The selected sites were provided with trained site support recruitment consultants who worked with the investigators and the site study teams to identify potential subjects for the study. In four weeks, over 1500 patients were identified and invited for pre-screening visits. It is expected that 10 percent of identified patients will pass through the "recruitment funnel" to become 150 evaluable subjects. This effort brought the study back on track to complete recruitment by the targeted deadline and is a good example of how careful site selection based on well-defined criteria, coupled with additional site support, can enable the site to fulfill its promise of productivity and data quality.

The Path Ahead

As a CRO, ECCRO has taken on the investment to develop clinical trial site capabilities at organizations where it has no ownership stake. There is a risk that the company may not achieve a full return on its efforts. However, a failure to make this investment in site capabilities would mean that clinical trial data could not be delivered in a consistent manner so as to meet customer expectations. Therefore, this investment is critical to its business. ECCRO seeks to build long-term relationships with sponsors such that they commit to working with ECCRO for their clinical trial needs, and can develop site capabilities to match their project pipelines. Such a partnership would not only mitigate risks but also ensure the best outcomes for all stakeholders.

Other emerging countries such as China and Russia also have resource-constrained healthcare environments with hospitals capable of being high-productive clinical trial sites. They too would benefit from site support as well as the development of their clinical trial site capabilities. Although lessons could be learned from this experience in India, the approach should be customized to meet the peculiarities of each country's healthcare system. It must be recognized that although global principles exist, site management remains a local endeavor. Understanding this and building the necessary working relationships are critical to success.

References

1. PricewaterhouseCoopers. *Emerging market report: Health in India;* 2007.
2. CIA World Factbook; 2010.
3. www.clintrials.gov; 2011 [accessed 15.02.11].
4. Varawalla N. India's growing clinical research sector: opportunity for global companies. *IDrugs* 2007;**10**:391−4.
5. Bhatt A. Clinical trials in India: pangs of globalization (Editorial). *Indian Journal of Pharmacology* 2004;**36**:207−8.
6. Varawalla N. Investigative sites unlock the door to success in India. *Applied Clinical Trials* 2007;48−54.

CHAPTER 8

Lessons Learned in China

Juncai (Jack) Xu*, Zhijie Xia[†]
*Shanghai Clinical Research Center, Shanghai, China
[†]ICU Department, Shanghai Huashan Hospital, Fudan University, Shanghai, China

INTRODUCTION

China has been proud of its system of traditional Chinese medicine (TCM) for thousands of years. However TCM suffered from 300 years of turbulence in China brought on by imperialism, invasion, and domestic wars, while Western countries enjoyed the rapid development of scientific civilization. There are few records of modern clinical trials before Western drugs were introduced into China during the past 100 years. It was not until 1949, when the People's Republic of China was established, that China began its scientific development. Good clinical practice (GCP) in China can be traced back to 1984, when the Law on Drug Administration included some regulations on clinical trials. In 1986, the Ministry of Public Health started to cooperate with the World Health Organization (WHO) and other international organizations to develop GCP awareness. Medical students were instructed in the provisions of the Declaration of Helsinki from that time. Afterwards, with the help of a number of global pharmaceutical companies, the International Conference on Harmonisation guideline for GCP (ICH-GCP) was introduced into China. The first version of GCP regulations was issued in 1998 by the Ministry of Health. After the establishment of the State Drug Administration — now the State Food and Drug Administration (SFDA) — new GCP regulations were issued on September 1, 1999.[1]

The current GCP guidelines were issued in 2003, after both the new Drug Administration Law (2001) and the new Drug Registration Procedure (2002) went into effect. The guidelines closely resemble the GCP guidelines (E6) of the International Conference on Harmonisation of Technical Requirements for Registration of Pharmaceuticals for Human Use (ICH), but with some modification to suit the specific circumstances in China. The guidelines consist of 13 chapters containing a total of 70 articles and two appendices (the Declaration of Helsinki and Essential Documents for Clinical Trials).[2]

China has attempted to streamline its regulation and align the country with international standards of practice; as a result, the country's legal system governing pharmaceutical research, production, and marketing was modified substantially in recent years. The SFDA is responsible for the evaluation and inspection of clinical trials of new drugs. On February 19, 2004, the SFDA issued a regulation specifying that all clinical trials (except Phase IV trials) to be registered in SFDA should be conducted at GCP-accredited sites that have been identified and ratified by the SFDA; all investigational new drug (IND) studies for SFDA submissions will be conducted at these accredited sites.[3]

As the trend for economic globalization continues to develop, the clinical trials market has been maturing in China. Several companies have successfully used clinical data generated in China to support their global clinical programs. First, since 1996, AstraZeneca has undertaken nine international multicenter clinical trials in the respiratory field in China, with the involvement of more than 130 domestic hospitals and institutions. The company recently conducted clinical trials for its asthma product (Turbuhaler) in China and used the data to support the drug application overseas.[4] Second, on November 23, 2005, Beijing SFDA approved Bristol-Myers Squibb's Entecavir product in China, only eight months after its first launch in the USA (on March 29, 2005), but seven months earlier than in Europe [approved by the European Agency for the Evaluation of Medicinal Products (EMEA), Paris, on June 28, 2006]. Third, Novartis has been conducting a chronic hepatitis B Phase III clinical trial, entitled the GLOBE study, at 112 clinical centers in 20 countries worldwide. It is the first international hepatitis B study to include clinical sites and patients in China, with an estimated 25 percent of the patients enrolled in the GLOBE study coming from Chinese centers. New data show telbivudine to be superior to lamivudine in treatment of Chinese patients with chronic hepatitis B.[5]

With more than 10 years' effort in strengthening intellectual property rights protection, and improvements to the regulatory environment, more and more global research and development (R&D) centers have come to China. Roche set up the first R&D center in the Zhangjiang area, Shanghai, in 1997; later, Eli Lilly followed. In 2003, Pfizer opened its clinical trial center and stated that the center would not only be concerned with developing drugs for local approval, but also form part of the company's global R&D network.[6] Now Shanghai Zhangjiang is becoming a drug development hub.[7] At the time of writing, AstraZeneca, Bayer, Bristol-Myers Squibb, Eli Lilly, GlaxoSmithKline, Merck, Novartis, Pfizer, and Sanofi-Aventis have all set up R&D centers in China.

Another big event is that the US Food and Drug Administration (FDA) has paid a lot of attention to China's food and drug quality. On November 19, 2008, the US FDA officially opened its China office in Beijing, the first for the FDA outside the USA.[8] The FDA has since set up three more working offices in China, two in Shanghai and one in Guangzhou. Their major responsibilities are to conduct capacity building for food and drug safety monitoring in China and the inspection of imported food and drugs from the USA.

Recent economic growth in China has led to increasing healthcare expenditure and a rising incidence of diseases linked to changing lifestyles; these are predicted to increase in the future.

In a recent report, financial analysts at Merrill Lynch estimated that China's pharmaceutical industry will grow at an annual rate of 24 percent between 2010 and 2020.[9]

As the Chinese pharmaceutical industry is expected to experience double-digit growth over the next few years and China offers tremendous opportunities relative to the availability of patients, low-cost clinical trials, and potentially huge market, more global clinical trials will be introduced in China during the twenty-first century and China will become a key player in global clinical trials in the future.

ADVANTAGES OF CONDUCTING CLINICAL TRIALS IN CHINA

There are many positive factors that encourage the conduct of clinical trials in China. The GCP environment is now maturing, and investigators, monitors, and pharmaceutical joint ventures have all been through the GCP education program. There are a number of endemic diseases in China that are less prevalent elsewhere (e.g. hepatitis B). For trials of drugs in these therapeutic areas, rapid recruitment will be ensured and may also help to secure rapid registration for products in the country where they have the greatest market potential. There are huge numbers of patients in the major hospitals in China, and in some hospitals there are even special patient pools available (such as the asthma patients' club in Shanghai 9th People's Hospital). An additional benefit is that many patients are either untreated or have not received previous treatment with particular drugs. The SFDA has encouraged foreign companies to bring early-phase clinical trials into the country so that the new drugs (especially for medically unmet needs) can be used as early as possible in the company's country of origin. The relatively low cost of performing trials in China is another attraction, particularly for trials that require a large number of patients.[10]

Global studies also have some positive impacts on Chinese doctors, by enhancing local researchers' skills and academic standing, strengthening international collaboration in the medical field, being at the leading edge of new treatments, and generating an additional income source for the hospitals.

Conducting later phase stage clinical trials in China for difficult-to-enroll indications with long enrollment periods will provide significant value to global sponsors. For many of these indications and therapeutic areas, the ability to recruit patients and complete enrollment is much faster in China than in the West.

CHALLENGES TO CONDUCTING GLOBAL CLINICAL TRIALS IN CHINA

Although there are so many advantages and benefits to conducting clinical trials in China, many challenges remain to conducting multinational clinical trials in China, such as non-transparent regulatory requirements, lengthy approval process for clinical trials, restrictive export of whole blood/DNA materials, unclear investigator's accountability, insufficient training for investigators, lack of qualified/experienced monitors and project managers, some local practices, cultural aspects, and the language barrier. Additional problems reported by foreign sponsors include inefficient patient referral networks (heavy patient load in large hospitals, inadequate infrastructure in some centers, less equipment and poor data management) and inconsistencies in GCP training. Logistical issues with long distances between laboratories and different time zones can make project communication difficult.

The main complaint of global sponsors is that it can take seven to 12 months, or more, to gain regulatory approval for a clinical trial from the SFDA. In October 2007, China's SFDA issued new guidance that established timetables for some parts of the review process, shortening the average review time by one to two months.

REGULATORY APPROVAL

History of Chinese Drug Regulation

China's drug regulation system can be traced back to 1962, when the Provisional Measures on the Administration of New Drug Products — the first central government regulations concerning drug administration (i.e. manufacturing, distribution, sales, and use) — were promulgated. In 1978, the State Council approved the Regulations on Drug Administration for trial implementation, which emphasized that R&D and the production of new drugs should be pursued according to the needs of disease prevention and treatment. In 1979, the Measures on the Administration of New Drug Products were promulgated, which clarified the definition of a new drug, the classification of new drugs, the materials required for the approval of new drugs, and the clinical practice procedures. On September 20, 1984, the first Law on Drug Administration was enacted. In 1986, the Ministry of Health established the Drug Evaluation Office in order to set up a drug registration system. Since 1990, increasing numbers of multinational pharmaceutical companies have entered China and there have been more and more new drug applications. In 1995, the Drug Evaluation Office was transformed into the independent Center for Drug Evaluation (CDE).[10]

It is useful to have an understanding of China's legislative body, which is divided into three different levels. The first level is the National People's Congress and Standing Committee. The laws and rules published at this level overrule legislation published at another level if the latter conflicts with the former. The second level is the State Council. The State Council publishes administrative statutes. It is important to point out that the Chinese courts decide cases relying only on the legislation published by these two levels. The third level consists of departments under the State Council (like the SFDA). These departments may also publish rules, orders, regulations, and circulations from time to time. The courts may also make reference to these rules as necessary, but will not rely on them when deciding cases.

In order to understand how to conduct good clinical trials in China, the reader could refer to the following laws and regulations:[11]

- Drug Administration Law of the People's Republic of China
- Provisions for Drug Registration
- Provisions for Drug Insert Sheets and Labels
- Provisions for Clinical Trials of Medical Devices
- Special Review and Approval Procedure for Drug Registration of the State Food and Drug Administration
- Application and Approval Procedure for Clinical Trials
- Application and Approval Procedure for Imported Drugs.

Regulatory Process for Clinical Trials Approval

China has improved its regulatory environment in recent years. The approval process is summarized in Figure 8.1.[12]

The documentation for an application for clinical trials can be prepared in line with the international IND package, including pharmacology and toxicology data. The SFDA may need details of the manufacturing process, specification information, and so on, which global companies may not be willing to provide.

Another regulatory consideration is that the SFDA will typically require some existing clinical data and/or long-term toxicology data before approving a clinical trial application. For a global company's IND study, China does not allow any global sponsor to conduct Phase I, first-in-human studies in the Chinese population without presenting human data for the original country. If a global company with R&D centers in China develops a new drug in China and

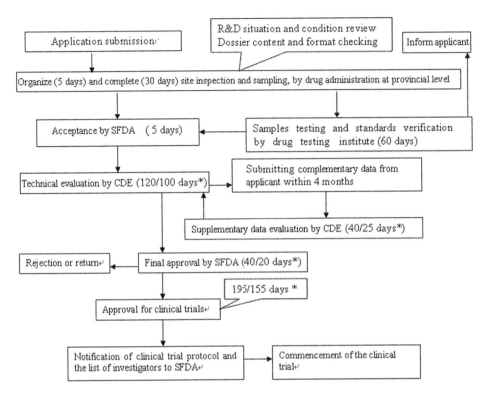

FIGURE 8.1

China's clinical trial approval process. SFDA: State Food and Drug Administration; CDE: Center for Drug Evaluation. *Note: Numbers before the slashed line refer to the timeline for ordinary approval and those after the line to the timeline for fast-track approval (all in working days).

follows China's IND process, providing research data generated from China, they can apply for their Phase I first-in-human study in China.[13]

Unfortunately, the long time for the process of regulatory review and approval of clinical trial applications has been a major hurdle when deciding whether or not to conduct a trial in China. It typically took approximately eight to 12 months for the SFDA to approve clinical trial applications, but in reality depended on the nature of the drug under trial. In the case of clinical trials that have not been previously approved, regulatory attitudes tend to be cautious, approval may take considerably longer, and timelines are often unpredictable owing to lack of manpower and additional regulatory requirements. If a drug to be trialed in China is already available on a Western market then SFDA approval is likely to be quicker. The SFDA is working closely with global industry leaders and regulatory bodies (e.g. the US FDA) to improve its processes. It is hoped that in the near future the approval process will become more favorable; in fact, some cancer studies were approved within four months in 2009 and 2010.

It should be noted that the ability to recruit patients in China more quickly than in any other region in the world may offset the initial regulatory delay. Depending on the study's enrollment period and/or the ability to submit an application early, this will have a considerable impact on what types of trials benefit most from being conducted in China.

HOW CAN CHINA PARTICIPATE IN GLOBAL MULTICENTER TRIALS?

Suppose that a global company is planning a multinational study with a total recruitment period of 12 months. Will China be included? Based on past experience, the answer would be no, since it would take at least six to nine months for IND approval. However, now that early

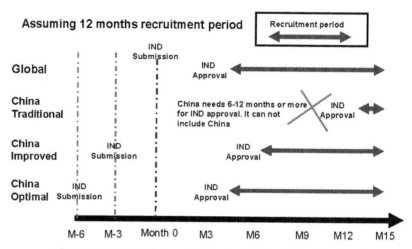

FIGURE 8.2

How to include China in a global study, by planning early: a practical strategy for investigational new drug (IND) study in China. (Please refer to color plate section)

initiation of IND submission is possible, if the sponsor has an early IND submission strategy, the answer could be yes. A practical strategy is summarized in Figure 8.2.

When planning their regulatory strategy, companies should consider designing the China component of the trial to position the drug for eventual market approval in China. When companies are interested in running a clinical trial in China, it is suggested that they:

- compile preclinical and available clinical documents at least six to nine months ahead of expected trial initiation
- draft a clinical trial protocol for submission; this can be finalized during independent ethics committee (IEC) approval
- conduct a quality control test; test samples and technical document transfer must be ready
- arrange a prereview meeting with the SFDA; this will be a key step towards conducting clinical trials successfully in China.

SOME PRACTICAL ASPECTS OF GLOBAL STUDIES IN CHINA

Good Clinical Practice-accredited Sites

GCP-accredited sites (called research bases in some literature) play a key role in promoting GCP implementation in China. The concept of GCP-accredited sites is unique. China produced generic drugs and initiated few IND studies before the 1970s. In 1983, in the hope of improving the quality of generic products, the Ministry of Health designated the first set of clinical pharmacology sites that were required to have essential training courses on GCP for clinical researchers and advanced facilities for clinical trials. The second and third sets of sites were approved in 1986 and 1990, respectively, for a total of 35 accredited sites that were responsible for bioequivalence studies for generic products and pharmacokinetics studies for new drugs.

In 1998, China reformed its central government system and, in order to manage medical products well, set up the organization that is now the SFDA, independent of the Ministry of Health. In the same year, the agency promulgated the Chinese GCP guidelines. Intending to popularize GCP in China, the agency invited principal investigators, ethics committee members, nurses, pharmacists, and clinical research coordinators (CRCs) nationwide to learn the guidelines. Through education, the agency re-evaluated the existing 35 clinical pharmacology sites, eventually approving them as well as some new sites as the country's GCP-accredited clinical trial bases.

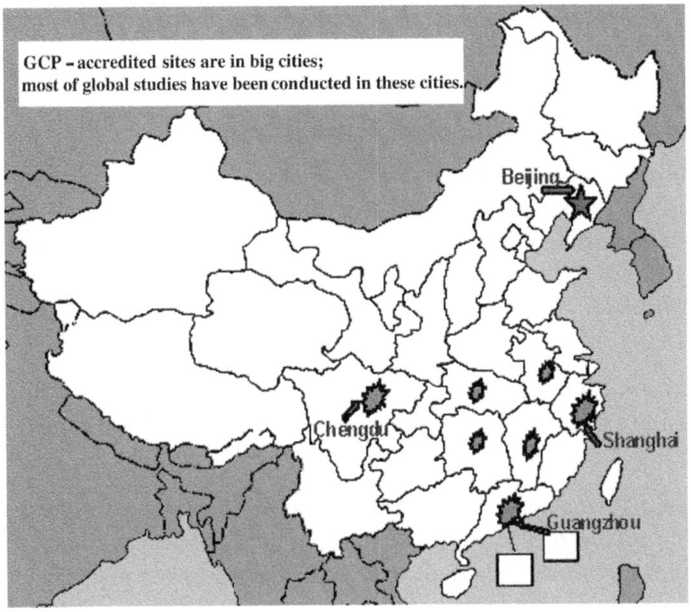

FIGURE 8.3
Main good clinical practice (GCP) sites in China. Most GCP-accredited sites are in big cities; most global studies have been conducted in these cities. (Please refer to color plate section)

Currently, there are 252 GCP-accredited sites for clinical trials on chemical-based medicines and 85 for those on TCM. All SFDA-registered clinical trials (except Phase IV trials) must be conducted at GCP-accredited sites.[3]

At present, 80 percent of medical resources in China are allocated to big cities, and 30 percent of these resources are focused in large hospitals. These include all the GCP-accredited sites. Beijing, Shanghai, and Guangzhou account for more than 60 percent of GCP sites (Figure 8.3). These big hospitals offer access to a large pool of eligible subjects, which greatly facilitates patient recruitment.[14]

Independent Ethics Committees

According to Chinese regulations, each GCP-accredited site must have an IEC. IEC members in China are selected on the same basis as is described by ICH-GCP. In China, every IEC must take the Declaration of Helsinki as its guide and operate in accordance with Chinese law and GCP guidelines. In a multicenter trial, the SFDA requires the sponsor to designate one principal GCP-accredited site from all the participating hospitals and the clinical trial must be approved by the IEC at this site. There is no requirement to obtain approval from the IECs of the other sites, but they must agree to use the central IEC. The principal investigator will be responsible for submitting the study materials to, and obtaining approval from, the principal IEC. Also unique to China is the fact that, when the principal investigator makes an application to the IEC, the research site will ask the applicant to gain SFDA approval first. Without SFDA approval, the research site will not accept the application. Usually, each research site will have one review meeting per month; therefore, it generally takes one to two months to obtain IEC approval.[10]

It should be noted that the ethics committee set-up in China principally follows ICH guidelines. However, at present, many of those who serve on ethics committees at Chinese hospitals are medical doctors from the same hospital. As they work for the very institution conducting the research they are reviewing, there is a potential conflict of interest.

91

Furthermore, they may feel influenced in their decision making by those senior to them in the institution.

Language Barrier and Document Translation

The importance of considering the language barrier is commonly underestimated in international clinical trials. The Chinese language can present a communication barrier, making it essential to have proper translation and interpretation to define the goals and clarify the expectations of all parties. Differences in patient literacy rates are another factor that must be considered, especially in the process of obtaining informed consent.

As with all global clinical trials, regulatory documents must be provided in the country's official language and patient-related materials must be translated into the patient's native language. Mandarin Chinese is used by the majority of the Chinese population.

Translators trained in translating documents for the pharmaceutical industry must follow a well-established process to ensure that translations are both accurate and culturally sensitive. This process will involve numerous steps that are performed systematically by translators who must be fluent in both the source language and the target Chinese language.

For important documents (e.g. protocol and drug safety information), back-translation is a critical part of the translation process as it helps to ensure that the meaning in the original text is not lost in the translation. However, in cases where languages differ significantly, such as English and Chinese, further comparison between the translated and original versions is required. In some cases, word equivalents may not exist at all, and translators must come up with the most acceptable functional equivalents in the target language that best represent words or phrases in the source language. Successful translations must therefore be reviewed by professionals who are native speakers, are familiar with the culture, and have a professional background in clinical research.

Study Sample Exports

China controls the export of whole blood and tissue samples of clinical trials to central laboratories outside China.

The growing importance of centralized laboratories for patient sample analysis generates a significant challenge for global sponsors in China, since permission is required for the export of all study tissues and samples. China set up a regulatory system to control the export of all research samples in the wake of some research scandals. Two regulations have to be followed:

- **Provisions for the Administration of Human Genetic Resources**, issued by the Ministry of Health and Ministry of Science and Technology (effective from June 10, 1998). The office of Human Genetic Resources Administration of China (hereinafter referred to as the HGRAC) is in charge of this regulation.
- **Provisions for Strengthening Management of Entry and Exit Health Quarantine on Medical Special Samples**, issued by the Ministry Of Health and General Administration of Quality Supervision, Inspection, Quarantine of the People's Republic of China (GAQSIQ) (effective from August 6, 2003).

Based on these regulations, the following samples require permits from the Ministry of Health:

- medical special samples associated with pedigrees or certain regions and populations, except for serum, plasma, and genetic resources
- more than 100 special medical samples
- special medical samples collected from new drug global multicenter clinical studies

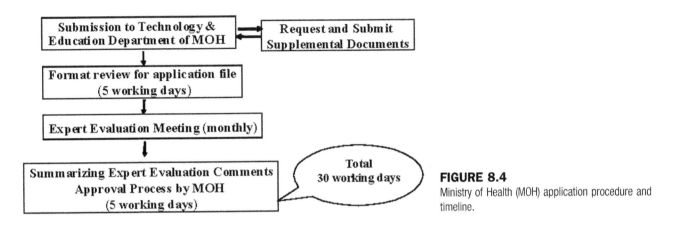

FIGURE 8.4

Ministry of Health (MOH) application procedure and timeline.

- special medical samples containing grade 3—4 disease-causing microorganisms (according to the risk classification standard for infectious substances based on the WHO Laboratory Health and Safety Manual).

The Ministry of Health application procedure is summarized in Figure 8.4. Applications for genetic materials export are sent for HGRAC approval. The process is shown in Figure 8.5.

Cultural Factors

Chinese cultural attitudes have a strong impact on medical practices and clinical research results. Each patient's perception of health, disease, and functioning as a result of disease depends on the individual and the society in which they live. It is therefore important for sponsors to account for any differences in cultural perceptions that can affect such things as patient reporting of disease symptoms and adverse events, or interfere with the diagnosis, treatment, and enrollment of patients in clinical trials.

For example, traditional herbal medicines and natural therapies have been in use for thousands of years. Many are commonly used today to strengthen the body, improve the immune system, relieve pain, reduce some symptoms, and treat diseases ranging from rheumatoid arthritis to gastrointestinal diseases. Two well-known examples, acupuncture and taking the herbal medicine ginseng, are common practice in China.

A comprehensive understanding of the culture from a social, economic, and government perspective also helps to maximize the roles of hospitals, doctors, monitors, government, and local partners. In China, there are significant differences among ethnic populations since there are in total 55 minorities plus the major population of Han in China. If a study involves any minority, it is useful to study their culture before starting the project.

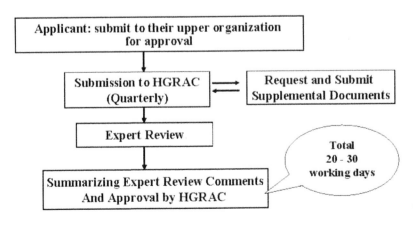

FIGURE 8.5

Human Genetic Resources Administration of China (HGRAC) application process and timeline.

93

COST OF CLINICAL TRIALS IN CHINA

It is generally believed that one of the main attractions of performing clinical trials in China is the relatively low cost, and this has been borne out by several reports. In terms of general running costs, it has been estimated that clinical trials can be conducted in China for around 10 percent of the equivalent cost in a Western country. More specific domestic estimates suggest that Phase I and Phase II clinical trials in China cost 15 and 20 percent, respectively, of the price in a Western country.[15]

An additional cost benefit is diagnostic procedure costs. When calculating the costs of a clinical trial, the impact of such costs is often underestimated and yet these procedures are essential to the trial from a scientific perspective. Estimates from one Chinese contract research organization (CRO) put these types of costs at between 10 and 30 percent of those for Western clinical trial centers.[16]

However, it may not always be the case that costs are lower in China. For example, the author had one case in which the site recruited only one patient in China, but the running cost for China was much higher than for any of the other countries involved. Over the past decade in China, wages and doctors' study grants have increased, and the trend towards higher cost fees is likely to continue.

CLINICAL TRIAL MONITORING IN CHINA

The key to success in conducting high-quality clinical studies in China is to have well-trained and conscientious clinical investigators and monitors who are of a good standard. Chinese monitors usually have a medical background as most of them have been hospital doctors (since young doctors' salaries are not high, some of them leave the hospitals to join companies as clinical research associates). They are very familiar with the Chinese medical system and can quickly and easily build a good cooperative relationship with the investigators. There is no difference between Chinese GCP and ICH-GCP regarding the responsibilities of the monitor. However, Chinese monitors usually have to do more work in the trial than their peers in the West because the supporting infrastructure is less well developed. During a routine monitoring visit, verification of source data is necessary. In general, direct access to subjects' medical records is permitted provided that it is specified in the informed consent form and approved by the IEC.

Good Clinical Practice Training and Training Hubs

As the clinical trial sector grows, it will need more qualified staff. On February 8, 2000, the SFDA set up six training hubs in Peking University, Fudan University, Sichuan University, Central South University, Zhongshan University, and Guangzhou University of TCM to improve the overall level of China's clinical research in relation to international standards. On August 9, 2001, another two institutions, China Academy of Chinese Medical Sciences (CACMS) and Chengdu University of TCM, were selected as GCP training hubs on TCM to cater for the growth in this area of clinical research.

As more companies enter the market, the clinical research industry will need to play its part in encouraging people to pursue relevant educational courses in the clinical research field. In order to implement high-quality studies, the companies are responsible for training the research team.[17] Shanghai Dr. J has provided professional education of GCP in Universities.

Regulatory Inspection

Along with lower costs, maintaining ICH-GCP quality and ethical compliance are the key industry concerns for conducting global trials in China. Global companies seeking to operate in China will need to ensure that their Chinese-based clinical trials can meet international standards, otherwise the data will be of no use in supporting product registration when dealing with regulatory agencies such as the FDA and EMEA.

Global companies need to select their development partners carefully (including investigators) and address quality concerns to ensure that the gap is filled for acceptance by the FDA and studies are conducted under ICH-GCP guidelines. Understanding the Chinese culture is critical in all aspects from establishing strong business relationships to ensuring that the patients, investigators, and research staff understand, adhere to, and execute the trials according to ICH-GCP and without bias.

In general, Chinese investigators willingly accept audits of their clinical sites. Quality assurance procedures are becoming familiar to them, since more and more international multicenter clinical trials are being conducted in China. According to Chinese GCP, the SFDA conducts inspections for GCP at some study sites for certain clinical trials.

The level of confidence regarding quality is rising quickly, as indicated by the increasing number of FDA IND products being tested in China. To ensure quality compliance, clinical trials are currently only conducted in hospitals that are China SFDA GCP certified. With regard to China, the FDA has stated that it is willing to accept foreign clinical data provided that the trials are conducted in an ethical manner, they are applicable to the US population, and the agency can inspect the trial sites if desired.

Based on the FDA's Clinical Investigator Inspection List database, as of June 20, 2011, the FDA had carried out 13 inspections in 10 cities in China. All inspections were of the "verification of study data" type. Four sites out of 13 had no major findings; the results were "no action indicated" (NAI, e.g. no objectionable conditions or practices were found during the inspection). Nine sites had some findings, with the result of "voluntary action indicated" (VAI, e.g. objectionable conditions were found but the problems do not justify further regulatory action. Any corrective action is left to the investigator to take voluntarily). The main findings at these nine sites were: Inadequate and inaccurate records (FDA code 06) (nine sites); Inadequate drug accountability (FDA code 04) (six sites); Failure to follow investigational plan (FDA code 05) (one site); and Failure to report adverse drug reactions (FDA code 16) (one site).[18]

Document Archiving

Chinese GCP requires the retention of documents for five years after a drug receives regulatory approval, while with ICH-GCP it is until the drug has been marketed in the last ICH country for two years. Most global pharmaceutical companies require documents to be retained for 15 years for practical purposes.

CLINICAL TRIALS OUTSOURCING IN CHINA

History of Contract Research Organizations

The CRO business in China dates back to 1995, when MDS became the first global CRO operation in China. Later, Covance, Quintiles, and Loudon set up operations, along with nearly all other global CROs (AAI, Apex, Consultech, EPS, Excel, ICON, Ingenex, Innapharma, Kendlewits, Medifacts, Omnicare, Parexel, Pharmanet, PPD, Siniwest, etc.). The CROs' presence has certainly helped to promote the concept of GCP in the pharmaceutical industry and in some major hospitals. These CROs have helped both international and domestic pharmaceutical companies to conduct international clinical trials, as well as local trials for drug registration or marketing in China.[10]

It is estimated that more than 100 CROs are now operating in China. Based on SFDA data, during 2005, pharmaceutical companies obtained approval for more than 4000 clinical trials in China. About 30 percent of this clinical work is believed to have been outsourced, suggesting that around 1200 clinical trial projects involved CROs in 2005.[14]

Selecting a Contract Research Organization

Evaluating a CRO in China seems like a daunting task. CRO options range from large, global companies with comprehensive services to small niche providers specializing in particular therapeutic areas or domestic CROs. CRO services and budgets often vary significantly with respect to details and assumptions, which makes comparisons very difficult since the CRO business is not maturing in China. The price for a project may vary by several-fold. The CRO employees who discuss proposals with clients may not be the same ones assigned to potential outsourcing projects, so a good step in finding a good CRO would be to interview the project management team.

A large or famous CRO may not be the right one for a sponsor in China. To find a suitable CRO, first, there is a need to identify a manageable number of appropriately experienced CROs in order to request their proposals. The CROs' capabilities and proposals must be compared to assess the most appropriate partner for possible outsourcing projects. In selecting a CRO, several questions need to be asked:

- Can the CRO offer the services that the sponsor needs?
- Does the CRO have related experience and a good track record (i.e. similar projects and references from satisfied clients)?
- Is the CRO financially stable?
- Does the CRO have a good system for employee training and a low staff turnover rate?
- Does the CRO have the key staff members and can it set up a team to deliver qualified results?
- Does the CRO have the required infrastructure?
- Does the CRO have a robust quality assurance system?

To ensure the integrity and success of a clinical trial, it is very important to use a CRO that is based in China and understands both ICH-GCP and China SFDA GCP requirements. In addition, the CRO should help the sponsor by having a thorough understanding of both Chinese and Western cultures and languages to ensure that trials are processed and executed with efficiency and to global standards.

INTELLECTUAL PROPERTY RIGHTS

Intellectual property rights (IPR) are very important to the economic development and the progress of modern society. Since China formally joined the World Trade Organization (WTO) on December 11, 2001, it has established a basic intellectual property rights legal system.

The current system includes laws and regulations on trademarks, patents, copyright, trade secrets, and unfair competition, most of which conform to the Trade-Related Aspects of Intellectual Property (TRIPS) Agreement. China's intellectual property laws have been amended and modernized essentially to meet the requirements outlined in the TRIPS Agreement and the General Agreement on Tariffs and Trade (GATT).

China has not only established a basic legal system to protect IPR but also made substantial efforts to improve judicial enforcement of its intellectual property laws. Two enforcement mechanisms, administrative and judicial, are used to protect intellectual property effectively.[19]

The year 2002 was a milestone in China for the promulgation of laws to improve intellectual property protection of pharmaceuticals. For example, as part of China's WTO accession, Chinese authorities promulgated legislation extending all patent coverage to 20 years. Other improvements include provisions for data protection and patent linkage. This is good news for foreign companies that want to introduce new drugs to China.

Although central government has made efforts to tackle the problem, the enforcement measures taken to date have not been sufficient to deter some IPR infringements effectively.

Several factors undermine enforcement measures, including China's reliance on administrative instead of criminal measures to combat IPR infringements, local protectionism at the provincial level, limited resources and training available to enforcement officials, and a lack of public education regarding the economic and social impact of counterfeiting and piracy.[20]

China's intellectual property protection is not perfect, but it has improved functionally. In 2006 alone, Chinese courts concluded nearly 2300 criminal cases involving IPR, sentenced over 3500 criminals, and resolved over 14,000 civil cases. China is making significant efforts to combat IPR violations, including patents and trademarks. Accordingly, companies doing business in or with China should be proactive in protecting their intellectual property in China.[21]

SUMMARY

China has become an important pharmaceutical market in its own right, so its clinical trial data are invaluable to global companies wishing to publicize their products worldwide. Population growth, increased life expectancy, urbanization, tobacco consumption, and the adoption of fatty dietary habits have all contributed to a higher incidence of modern life diseases among Chinese people; therefore, the main clinical trials in China are being conducted in related therapeutic areas, including cardiovascular diseases, cancer, diabetes, obesity, hepatitis, and respiratory diseases.

No global company can ignore China in its global strategy. Although China's IND strategy has some unique concepts (e.g. GCP-accredited sites, minimal study subjects in IND studies, IEC approval after SFDA regulatory approval), its main content is similar to the international IND scheme (Figure 8.6).

Any company looking to conduct clinical research in China is strongly advised to work with a well-established team, local partner, or contract research organization that has knowledge of the local regulations, testing facilities, etiquette, and culture. This will not only smooth things along and help to absorb some of the frustrations, but also make conducting research work in China more interesting and rewarding.

97

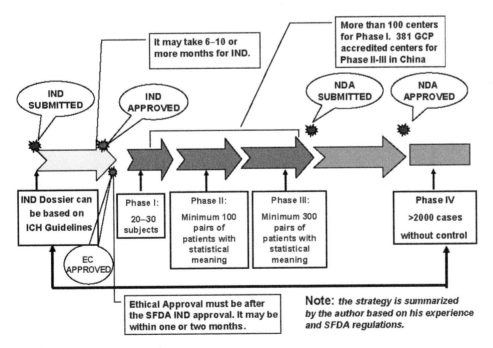

FIGURE 8.6
Investigational new drug strategy (IND) in China (manufacturing drug in China). (Please refer to color plate section)

Acknowledgments

The author sincerely thanks Dr. George Li, BD director of Quintiles China, for drafting the process of blood sample export application, and Sophia Li, CRA of Shanghai Clinical Research Center, for reference checking and organization.

References

1. Guo-wei S. Current status of clinical trials on drugs and GCP in China. *Drug Information Journal* 1997;**31**:1109−25.

2. http://www.rdpac.org/misc/news2.php?cid=77&page=3 [accessed 22.06.11].

3. Kong L. Clinical trial opportunities in China. *Applied Clinical Trials*; 2007. April 1.

4. Anon. *AstraZeneca and China Medical Association jointly initiate research fund for chronic respiratory diseases.* AstraZeneca China Press Release; 2006. March 27.

5. Novartis. *New data show telbivudine superior to lamivudine in treatment of Chinese patients with chronic hepatitis B.* Novartis Press Release. March 27. http://dominoext.novartis.com/NC/NCPrRe01.nsf/ 44aff02a639be034c1256b4b007b5f4d/095509fa24122580c125713e0026fb4d?OpenDocument; 2006 [accessed 23.12.11].

6. Anon. Shanghai to get new Pfizer clinical trial center. *China Daily*. November 5. http://www.chinadaily.com.cn/ en/doc/2003-11/05/content_ 278834.htm; 2003 [accessed 23.12.11].

7. http://www.zjpark.com/ (Chinese version) [accessed 23.12.11]

8. http://english.peopledaily.com.cn/90001/90776/90883/6537942.html [accessed 22.06.11].

9. http://www.globalintelligence.com/insights-analysis/asia-news-update/asia-news-update-january-28-2011/ #ixzz1EEpfIQ3X [accessed 23.12.11]

10. Xu J, Lee G, Guo X, Xin D. A bright outlook for clinical trials in China. *Clinical Researcher* 2002;**2**(12):12−9.

11. http://eng.sfda.cn/WS03/CL0769/ (English version) [accessed 19.06.11].

12. http://eng.sfda.gov.cn/WS03/CL0769/61659.html [accessed 23.12.11]

13. http://eng.sfda.cn/WS03/CL0769/ (English version) [accessed 19.06.11].

14. UKTI. *The Chinese biotechnology, life science & pharmaceutical industry.* January. http://www.uktradeinvest.gov.uk; 2007 [accessed 23.12.11].

15. Reymond E. China lives up to outsourcing hype. *In-Pharma Technologist 16.* January. http://www.drugresearcher. com/news/ng.asp?n=73400-ukti-pfizer-china-clinical-trials-outsourcing; 2007 [accessed 23.12.11].

16. Engel M. *Drug development in China: opportunities and challenges − a clinical trial perspective.* Beijing: China Life Sciences Partnering Forum; 2006. January 16.

17. Xu J, Liu M. An update on GCP education and training in China. *Monitor*; 2011. February, 44−8.

18. http://www.accesSFDAta.fda.gov/scripts/cder/CLIIL/index.cfm?fuseaction=Search. Search [accessed 20.06.11].

19. Yang D. The development of intellectual property in China. *World Patent Information* 2003;**25**(2):131−42.

20. http://www.mac.doc.gov/china/docs/businessguides/intellectualpropertyrights.htm [accessed 23.12.11]

21. http://www.highbeam.com/doc/1G1-190365015.html [accessed 22.06.11].

CHAPTER 9

Lessons Learned in Eastern Europe

Jakub Hort[*†], **Bogdan O. Popescu**[**], **Philip Scheltens**[‡]
*2nd Medical Faculty, Charles University and University Hospital Motol, Prague, Czech Republic
†International Clinical Research Center, St. Anne's University Hospital Brno, Brno, Czech Republic
**University Hospital, "Carol Davila" University of Medicine and Pharmacy, Bucharest, Romania
‡VU University Medical Center, Amsterdam, The Netherlands

INTRODUCTION

There are differences in organizing randomized controlled trials (RCTs) across Europe. Clinical trials on Alzheimer's disease (AD) are frequently performed in Western, Central, and Eastern Europe. The Czech Republic and Romania are referred to here to represent several specific issues that can occur within RCTs. Both countries offer a very good infrastructure within the public health system as well as university hospitals and private practices with huge experience in performing RCTs. There are differences, however, in contracting, investigators' motivation, site selection, and qualification for performing RCTs. Organizing RCTs on AD may represent a specific field to reflect these differences.

CONTRACTING

A specific situation in the Czech Republic and Romania, as well as probably all Eastern European countries, comes from the fact that the salaries of the doctors working in the hospitals lag behind both the domestic private sector and Western European countries. This issue led to a mass resignation of hospital employees in early 2011.[1] Despite slight salary increases during the past few years, the proportion of income received from hospitals and the possibility of earning considerably more money from RCTs remain unchanged. However, in

Global Clinical Trials Playbook. DOI: 10.1016/B978-0-12-415787-3.00009-6

the Czech Republic, hospitals tend to control the flow of money and charge an overhead of 30–70 percent when doctors are contracted through hospitals. This has led to a drop in the income from RCTs among hospital doctors below motivational levels, and a tendency to demand two contracts, one with the hospital and another with a contract research organization (CRO) or directly with a sponsor to bypass the overheads charged by the hospitals. Since this two-contract practice may be against hospital or sponsors' policy and therefore unfeasible, many principal investigators (PIs) decline to take part in RCTs. This situation is different from that in many Western European countries, where doctors earn satisfactory salaries from the hospitals and conducting RCTs may be part of their contract with the hospital. Two-contract practice is legal and a tax-official approach which complies with the law in Central and Eastern Europe, but may be conflicting for hospitals, or CROs' or sponsors' policy.

In Romania, CROs have different contracts with the hospital, with the PI, and with the subinvestigators. On average, from the amount paid for one patient, 10 percent goes to the hospital, 50–60 percent to the PI, and 30–40 percent to the subinvestigators. Sometimes, the subinvestigators are not offered a contract for their clinical trial work and do not receive any money. Although this demotivating practice was the norm in the early years of RCTs in Romania, it is becoming less and less frequent. Therefore, in contrast to the Czech Republic, in Romania PIs prefer to conduct RCTs in the hospital and not in private practices.

ROLE OF THE HEAD OF THE DEPARTMENT

There is a difference between the USA, Great Britain, and the other countries on the one hand and, for example, Germany, Austria, the Czech Republic, and Romania on the other. In the latter group of countries, a very strong role is played by the head of the department and weaker roles by heads of the particular units. An analogy is that there is a strong king or queen and weak dukes in these countries. In many hospitals, the head of the department is the PI in 10 or even more RCTs at the same time. There are examples of the head of the department being the PI in all the RCTs running in his department. However, it is the head of the particular unit (multiple sclerosis unit, stroke unit, memory clinic, movement disorders clinic, etc.) who actually looks after the patients. The heads of the units may become demotivated under these circumstances. It is practically impossible to run so many clinical trials at the same time and there have been examples in the Czech Republic of PIs who were involved only financially, but not practically, in the RCTs. In Romanian hospitals, only the heads of the departments are appointed as PIs. Therefore, some doctors use their private practice for RCTs, where they can qualify for the PI position and gain better income from the same work. In Germany and Austria, there may be situations where the finances earned from RCTs can be used only for hiring new residents or, for example, neuropsychologists. Under these circumstances, the subinvestigators receive no payment for conducting RCTs.

SITE SELECTION

In many Czech hospitals with difficult contracting environments or dominant roles of department heads, investigators either resign from conducting RCTs within the hospitals or convert the RCTs to their private practices when possible. This solution is relatively frequent as it is allowed to have a concurrence of private and hospital or academic affiliations. Since CROs and sponsors have been mainly interested in high recruitment, they have complied with this trend and have transferred RCTs to private practices. They appreciate the direct financial motivation of the personnel in these sites and the more flexible and faster contracting process. Complicated negotiations with a hospital can last for many weeks, which puts hospital sites at a disadvantage in an environment of competitive enrollment. However, not all experts open their private practices and, also, patients cannot be easily transferred out of the hospitals as they must remain to be managed in the hospitals for economic, logistic, safety, and insurance policy reasons. Therefore, in many cases, RCTs were moved to private practices with less educated, less skilled, and less specialized personnel, or sites with ethically weaker backgrounds. These sites do not look primarily after patients, nor diagnose and treat them routinely. Therefore, they have to gather patients primarily for the purpose of the RCT. These facts have been repeatedly discussed within scientific societies and ethics committees. Many notions of lower accuracy and lower compliance in these private practices were discussed. Among them, it is important to mention false referrals (when a main private practice site owns the other economically dependent subsidiaries), lower ethical background (when local ethics committees are founded to become even more independent from regulatory organs), and lower diagnostic accuracy (when employees of these sites are not key opinion leaders or skilled experts).

SPECIFICS OF RANDOMIZED CONTROLLED TRIALS IN ALZHEIMER'S DISEASE

The previous diagnostic criteria on AD comprised a subjective and less accurate approach for the establishment of a diagnosis.[2] New diagnostic criteria have introduced biomarkers which make the diagnostic process more reliable.[3] However, these biological markers, such as cerebrospinal fluid assessment, magnetic resonance imaging volumetry, single-photon emission computed tomography (SPECT), and positron emission tomography (PET), together with extensive neuropsychology, are not easy to perform and their wider use depends on many interfering factors. Therefore, these procedures are usually not applied to all patients recruited to RCTs. For example, spinal tap may limit the recruitment rate. If the biomarkers are not applied in all recruited subjects in the RCT, the recruitment rate is likely to be higher but diagnostic accuracy lower. In cases where diagnosis is based on more subjective and old criteria,[2] or the incomplete use of novel methods, subjects who are less affected by AD, and even those with no dementia, are more likely to be recruited. These individuals may have only subjective memory complaints, depression, or mild cognitive impairment. In the case of RCTs on AD, when patients with no dementia are enrolled, the placebo arm cannot deteriorate, which is crucial to the outcome. Subjects may also be recruited who suffer from ailments other than AD dementia, mainly vascular cognitive impairment, which can corrupt the outcome of the RCT. Clinical diagnosis of AD remains difficult and may differ from the diagnosis made at autopsy. There is higher accuracy in specialized memory clinics and the use of novel biomarkers can further increase the confidence in clinical diagnosis as these procedures have a higher sensitivity and specificity for AD.[4] Further to the lower diagnostic accuracy, when biomarkers were not used, extreme cases have been reported to the ethics committees; these included suspicions of malpractice and violations of good clinical practice (GCP) and were related mainly to RCTs being transferred from specialized clinics to obscure and dubious private sites.

PREVENTIVE MEASURES

Diversity and problems present in the performing of RCTs have been repeatedly discussed within the scientific community and several measures have been suggested:

- The field of AD research could profit from performing fewer, better designed studies at well-established sites.
- These sites should preferably include specialized clinics or sites recommended by national key opinion leaders or scientific societies. These bodies and experts should provide references and positive lists of the sites should be available.
- Performing RCTs at academic sites may be more expensive because of the higher overheads, but diagnostic accuracy and compliance to GCP are more likely at these sites.
- Patient histories should be well documented and referrals from GPs or other experts, or previous history in the case of patients on file should be available. Histories are usually better documented in specialized clinics or academic sites as the patients come primarily to seek care, not solely for the purpose of the RCT. In the case of external referrals, it should be clear that the referring subject is not economically dependent on the PI.

- A PI should run only a reasonably small number of RCTs at one time.
- In the case of AD, the use of biomarkers can increase diagnostic accuracy.
- If computed tomography (CT) and MRI are used, then there should preferably be a central or blinded reading of the images.
- One should avoid repeatedly recruiting the same patient in subsequent RCTs.
- Scientific papers should list information on how many patients were recruited from which sites. Detailed lists with the number of patients per site should be available.

CASE STUDIES

How Easy is it to Cheat?

A 67-year-old man has been observed in an academic center since 2006 for subjective memory complaints and depression. He has a history of hypertension and three hospitalizations in the intensive care unit for transient ischemic attacks. An MRI at the academic site performed for research purposes revealed extensive vascular changes subcortically and in the basal ganglia. Neuropsychology showed executive dysfunction, depression, and slowness of thought. His apolipoprotein E genotype was E3/E3. The patient attended annual check-ups at the university hospital and was treated with aspirin, antihypertensives, statins, and vasoactive substances. He did not match the criteria for prescription of cholinesterase inhibitors.

During a well-documented visit to a memory clinic in September 2009, an extensive neuro-psychological assessment was again performed, revealing executive dysfunction, normal memory, depression, Geriatric Depression Scale (GDS) 8, and Mini-Mental State Examination (MMSE) 29/30. The patient's wife said that he had been started on donepezil at a private site three weeks earlier, since when he had suffered from nausea and diarrhea. He had mild hemiparesis but was functioning independently. His Hachinski Ischemia Score was 8, the clinical dementia rating score was 0.5, and the activities of daily living scale was normal. He was prescribed antidepressive medication at the academic site and was advised to stop taking donepezil immediately.

In October 2009, the wife informed the academic center that her husband was enrolled in a clinical trial on AD, with a screening period that had started in August 2009. She had been afraid to report it earlier but decided to mention it when her husband was unable to tolerate donepezil.

This case study demonstrates a violation of two exclusion criteria: measuring the National Institute of Neurological and Communicative Disorders and Stroke—Association Inter-nationale pour la Recherche et l'Enseignement en Neurosciences (NINCDS—AIREN) for vascular dementia with a score of 8, and exceeding the allowed Hachinski score of 6. At the same time, there was a violation of five inclusion criteria: not demented [Diagnostic and Statistical Manual of Mental Disorders (DSM) IV)], not probable AD [NINCDS—Alzheimer's Disease and Related Disorders Association (ADRDA)], not on a stable dose of donepezil for six months, depression (GDS 8), and vascular changes on MRI. Independent referrals in this case were biased as the site bought six other private practices, which may provide their own and biased referrals. The private site did its own neuroimaging. However, it was a CT scan performed at another private facility that was again economically related to the PIs. An official description of this CT scan did not mention any vascular changes.

Knowing this information, the academic center immediately recommended that the patient leave the clinical trial on AD, and reported to the ethics committee, which further reported to the sponsor. Unfortunately, the response of the sponsor was lukewarm and a local subsidiary swept the case under the rug (the site reported the patient as withdrawn informed consent). The ethics committee could not prove malpractice as the PI insisted that he had not known that the patient was being observed in the academic center. Since this case was not the only reported suspicious case, one idea would be to boycott the site involved in many other RCTs on AD. Well-documented histories would be of little help, as the diagnosis of AD according to

NINCDS—ADRDA criteria is a very subjective diagnosis and the private site claimed that documentation from the academic center was not available. There was no motivation by the CRO or the local subsidiary of the sponsor to investigate this case and they claimed that the mentioned site recruits many patients and has plenty of experience. At the same time, they claimed that the paperwork was always in order when monitoring the site. Several audits at this site found that the paperwork was completed very well, and there were good referrals and appropriate CT descriptions.

Differences Among Study Centers

A large international RCT on AD treatment included a few different study centers in one country. One of the inclusion criteria was the complete absence of any vascular brain lesions on the CT scan (including lacunae and white matter changes). At that time, the study protocol for the CT scan examination was not standardized, and therefore the data collected in different centers were heterogeneous. In the study center with the highest experience with AD patients, 10 patients were screened and all were declared screening failures, most of them due to minor brain vascular lesions; in a different center with a low-performance CT scan and non-specialized radiologists, seven patients were screened, five of whom were included in the study. This case raises the issue of uniform performance capabilities among different study centers.

References

1. Holt E. Czech doctors resign en masse. *Lancet* 2011;**377**:111—2.

2. McKhann G, Drachman D, Folstein M, Katzman R, Price D, Stadlan EM. Clinical diagnosis of Alzheimer's disease: report of the NINCDS—ADRDA Work Group under the auspices of Department of Health and Human Services. Task Force on Alzheimer's Disease. *Neurology* 1984;**34**:939—44.

3. Dubois B, Feldman HH, Jacova C, Dekosky ST, Barberger-Gateau P, Cummings J, Delacourte A, Galasko D, Gauthier S, Jicha G, Meguro K, O'Brien J, Pasquier F, Robert P, Rossor M, Salloway S, Stern Y, Visser PJ, Scheltens P. Research criteria for the diagnosis of Alzheimer's disease: revising the NINCDS—ADRDA criteria. *Lancet Neurology* 2007;**6**:734—46.

4. Hort J, O'Brien JT, Gainotti G, Pirttila T, Popescu BO, Rektorova I, Sorbi S, Scheltens P, EFNS Scientist Panel on Dementia. EFNS guidelines for the diagnosis and management of Alzheimer's disease. *European Journal of Neurology* 2010;**17**:1236—48.

CHAPTER 10

Lessons Learned in Singapore

James (Dachao) Fan*, Quintin van Wyk[†], Jing Yin**
*ICON Clinical Research Pte Ltd/Asia Pacific, Singapore
[†]ICON Clinical Research Pte Ltd, Hampshire, UK
**ICON Clinical Research Pte Ltd, Singapore

105

INTRODUCTION

Singapore is a South East Asian country comprising an area of 712.4 square kilometers. The total population is 5.08 million, including 3.23 million citizens, 0.54 million permanent residents, and 1.31 million foreigners.[1] Since its independence from Malaysia in 1965, the city-state has achieved great success in economic development and has become one of the wealthiest countries in the world. Because of its small population and limited natural resources, insightful policy making and strategic development planning have always been crucial to the country's success. In the second half of the twentieth century, Singapore established its competiveness in electronics and chemical manufacturing. At the beginning of the twenty-first century, as the low cost-advantage of the economy slowly began being lost to neighboring developing countries, Singapore focused on transforming into a knowledge-based economy in order to sustain growth and development. One of the nation's current efforts is to establish the biomedical sciences as the fourth pillar of the country's industries, alongside electronics, engineering, and chemicals. Within the short span of one decade, Singapore has made tremendous achievements in a number of segments within the biomedical sciences industry, including clinical research. It has emerged as an attractive destination for the performance of clinical trials as well as a regional management center for global clinical trial activities in Asia Pacific. This article reviews how Singapore has successfully built up capabilities and capacity in the clinical trials arena.

OVERVIEW OF THE HEALTHCARE SYSTEM IN SINGAPORE

Singapore's healthcare system is generally considered one of the most advanced and well-established systems in the world. The Singapore Ministry of Health website has listed the various accolades its healthcare system has claimed over the years. This includes being ranked sixth of 191 countries for overall health system performance by the World Health Organization in 2000, being recognized as the third best healthcare system in the world and the country best prepared to deal with a major medical crisis in Asia by Political and Economic Risk Consultancy (PERC) in 2003, being ranked third of 55 countries by IMD's World Competitiveness Yearbook in 2007, and being ranked second for infant mortality rate and ninth for life expectancy at birth in World Health Statistics 2010.[2] The healthcare system in Singapore has also been acclaimed for its cost-effectiveness, which has been achieved by emphasizing individual responsibility towards the cost of healthcare while providing government subsidies for basic medical services and promoting preventive healthcare programs.

In Singapore, primary healthcare services are provided by 18 outpatient government polyclinics and approximately 2000 private medical practitioners' clinics.[2] It is estimated that private practitioners provide 80 percent of primary outpatient healthcare and 80 percent of the hospital care is provided by public hospitals. Currently, there are eight public hospitals and six national speciality centers providing high-quality secondary and tertiary care. There are plans to build another public hospital by 2014 to enhance health service capabilities. All of the public health institutions have robust facilities and are well suited to be used as investigative sites for clinical trials. The majority of industry-sponsored clinical trials are conducted in the public hospitals. In addition, the public hospitals conduct investigator-initiated trials, mainly financed through government funding.

Before 2000, the Ministry of Health directly ran the public healthcare institutions in Singapore. Now the public healthcare facilities are run as private companies wholly owned by the government, which enables management autonomy and flexibility to respond more promptly to patient needs. They are managed like not-for-profit organizations and receive annual government subventions or subsidies, thereby providing affordable medical services to patients. The public healthcare institutions were divided into two "clusters": National Healthcare Group (NHG) and Singapore Health Services (SingHealth), until a recent restructuring in 2008. The two-cluster system was revamped into a pyramid model, whereby the base of primary care is anchored by regional hospitals serving the north, west, east, and central zones, and two Academic Medicine Centers (AMCs) at the Outram and Kent Ridge campuses occupy the apex.[3] The new model is now run by five companies to better facilitate integration of primary and secondary care in each region (Table 10.1).

ROLE OF GOVERNMENT
Biomedical Sciences Initiative

In June 2000, the Singapore government launched the Biomedical Sciences (BMS) initiative to build capabilities across the entire value chain in the BMS industry, which comprises four key sectors: pharmaceuticals, biotechnology, medical technology, and healthcare services.[4] The first phase of the BMS initiative (2000–2005) focused on establishing a strong foundation in basic biomedical research. During this period, Singapore's Agency for Science, Technology and Research (A*STAR) built five new public biomedical research institutes. Biopolis, a research center with state-of-the-art infrastructure, was built to house the public biomedical research institutes and the industry research centers. The country also attracted a large number of international biomedical research experts and reshaped the academic curriculum to promote

TABLE 10.1 Public Healthcare Facilities in Singapore	
Cluster	**Healthcare Facilities**
Alexandra Health Pte Ltd	Khoo Teck Puat Hospital
	Jurong Medical Center
Jurong Health Services	Alexandra Hospital
	Jurong General Hospital (scheduled to open in 2014)
National University Health System	National University Hospital
National Healthcare Group (NHG)	Tan Tock Seng Hospital
	Institute of Mental Health
	National Skin Center
	The Eye Institute
	NHG Polyclinics
Singapore Health Services (SingHealth)	Changi General Hospital
	KK Women's and Children's Hospital
	Singapore General Hospital
	National Cancer Center Singapore
	National Dental Center
	National Heart Center
	National Neuroscience Institute
	Singapore National Eye Center
	Polyclinics SingHealth

the study of life sciences among students from diploma to postdoctoral levels. The expanded talent pool, a strong science base, and advanced infrastructure have become Singapore's core capabilities in biomedical sciences.

The second phase of the BMS initiative (2006–2010) focused on building new capabilities in translational and clinical research, while strengthening basic biomedical sciences research capabilities. Public research institutes and consortia established during this period were aimed at facilitating the translation of scientific discoveries from bench to bedside and marketplace. Milestones in the effort to enhance Singapore's clinical trial capabilities included the establishment of the Singapore Clinical Research Institute at Biopolis and two Investigational Medicine Units within each of the new AMCs at the Outram and Kent Ridge campuses. Programs have also been developed to nurture more clinician scientists in the country.

After 10 years of development, Singapore has achieved greater capabilities in the BMS industry. The third phase of the BMS initiative will see a stronger focus on economic and social outcomes by promoting multidisciplinary and multiagency research collaborations and emphasizing translational and clinical research. The government is committing an investment of S $3.7 billion, which is a 12 percent increase over that of the previous phase.[5] The multidisciplinary capabilities offered by Singapore with strong government support set an excellent environment for conducting clinical trials.

Tax and Financial Incentive Schemes

To enhance the country's capabilities in managing clinical trials, the Singapore government has given strong incentives to global pharmaceutical companies and contract research organizations (CROs) to operate in the country. The corporate income tax rate of Singapore is one of the lowest in the region and the rate continues to reduce, currently being 17 percent. There are further tax incentive schemes for research and development (R&D) activities and for locating headquarters in Singapore. Pharmaceutical companies and CROs have also been able to obtain financial incentives from the Singapore Economic Development Board (EDB) such as cofunding of set-up expenditures, and have formed partnerships with EDB.[6]

Regulatory Environment

In Singapore, clinical trials are regulated by the Health Sciences Authority (HSA). Whereas in most Asian countries the diverse and often changing regulatory environments produce an obstacle in conducting clinical trials, in Singapore the regulatory processes are relatively streamlined, fast, and predictable. The conduct of clinical trials in Singapore is regulated by the Medicines Act 1975 and the Medicines (Clinical Trials) (Amendment) Regulations 1998. A clinical trial certificate (CTC) must be obtained from HSA by the principal investigator and is specific for each study protocol and each site. Parallel submissions to the institutional review board (IRB) and HSA are allowed, greatly shortening the lead time to commence a trial. The target processing timeline for a CTC application is 30 working days; and it is even faster (15 working days) to obtain a CTC for Phase I clinical trials that solely evaluate bioequivalence, bioavailability, food effect, or drug–drug interaction. Other administrative changes have been adopted by HSA to further facilitate the clinical trial process, including using an online system for the submission of a CTC application and issuing an electronic CTC. The list of supporting documents has also been reviewed to reduce unessential document submission.[7]

The conduct of clinical trials in Singapore must also comply with the Singapore Guideline for Good Clinical Practice (SGGCP). SGGCP was established in 1998 by adapting International Conference on Harmonisation Good Clinical Practice (ICH-GCP). Singapore has set up a Coordinating Center for GCP for APEC countries (APEC CCG). In 2009, HSA started the implementation of GCP Compliance Inspection Framework, aimed at improving regulatory oversight of clinical trial sites, sponsors, and CROs, and ensuring a high standard of GCP compliance in Singapore.[7] HSA constantly reviews its guidelines to provide an attractive regulatory approval environment while maintaining the quality of trials. Singapore is thus a good example of how to enhance clinical trial site capability from the regulatory aspect.

SINGAPORE AS A CLINICAL TRIAL CENTER IN ASIA PACIFIC

Clinical Trial Management Center

Most global pharmaceutical companies and CROs base their Asia Pacific hub in Singapore. In the globalization trend of industry-sponsored clinical trials, more trials are now being conducted in emerging regions such as Asia because of lower costs and faster patient recruitment. Although the small population of Singapore represents a ceiling in terms of clinical trial capacity, Singapore has aimed at becoming a regional clinical trials management center. Nowadays, CROs are an integral part of the drug development process and pharmaceutical and biotech companies are outsourcing increasing numbers of trials to CROs. Leading CROs have also been forming strategic partnerships and functional service provider agreements with pharmaceutical and biotechnology companies. Coupled with a strong international management team of those global CROs in Singapore, the management covers most of the sites in Asia Pacific countries. This is attractive to the clinical trial talent relocated to Singapore, and increases the overall capacity of clinical trial expertise and staff for the country.

In 1995, Quintiles opened its office in Singapore as the first CRO. One year later, Covance, another major player in the CRO market, also started clinical development operations in Singapore. Subsequently, more leading global CROs established a presence, such as ICON, PPD, and Parexel. The service range of these CROs in Singapore also expanded from solely clinical development to central laboratory services and discovery services, and the CROs are continuing to expand. A Covance central laboratory officially opened in Singapore in 2000 and expanded in 2006 to four times its former capacity, making it one of largest central laboratories in South East Asia. Covance's clinical development services in-country team in Singapore doubled in size from 2009 to 2011. In 2009, Quintiles doubled the size of its regional headquarters and reserved additional room for future growth.[8] In the same year, ICON's central laboratory moved to a larger facility for expansion of services and PPD opened its global central laboratory facility in Singapore.[9] These are clear signals that Singapore will continue to be the regional hub for managing clinical trials in Asia Pacific countries.

Besides the strong presence of global CROs, Singapore has also grown its local capabilities in clinical trial management. An example of success is GleneaglesCRC. GleneaglesCRC was founded in Singapore in October 1999 and it is a wholly owned subsidiary of Singapore Stock Exchange listed Parkway Holdings.[10] This regional CRO has tapped on the large network of private hospitals of its parent company, ParkwayHealth, and managed clinical trials from eight branch offices in the Asian–Australasian region. The key strength of GleneaglesCRC is providing local solutions in the diversified and complex regulatory environment in the region.

According to a Frost & Sullivan analysis, the estimated revenues of Asian CRO market for clinical services (excluding drug discovery) were US $1 billion in 2009, and Singapore has a 12.8 percent share of the CRO market in Asia (Table 10.2).[11] Singapore is a key player in the region despite its small population. Eighty percent of the trials performed there are international. It is worth noting that the Phase I and II market sizes are increasing more rapidly than Phase III, while Phase IV is likely to decrease (Table 10.3).[11] The shift in CRO market size from later phase to earlier phase is concurrent with the increase in the number of early-phase trials (see Table 10.5).

Transportation and Logistics Center

Clinical trials involve logistic processes throughout most of their duration. Clinical trial supplies require import/export of investigational drugs, coordination of drug supplies from manufacturers, distribution of drugs to trial sites, return and destruction of drug products, and inventory management. Laboratory sample shipping requires distribution of patient forms and sample collection kits and transportation logistics for laboratory testing samples. For complex trials, sponsors have to overcome the clinical supply and logistic obstacles to deliver supplies to multiple locations around the world.

Singapore has great logistic connectivity which pharmaceutical companies or CROs can leverage. There are sophisticated road, rail, and air transport systems within Singapore. The

TABLE 10.2 Market Size of Contract Research Organizations in Seven Key Markets in Asia, 2009, by Trial Phase[11]

	Phase I ($US Million)	Phase II ($US Million)	Phase III ($US Million)	Phase IV ($US Million)	Total Market Size ($US Million)
India	48.0	99.0	234.0	52.0	433.0
China	30.0	52.0	85.0	88.0	255.0
South Korea	14.0	14.0	23.0	14.0	65.0
Taiwan	11.0	34.0	53.0	2.0	100.0
Singapore	20.3	33.8	47.3	27.0	128.4
Thailand	0.2	0.9	5.7	1.8	8.6
Philippines	3.6	9.5	22.5	9.5	45.1

TABLE 10.3 Market Size of Contract Research Organizations in Singapore, 2009–2010, by Trial Phase[11]

	Phase I ($US Million)	Phase II ($US Million)	Phase III ($US Million)	Phase IV ($US Million)	Total Market Size ($US Million)
2009	20.3	33.8	47.3	27.0	128.4
2010	22.3	36.6	48.4	25.3	132.6

country has worked for years on the vision to become a leading global integrated logistic gateway and is well established as a world-class port. It is also becoming more competitive as a leading logistics hub for the clinical trials sector of Asia by improving the cold-chain logistic management expertise, information technology, and telecommunications infrastructure. Major logistic service providers have set up dedicated regional life sciences facilities in Singapore. For example, DHL located its new regional headquarters in Singapore in 2007, aiming to leverage Singapore's excellent location to support Asian markets, including growing clinical trial logistic needs.[13] In March 2011, Marken announced the opening of a directly owned clinical trial supply depot in Singapore. The new clinical trial supply depot is a good manufacturing practice (GMP)-compliant facility and has the capacity for kit building and drug distribution in addition to full-range storage conditions for investigational drugs and biological specimens.[14] The increased presence and capability of logistic service providers in Singapore add to the country's ability to accommodate its expanding clinical trial activities.

CLINICAL TRIAL SITE CAPABILITIES IN SINGAPORE
Clinical Trial Sites

All the public hospitals and speciality centers in Singapore have established their own dedicated clinical trial units or clinical trial resource centers to coordinate high-quality trials in the hospital. These units act as supporting departments for the principal investigators and sponsors by providing guidelines and advice, archiving study-related documents, and maintaining a database of ongoing trials in the hospital. They also coordinate training for principal investigators and study coordinators and may give secretarial support to the hospital's IRB. Some clinical trial units have the infrastructure and capabilities to house pharmacokinetics, pharmacogenetics, and bioequivalence studies. An example is Changi General Hospital's Clinical Trial Research Unit, which occupies an entire ward of 835 square meters and has the capacity to house 20 clinical trial subjects for overnight stays.[15] The expertise of clinical trial units or resource centers makes it easy to set up clinical trials within hospitals in Singapore.

Central Institutional Review Board

Since 1998, the Singapore Ministry of Health has required all public hospitals to establish IRBs, and the IRBs are required to comply with the Ethical Guidelines on Research Involving Human Subjects (NMEC Guidelines) issued by the National Medical Ethics Committee (NMEC) in 1997. The Bioethics Advisory Committee (BAC) has also issued reports to make recommendations on the ethics governance of human biomedical research.

Singapore has a unique central IRB model: domain-specific review boards (DSRBs). In 2004, NHG, one of the main healthcare clusters, reorganized the individual IRBs in its member institutions into four DSRBs which function like a central IRB for all its member institutions.[16] The DSRBs are divided by broad disease groupings or disciplines, and each DSRB conducts ethics reviews of clinical trial protocols relevant to its respective domain of diseases throughout the entire cluster. Such an arrangement ensures that each domain has specialized expertise and capability to assess the scientific merits and ethical concerns of submitted protocols. The innovative and efficient approach of DSRBs, together with other efforts in the Human Subject Protection Program, won NHG recognition from the Association for the Accreditation of Human Research Protection Programs, Inc. (AAHRPP). In 2007, NHG was awarded full AAHRPP accreditation for its high ethical standards, making it the first public healthcare institution accredited outside North America.[16] There was a regrouping of specialities in NHG DSRBs in 2008 to optimize their capabilities, and currently there is a group of five DSRBs in NHG covering 27 medical specialities (Table 10.4). Each DSRB has 13–15 members and is constituted in compliance with the SGGCP guidelines. There are also two or three coordinators assisting the administrative functions in each DSRB.[16] SingHealth adopted the same approach in 2009 and has set up the Centralized Institutional Review Board (CIRB) for its member

TABLE 10.4 National Healthcare Group Domain-Specific Review Boards and their Specialities[16]

Domain A	Domain B	Domain C
Ophthalmology	Oncology	Cardiovascular science
Psychiatry	Hematology	Pharmacology
Neurology/neurosurgery	Pathology	Emergency medicine
Genetics	Pediatrics	Endocrinology
Geriatric medicine	Respiratory medicine	Diagnostic imaging

Domain D	Domain E
Obstetrics/gynecology	Infectious disease
Anesthesia	Gastroenterology
Surgery	Renal Medicine
ENT	Rheumatology/immunology
Dentistry	Dermatology
Sports & rehabilitation medicine	
Allied health	

institutions.[17] The SingHealth CIRB has five review boards similar to NHG's DSRBs, each to review a group from 30 classified medical specialities.[17] Currently, both NHG and SingHealth IRB reviews have a timeline of about 30 days. The centralized, yet domain-specific IRB review allows for standardized and strengthened research ethics in public healthcare institutions with better efficiency, and enhances clinical trial capabilities in Singapore.

Nurture of Clinician Scientists

Clinician scientists play an important role in translational and clinical research. Singapore has been investing in nurturing clinician scientists to build up human capital for clinical research. In 2008, the Translational and Clinical Research (TCR) Flagship Program was launched, focusing on the five key disease areas of cancer, metabolic disorders, infectious diseases, neurosciences, and eye diseases. Each was funded with a five-year budget of S $25 million. These areas were chosen because of their relevance to Singapore's healthcare challenges; clinician scientists are encouraged to work with researchers to identify the causes of the diseases and improve treatment by designing and conducting clinical trials. In addition, the Clinician Scientist Award (CSA) and Singapore Translational Research (STaR) Investigator Award were created to recruit and nurture clinician scientists to drive translational and clinical research in Singapore. Talent development programs, such as the Duke-NUS Graduate Medical School, have been put in place to develop a new generation of clinician scientists. The country aims to double the number of clinician scientists from around 80 currently to 160 by 2015, to reinforce its leading position in translational and clinical research in Asia.[18]

Patient Resources

In terms of patient resources, the small population of Singapore limits its capacity at clinical trial sites. However, since the population is multiracial, it is easy to recruit study subjects of Chinese, Indian, and Malay origin within the same country, and this can be beneficial to some types of trial. Another opportunity in increasing Singapore's patient resource capacity is by attracting patients from neighboring countries. In 2003, the Singapore Medicine program was launched jointly by EDB, Singapore Tourism Board, and International Enterprise Singapore as a multiagency effort to develop Singapore as a leading destination for healthcare services in Asia.[19] The program aims to attract patients in regional countries to come to Singapore for high-quality and reliable medical services. These patients are further encouraged to take part in clinical trials in Singapore by gaining access to novel treatment options. The number of

TABLE 10.5 Number of Clinical Trial Certificates* Issued in Singapore, 2000–2010, by Trial Phase[7]											
Phase	2000	2001	2002	2003	2004	2005	2006	2007	2008	2009	2010
I	21	19	20	24	31	44	48	47	54	54	55
II	44	50	52	19	49	50	35	45	61	61	46
III	63	68	97	91	88	90	116	135	140	108	95
IV	29	28	26	26	32	17	18	26	31	39	38
Total	157	165	195	160	200	201	217	253	286	262	234

*A clinical trial certificate is issued for each participating site in a clinical trial.

international patients increased from about 200,000 in 2002 to 570,000 in 2009.[19,20] The target is to attract one million international patients annually by 2012.[19]

Status and Statistics of Clinical Trials

The total number of clinical trials in Singapore increased from 2000 to 2008, but declined in 2009 and 2010 (Table 10.5). The main reason is the decreasing number of Phase III trials, which may arise from the general slowdown of clinical trial activities worldwide during these two years, and shifting of those large-scale trials to places where there are large numbers of patients with lower cost, such as China and India. Nevertheless, the number of Phase I clinical trials keeps growing, although the growth slowed down in 2009 and 2010, a challenging time for the whole pharmaceutical industry. It is likely that early-phase clinical trials will continue to rise in Singapore when the market recovers because of the quality data that Singapore can provide and the strategic governmental focus on the early-phase trials. Early-phase studies involve a small number of subjects and can be completed within a shorter period in a single site. Phase I trials and proof-of-concept trials are usually complex and medically challenging, and require dedicated resources and facilities providing the full range of scientific and technological expertise. Singapore's strength in research and the medical expertise of clinicians are definite advantages for conducting early-phase studies. The initiatives to nurture clinician scientists and establish academic medicine centers boost its early-phase trial capabilities further. The stringent GCP guidelines ensure credibility in clinical trial data. In addition, the diverse ethnic population allows easy recruitment of different ethnic groups according to the trial's needs. In early-phase trials, Singapore can maximize its strength and minimize the population constraint. Singapore has become and will continue to be an attractive location for conducting early-phase trials.

Figure 10.1 shows a breakdown of clinical trials by therapeutic areas in Singapore. Oncology is the most popular therapeutic area, followed by clinical pharmacology and cardiology.

Sponsor–site Partnership Model for Phase I Trials Unit

The BMS initiative has enabled pharmaceutical companies to set up dedicated Phase I centers, such as the Lilly–NUS Center for Clinical Pharmacology and Pfizer's Phase I clinical research unit at Raffles Hospital. The country is also building up new infrastructure such as the two investigational medicine units (IMUs) set up at the Outram and Kent Ridge campuses in 2009. The IMU at Outram campus is the largest public early-phase clinical research unit and is funded with S $20 million over five years by the Singapore Ministry of Health. It has already hosted more than 20 clinical trials, with 40 percent of trials led by local clinician scientists.[21] The establishment of advanced infrastructure will further enhance Singapore's capabilities with early-phase clinical trials and its reputation as an attractive place for early drug development outsourcing.

CONCLUSION AND FUTURE ASPECTS

Singapore's ambition is to be a regional medical research hub. The Singapore government has given strong support to global pharmaceutical, CRO, and logistics companies to operate there,

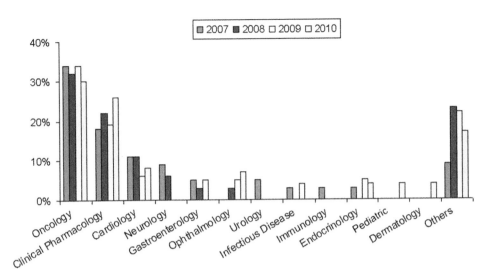

FIGURE 10.1
Percentage of clinical trials by therapeutic area in Singapore, from 2007 to 2010.[7] (Please refer to color plate section)

using tax and financial incentive schemes for performing R&D activities and for locating headquarters in Singapore. This strategy has made Singapore the center for clinical trial management, logistics, and transportation.

The globalization of industry-sponsored clinical trials is still ongoing, but it has matured into a more stable and predictable process. Given its small population compared with many other Asian countries such as China and India where clinical research is carried out, Singapore is unable to contribute a large patient pool for global trials. How can it find a niche market for clinical trials? Singapore's answer is by tapping on its strength in biomedical research and medical expertise to attract early-phase studies, which do not require a large patient pool but do require a high level of medical and clinical research sophistication because of the complicated monitoring and assessment processes. The successful execution of this kind of trial has been seen by many as an indication of the maturity of the Singaporean early trials capabilities.

To stay ahead in the competition of clinical trials management, Singapore needs to continue building on its strength of infrastructure and regulatory framework. There should be continual support from the government to the BMS industry. As the local talent pool is relatively young in conducting clinical trials compared to that of USA and Europe, in response to the market need for clinical trial personnel, there is a need to systematically train a workforce in clinical trials and to build bridges between academia and industry. In June 2010, Singapore launched two workforce capability-building initiatives for clinical research.[22] The first is to develop a specialist track for clinical research professionals under the national competency-based training and assessment system, known as the Workforce Skills Qualification (WSQ) scheme. The Singapore Workforce Development Agency (WDA) is currently collaborating with the clinical research industry, government agencies, and training providers to develop WSQ programs for clinical research coordinators and clinical research associates. Five levels of structured trainings have been planned in the clinical research coordinator training frame-work, which support the career progression from an assistant clinical research coordinator up to a clinical research manager.[22] The first level in the series was rolled out in October 2010 in Nanyang Polytechnic. Similarly, three levels of training have been identified for the clinical research associates progression pathway. In June 2011, WDA announced a collaboration with Edinburgh Napier University, UK, to offer the WSQ Diploma in Clinical Research, WSQ Specialist Diploma in Clinical Research, and WSQ Graduate Diploma in Clinical Research. Clinical research associates who finish all three levels of the training program can also obtain a Master of Science degree in clinical research upon completion of a dissertation component.[23] The various training programs will train fresh graduates and mid-career professionals with a background in life sciences, pharmacy, or nursing, and at the same time provide opportunities for existing clinical research workers to upgrade their skill sets. It is anticipated that over the next five years, more than 150 new clinical research coordinators will be trained and the number of clinical research associates will also grow at 10–15 percent each year from the current pool of 400.[22,23] The training programs are supported and ascertained by the formation of an industry-led Clinical Research Consortium, the second of the workforce capability building initiatives for clinical research.[22] Clinical research organizations and industry players in pharmaceutical and biotechnology are brought together to identify training gaps, set training standards that reflect best practices in industry, and advance industry knowledge through industry forums, networking sessions, and other programs.

On the academic level, the National University of Singapore Academy of GxP Excellence (NUSAGE) also offers an online self-learning course on good clinical practice. "GxP" is the general term to denote the quality guidelines for the pharmaceutical industry: "G" stands for "good", "P" for "practice", and the "x" in between is the specific practice descriptor. In all, "GxP excellence" is about establishing the best regulatory systems to ensure that all medical products and solutions produced are safe, high quality, and efficacious for the consumers. This course is designed for health professionals with little or no prior experience in clinical trials, and prepares doctors and other health professionals to become proficient in the ICH-GCP, so as to undertake the role and responsibilities of an investigator confidently in future. Upon completion, they will have the basic knowledge and understanding in the conduct of a clinical trial; for example, the course consists of a wide range of clinical trial topics incorporated into a case study. Each topic has a quiz associated with it that addresses a specific aspect of GCP covering practical interpretation and implementation of the GCP regulations. At the end of the topics, applicants must pass a test consisting of 50 multiple choice questions in order to receive the certificate of completion, which will be valid for a two-year period.

The Singapore Medical Council (SMC) has approved the online iGCP course as a Category 3B activity. Doctors who successfully complete the program will be awarded 18 non-core CME points; pharmacists who successfully complete the program will be able to claim 18 CME points under category 3A as well.

These initiatives undoubtedly will raise the standards of the clinical research workforce in Singapore and further enhance the country's capability in clinical research.

References

1. Department of Statistics Singapore, http://www.singstat.gov.sg/stats/keyind.html. Key Annual Indicators 2010 [accessed 24.04.11].

2. Singapore Ministry of Health. Healthcare System, http://www.moh.gov.sg/mohcorp/hcsystem.aspx. [accessed 24.04.11].

3. Singapore Healthcare System. MOH Holdings, http://www.ahp.mohh.com.sg/singapore_healthcare_system. html. [accessed 24.04.11].

4. Biomedical Sciences Initiative. Agency for Science, Technology and Research, http://www.a-star.edu.sg/ AboutASTAR/BiomedicalResearchCouncil/BMSInitiative/tabid/108/Default.aspx. [accessed 24.04.11].

5. Agency for Science. Technology and Research and Ministry of Health. *Singapore's Biomedical Sciences R&D effort gets boost of S$3.7 billion.* Press Release at the 15th Biomedical Sciences International Advisory Council Meeting; October 8, 2010.

6. Singapore Economic Development Board, http://www.sedb.com. [accessed 24.04.11].

7. Health Sciences Authority. Clinical Trials, http://www.hsa.gov.sg/publish/hsaportal/en/health_products_ regulation/clinical_trials.html [accessed 30.04.11].

8. *Quintiles opens expanded Asia-Pacific headquarters in Singapore.* Quintiles Press Release, http://www.quintiles.com/ news/press-releases/2009-11-6/quintiles-opens-expanded-asia-pacific-headquarters-singapore/; November 6, 2009 [accessed 30.04.11].

9. *PPD opens global central lab in Singapore.* PPD Press Release, http://investor.ppdi.com/releasedetail.cfm?ReleaseID=409432; September 15, 2009 [accessed 30.04.11].

10. *BioSpectrum Asia Pacific Awards: GleneaglesCRC,* http://www.biospectrumasia.com/Content/100309OTH8796.asp; 2009 [accessed 30.04.11].

11. *The rising dominance of the Asian CRO market,* http://www.biospectrumasia.com/content/051010CHN14153.asp; October 2010 [accessed 30.04.11].

12. Frost & Sullivan. *Singapore Shifting to a Specialized CRO Market,* http://www.frost.com/prod/servlet/market-insight-top.pag?docid=213988299; November 3, 2010 [accessed 30.04.11].

13. *DHL's new Asia Pacific Logistics Division headquarters complements Singapore's mission to be leading regional hub.* DHL Press Release, http://www.dhl.com.sg/en/press/releases/releases_2007/local/160407.html; April 16, 2007 [accessed 07.05.11].

14. *Marken announces the opening of a directly owned clinical trial supply depot in Singapore.* Market Press Release, http://www.marken.com/pdf/Marken%20announces%20the%20opening%20of%20its%20newly%20expanded%20Singapore%20office.pdf; March 4, 2011 [accessed 07.05.11].

15. Changi General Hospital. Clinical trial facility, http://www.cgh.com.sg/Medical_Specialities/CTRU/Pages/ctru.aspx [accessed 07.05.11].

16. National Healthcare Group. Research and Development Office, http://www.research.nhg.com.sg [accessed 07.05.11].

17. SingHealth Research. http://research.singhealth.com.sg [accessed 26.05.11].

18. *Transforming health through research and innovation.* Singapore National Medical Research Council Annual Report; 2010.

19. SingaporeMedicine. http://www.singaporemedicine.com [accessed 26.05.11].

20. Annual Report 2009/2010. Singapore Tourism Board.

21. *Minister for Health opens $20million clinical research unit on SGH Campus.* SingHealth Press Release; July 30, 2010.

22. *New WSQ training for support personnel in clinical research.* Singapore Workforce Development Agency Press Release, http://app2.wda.gov.sg/web/contents/contents.aspx?yr=2010&contid=1127; June 24, 2010 [accessed 26.05.11].

23. *First Master of Science and three new WSQ courses in clinical research among new initiatives for clinical research professionals.* Singapore Workforce Development Agency Press Release, http://app2.wda.gov.sg/web/contents/contents.aspx?yr=2011&contId=1234; June 6, 2011 [accessed 20.06.11].

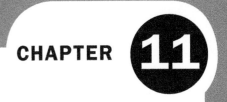

CHAPTER 11

Lessons Learned in Turkey

Mehtap Asenaoktar, Serdar Asenaoktar
Kuantum CRO and Logistics, Izmir, Turkey

INTRODUCTION

Turkey is situated where Europe and Asia meet. It is made up of the European part (Thrace) and the Asian part (Anatolia). The country is located in south-eastern Europe and south-western Asia, bordering both the Black Sea, between Bulgaria and Georgia, and the Aegean Sea and Mediterranean Sea, between Greece and Syria. It has an area of 785,347 square kilometers and had a total population of 74.8 million in 2010.

Present-day Turkey was created in 1923 from the Turkish remnants of the Ottoman Empire. Soon afterwards, the country instituted secular laws to replace traditional religious fiats. In 1945 Turkey joined the United Nations, and in 1952 it became a member of the North Atlantic Treaty Organization (NATO).

On March 5, 1995, Turkey and the European Foreign Ministers decided to implement the final phase of the Ankara Agreement to establish a Customs Union with Turkey. In this framework, a Customs Union Agreement came into force on January 1, 1996. The Customs Union between Turkey and the European Community (EC) provides the free circulation of goods, capital, services, and people, as well as coordination of economic and financial policies. The Union also involves the elimination of all custom duties and the abolition of all quantitative restrictions.

The Turkish economy has shown remarkable performance with its steady growth over the past decade. A sound macroeconomic strategy in combination with prudent fiscal policies and major structural reforms, in effect since 2002, has integrated the Turkish economy into the globalized world, while transforming the country into one of the major recipients of foreign direct investment in the region.

Global Clinical Trials Playbook. DOI: 10.1016/B978-0-12-415787-3.00011-4

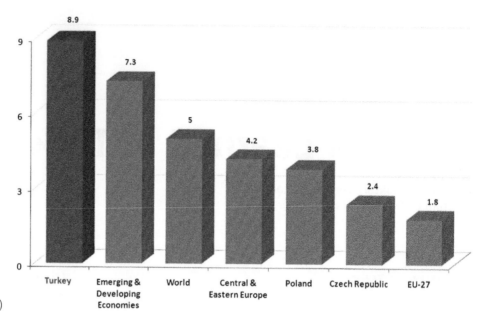

FIGURE 11.1
Real gross domestic product growth (%), 2010. (Please refer to color plate section)

Significant improvements over such a short period have registered Turkey on the world economic scale as an exceptional emerging economy, the 16th largest economy in the world and the sixth largest economy when compared with the European Union (EU) countries, according to gross domestic product (GDP) figures (at purchasing power parity) in 2010 (Figure 11.1). Turkey, with such a robust economic performance, stood out as the fastest growing economy in Europe and one of the fastest growing economies in the world.

Moreover, according to the OECD, Turkey is expected to be the fastest growing economy of the OECD members during 2011–2017, with an annual average growth rate of 6.7 percent (Figure 11.2).

OVERVIEW OF THE TURKISH HEALTHCARE AND PHARMA SECTOR

Turkey accounts for around 42 percent of the total Middle Eastern pharmaceutical market, owing to its population and GDP. The Turkish pharmaceutical market is expected to grow by a moderate compound annual growth rate in US dollar terms between 2011 and 2016. While the overall pharmaceutical market size is among the top 30 largest in the world, per capita spending on pharmaceuticals in Turkey remains low, and given the possible accession to the EU (though this is still at least a few years away) the potential for growth is very promising, compared with more established and mature markets in Western Europe.

PHARMACEUTICAL INDUSTRY

Pharmaceutical preparations were produced on a small scale in Turkish laboratories between 1928 and 1950. Production increased with the establishment of local and foreign-invested plants from 1952, which is seen as the start of the "fabrication period" of the Turkish pharmaceuticals industry.

Investments by foreign capital companies have increased since 1984, and 19 foreign capital firms have entered the Turkish pharmaceuticals market since 1990. Today, there are approximately 300 entities operating in Turkey. Out of 42 manufacturing facilities, a quarter are multinational firms. Social Securities Institution Pharmaceuticals Plant and Ministry of Defense Army Pharmaceuticals Plant are publicly owned, while the others are private enterprises.

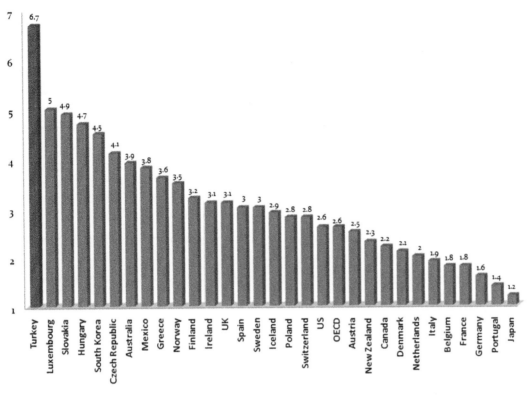

FIGURE 11.2
Annual average real gross domestic product growth (%) forecast in Organisation for Economic Co-operation and Development (OECD) countries, 2011–2017. (Please refer to color plate section)

The Turkish prescribed pharmaceutical market reached €6.54 billion and 1.42 billion units by volume in 2009. The growth rate of the market is 3.1 percent in terms of euros and 3.9 percent by volume. The market size for original drugs in Turkey was US $4.1 billion in 2009 and US $4 billion in 2010.

The production structure of the pharmaceutical industry has a high level of technology and automation. Approximately 25,000 people are employed in the sector. Owing to its nature, this industry employs a high proportion of personnel (50 percent) with a university education. The distribution of highly educated employees is: pharmacists 4.5 percent, doctors 3 percent, chemical engineers 7.5 percent, chemists 7 percent, and biologists 9.5 percent.

Production

Pharmaceutical production trends are closely related to domestic and foreign demand. There were 7413 pharmaceutical products on the market in 2009, 4928 of which were prescribed products. In 2009, 6.8 percent of pharmaceuticals were local on the Turkish pharmaceutical market; 24.9 percent of these were reference products and 75.1 percent were generic products.

In 2008, there were 1350 hospitals in Turkey with a total bed capacity of 188,065. There is an important new trend towards receiving incoming patients from European (mainly UK) or Middle East countries for treatment in Turkish private hospitals.

Turkish companies have started new product development. İlsan İltaş has a sound worldwide knowledge and technology in pellet development and production; the company has been granted process patents for omeprazol pellet production in Europe, Canada, and South Korea, and has also been granted Food and Drug Administration (FDA) approval for the finished product. Mustafa Nevzat plants have been approved in the active pharmaceutical ingredient and finished dosage forms by the FDA. This is a first for the Turkish pharmaceutical industry. Mustafa Nevzat has signed strategic partnership agreements with several leading US generic companies for the marketing and sale of its products.

Pharmaceutical consumption in Turkey, by therapeutic class, includes antibiotics, and cardiovascular, antirheumatic, nervous systemic, and oncological agents. The consumption of antibiotics decreased from 20.6 percent in 2004 to 15.6 percent in 2009, whereas the consumption rate of oncologics increased from 4.1 percent in 2004 to 7.1 percent in 2009.

The production of raw materials in Turkey concentrates on the active ingredients of antibiotics and analgesics, using the methods of fermentation, extraction, and synthesis. In the Turkish pharmaceutical raw materials sector, 11 plants are in the private sector. The production and marketing of all pharmaceuticals must be authorized by the Ministry of Health, and pharmaceutical products and firms must be registered with the Ministry.

The Turkish government has implemented a number of regulations to bring its pharmaceutical laws into line with those in the EU:

- patent protection
- data exclusivity
- pricing
- registration
- good manufacturing practice (GMP)
- good laboratory practice (GLP)
- good clinical practice (GCP)
- bioavailability/bioequivalence
- packaging labeling
- promotion/advertising
- drug research and medicinal product registration
- stability requirements
- regulation on good distribution and storage practices
- pharmacovigilance.

Since 1995, pharmaceutical manufacturers have had to abide by regulations specifying GMP, GLP, and GCP, necessitating significant investment by local industry companies. The necessary investments for the development of technology in the industry have been accelerated and today production technology in the Turkish pharmaceutical industry has reached world standards.

Exports

Turkish companies have seen a steady increase in their exports in recent years. In 2010, the total value of pharmaceutical industry exports reached US $612 million. Turkey exports various pharmaceutical products to 144 countries, including developed countries such as Germany, the USA, Switzerland, the UK, Belgium, and the Netherlands.

The healthcare system in Turkey has entered a long period of development under the 2003−2013 Health Transformation Program. The purpose of the program is to increase the quality and efficiency of the healthcare system and enhance access to healthcare facilities.

Turkey is one of the fastest growing pharmaceutical markets in Europe and ranks as the 16th largest pharmaceutical producer in the world, and the sixth largest pharmaceutical market in Europe, following Germany, France, the UK, Italy, and Spain.

CLINICAL TRIALS

Turkey is considered among the top 10 countries in terms of potential study subject population, the others being the USA, China, India, Brazil, Russia, Japan, Mexico, Germany, Turkey,

120

and Thailand. The potential for conducting clinical trials in Turkey is huge. There are 94 universities, 59 medical schools, 1190 hospitals, 200,000 hospital beds, and 95,100 practicing medical doctors, 46 percent of whom are specialized.

The most important advantages are the presence of well-equipped and high-level university and state hospitals; well-trained specialized clinicians; lower costs associated with ethical reviews, regulatory approvals, and investigator compensation; and good success rates for patient recruitment.

The history of clinical trials in Turkey dates back to the beginning of the twentieth century, but for many years studies did not comply with GCP guidelines. This was not due to a lack of legal documents; on the contrary, clinical trials were first mentioned in a legal document in 1926: "The Code of Pharmaceutical Products and Preparations No. 1262" law carried the statement: "Experimental drugs can be used in a patient only by his/her permission".

After decades of badly conducted and ill-designed studies, the modern era of clinical trials began in 1993 with the introduction of the Drug Research Bylaw. It was directly influenced by the initial drafts of the International Conference on Harmonisation (ICH)-GCP Guidelines, and some parts were very similar. A GCP guideline document was added in 1995, followed by GLP and GMP guidelines, issued and published by the Ministry of Health. Although these were quite early and impressive achievements, the growing number of different clinical trials and clinical investigators over time increased the need for new and updated regulations. This demand was partly covered by documents such as regulations on compassionate use, observational trials, patient rights, and articles in the Turkish penal law. During that time, major changes in Turkey's national policies occurred, as it turned dramatically towards the EU, and a new period began that required a complete revision of all legal documents and adaptation to EU rules and principles.

CLINICAL TRIALS IN TURKEY DURING THE TRANSITION PERIOD

The main regulations in Turkish law regarding clinical trials are the provisions of the Constitution on Body Immunity and Convention for the Protection of Human Rights and Dignity of the Human Being with regard to the Application of Biology and Medicine, to which Turkey is a party. Other related substantive legislation includes Article 90 of the Turkish Criminal Code, which stipulates the eligibility requirements for experiments on people; the Regulation on Clinical Trials; Article 13 of the Regulation on Medical Devices; and the Regulation on Patient Rights and Regulation on Medical Deontology. The Helsinki Declaration of the World Medical Association and EU Directives 2001/20/EC and 2005/28/EC are considered reference legislation for Turkish law.

Among the above-mentioned regulations, the Regulation on Clinical Trials (No. 27089, published in the Official Gazette on December 23, 2008) includes substantive provisions regarding clinical trials in Turkey. Regulation was prepared by the Ministry of Health by taking into consideration the EU Directives. Recently, the Turkish Medical Association (TMA) has filed a lawsuit against the Ministry of Health before the Council of State and requested the cancellation and stay of execution of certain provisions of the Regulation, based on the allegation that it contains provisions against the Constitution, the Helsinki Declaration, and the EU Directives.

A motion for a stay of execution has been partly granted by the relevant chamber of the Council of State and the TMA has appealed this interim decision before the Board of Chambers of the Council of State (BCCS). The BCCS has primarily reviewed the procedural aspects of the Regulation without going into its merits. It ruled that the provision regarding the human body immunity which is protected by the Constitution should be regulated by a statute to be enacted by the parliament and should not be set forth with a regulation which is an administrative act of the Ministry of Health, and therefore granted the motion for a stay of execution on the Regulation provisions as requested by the TMA.

In order not to interrupt the clinical trials, the authorities took immediate action to resolve the problem in the short and long term. Immediate patches and adaptation to the working procedures of the EC and RA have been provided until the new law is in force. As a long-term resolution, an amendment to the law has been prepared and has been accepted (No. 27916, published by the Official Gazette on April 26, 2011).

The Article states that:

> 8 – Fundamental Law #3359 on Health Services of 07.05.1987 is appended with the following article:
> "SUPPLEMENTAL ARTICLE 10 – For any therapeutic tools or methods, or medicinal products or preparations, traditional herbal medicinal products or medical devices to be used in humans for scientific research purposes, even if licensed or authorized, the permission of the Ministry of Health must be obtained".

This new law fills this gap and describes the role of the Ministry of Health as an authority.

On August 19, 2011, a Clinical Research regulation was published in the Official Gazette. This led, in September 2011, to the formation of ethics committees and completion of the required procedures and forms.

CLINICAL TRIAL LOGISTICS

While faster patient recruitment offers significant benefits to clinical trial industry, it is important to take other factors into consideration when planning a clinical trial in an emerging market. Clinical trial logistics (getting medication to patients and samples back for analysis) in these regions is a key area of concern. The main issues are listed below.

- Import licenses are required for each shipment of drug into Turkey if batch numbers are different. As a result, direct to-site shipments from a centralized warehouse outside the country can become impractical. Sometimes, the qualifications of importers (e.g. pharmacists) and the type of company performing the import [e.g. sponsor, distributor, or contract research organization (CRO)] can complicate the process.
- There are complex customs regulations for investigational medicinal products (IMPs) and these are strictly adhered to by customs staff. Any issues with the shipment itself, or the accompanying paperwork, can result in material being held in customs for prolonged periods. With the current growth in temperature-sensitive products and time-sensitive shipments, a strategy to avoid these issues is essential. It can take a considerable time to reach the country if material is shipped from a depot in Europe or the USA, and one may need to allow for significant additional time once the drug reaches the country.
- Inadequate training of site staff in the correct procedures for receiving medication and returning samples can also lead to supply chain problems. Local knowledge of the regulations and import procedures related to clinical trials is essential. Some companies have used their own affiliate companies in Turkey to assist in the process. While this strategy has undoubtedly worked for some companies, there has also been a rethink towards this approach on the basis of affiliates' lack of appropriate storage capacity, storage conditions, or trained staff.

Local CROs, and international organizations with a strong local presence, can provide an answer. As the clinical trial market grows, the number of CROs with local knowledge is also increasing. While these companies may offer strong assistance in gaining regulatory approvals and may be able to advise on logistical issues, only a minority of these companies can perform logistical services themselves. Most CROs provide a service to obtain an import license, but for logistical issues it may be necessary to also identify a local logistics company with appropriate pharmaceutical and clinical trial experience to support the activities of the CRO.

Clear Identification of Roles and Responsibilities

It is important that sponsors clearly define their expectations from a third party company, and that all third parties are realistic about the level of service that they are able or willing to offer.

If the sponsor and all third parties agree in advance who is responsible for what, and whether this arrangement is possible, problems can be avoided. If a trial sponsor with limited experience of Turkey is to conduct a clinical trial, it is important that planning and identification of potential issues start as early as possible. Items such as power of attorney documentation can take several weeks to obtain, so this needs to be planned in advance.

Depot Strategies

For maximum visibility of inventory levels and maximum flexibility of drug supplies, a centralized distribution strategy is ideal. However, shipping medication directly from these hubs to study sites within Turkey with difficult import regulations can be subject to delays. A local drug repository within Turkey limits the occasions on which a drug passes through customs, minimizing the administration associated with imports and reducing the risk of delays. Communication of inventory levels between regional hubs, local depots, and the sponsor or contractor is essential if a reliable supply of drug is to be maintained. This can be achieved via a simple paper-based system, through which the sponsor or contractor receives regular reports of on-site inventories. Sponsors and contractors can then resupply depots when inventory levels reach a predetermined trigger level that takes into account the time required to ship fresh stock to a depot and projected recruitment rates. Although this approach works, telephone- and web-based tools, such as an interactive voice response system (IVRS), allow real-time monitoring of recruitment and inventory levels in each location. Some IVRS companies (e.g. ICTI, Clinphone) also offer demand-forecasting tools that can assist this process.

Other Considerations

It is critical not to underestimate the importance of training site personnel in correct receiving processes for clinical trial medication. The reasons for this are self-explanatory for cold-chain shipments. Delays in receiving these materials, stopping temperature recorders, and transferring to appropriate storage areas remain a key reason for "out of specification" shipments of refrigerated and frozen materials. Confirmation that shipments are received is another important issue. As mentioned above, accurate visibility of an inventory held on site and in depots is critical to supply chain management. If sites do not confirm receipt of medication, this can have an impact on the entire process.

The return of clinical samples to central laboratories for testing is another key issue. Returned or unused IMPs should be destroyed in the Ministry of Health approved destruction facilities or should be exported back for destruction; then, a certificate of destruction from the authorized facility should be submitted to the Ministry. It is not possible to arrange these shipments directly from sites. This can have serious legal and cost implications for the sponsor.

When planning shipments, it is also important to ensure that any supply chain includes the management of inventory of items such as specialized shipping systems, training of depots/sites to use these correctly, and even whether items such as dry ice can be easily obtained locally. For example, if a cold-chain shipment requires the use of a validated shipping system established by the sponsor, it may be necessary to supply depots with these materials.

Delays can also be caused by the process of paying import duties. One way of preventing such delays is to lodge money with the chosen importer, so that these fees can be paid as and when they arise. Local support is needed for the management of customs clearance. This can have a severe impact on shipment timelines, especially where cold-chain and time-sensitive shipments are involved.

CONCLUSION AND LESSONS LEARNED

With the current amendment to the law, the biggest cornerstone has been laid with respect to the adaptation of the regulations in accordance with EU regulations and global guidelines.

The Ministry of Health of Turkey, General Directorate of Pharmaceuticals and Pharmacy, has achieved remarkable success in adapting the clinical trial regulations in the past few years, and by acting proactively they have provided maximum support to the newly developing CRO sector. They have implemented inspection processes for CROs, Phase I units, and depots managing study drugs; implemented and updated the various guidelines, including the Guideline for the Storage and Distribution of Investigational Medicinal Products; and organized frequent updating and training meetings.

Although the period for the adaptation of the regulations was quite long, it is a good indicator of the sensitivity of the Ministry of Health and all the other related parties to clinical research in Turkey. It will bring advantages with regard to the reliability of clinical research data from Turkey in the near future. During this transition period, the Ministry of Health has built close ties with the local sector. The Ministry has always had a very strict approach towards clinical trials in Turkey, which may not be perceived as highly favorable, but this consistency is actually the strength of the Turkish market in the long term. In this way, the quality of data produced by clinical trials conducted in Turkey is and will remain high and acceptable to the global authorities.

The Turkish Association of CROs, founded in 2009, is working very closely with both the Ministry of Health and the pharmaceutical sector, both of which have a large input in providing ICH-GCP training to investigators, site staff, and the research sector.

The number of experienced and trained CRAs, other research employees and investigational site staff has increased tremendously over the past decade. In previous years it was not possible to find experienced personnel. For example, a CRO had to invest in a clinical research associate (CRA) candidate and wait for a minimum of one year before that CRA was acceptable globally. Today, it is quite common to recruit experienced personnel. In addition, a pool of freelance CRAs has developed over the years. Some global CROs still prefer to work via freelance CRAs; however, the Ministry prefers the local company to be present at the clinical trials.

When selecting a local CRO in this emerging environment of Turkey, experience is important and the choice of CRO should be evaluated carefully. In this respect, one important evaluation should be the CRO's area of focus. Since the local CROs are still small on a global scale, quality can be maintained by focusing on the business tasks covered, e.g. medical writing, data management, or monitoring management. The percentage of global trials, national trials, and market research should be noted.

It is not easy for a CRO to survive in a fluctuating emerging market. In Turkey, as in other countries, obstacles arising from new clinical trial regulation and the global crisis have led to local developing CROs searching for alternative business areas. Some CROs have started to provide services in, for example, postmarketing activities and publication management, while some have reduced the number of staff and costs in order to survive. Global CROs have delayed their plans to open subsidiaries and continued working via local CROs. This picture will change soon, with the resolution of the regulatory infrastructure. Current local CROs and suppliers will remain the main service providers for the new global sector. The reason for this is that close follow-up to the changes in the regulations is crucial. The forms and guidelines are being changed very frequently, making the application and follow-up process hard even for experienced parties. Under such conditions, the involvement of a local supplier is mandatory. However, the availability of experienced staff in CROs may still be limited. As a solution, it has been observed recently in Turkey that global companies running clinical trials prefer to work with two local CROs, depending on the number of projects.

A local CRO has a challenge to keep three parameters in balance:

- an adequate and acceptable workforce
- sustainable quality
- cost-effectiveness.

There is always a high possibility of the loss of a client or a decrease in staff in emerging market conditions as seen in Turkey. Only those who are able to balance these three parameters will be able to survive in the long term.

With all the experience gained over the years by the government, pharmaceutical sector, and study sites, Turkey stands as a reliable, efficient, and cost-effective emerging region.

The country's most important advantages are the presence of well-equipped and high-level university and state hospitals; well-trained specialized clinicians; lower costs associated with ethical reviews, regulatory approvals, and investigator compensation; and good success rates for patient recruitment.

If pharmaceutical and biotechnology companies are not already performing clinical trials in emerging countries such as Turkey, all the indications are that they soon will be. While these regions offer significant advantages in terms of large populations and increased speed of recruitment, they also bring complexity to the clinical trials planning process. Much of this complexity is manageable, and will become less of an issue as the industry becomes more familiar with operating in these locations. In the meantime, assistance is available from a range of local and international service providers who have already experienced the highs and lows of managing trials in emerging markets.

References

1. Turkish Statistical Institute (TurkStat). *Turkey in Statistics*; 2010.
2. Turkish Statistical Institute (TurkStat). *IMF World Economic Outlook*; April 2011.
3. Organisation for Economic Co-operation and Development. OECD Economic Outlook No. 86.
4. Espicom. *Turkey world pharmaceutical market*; 2010.
5. Tascioglu H. *Pharmaceutical industry.* Export Promotion Center of Turkey; 2011.
6. Republic of Turkey Prime Ministry Investment Support and Promotion Agency. Invest in Turkey, www.invest.gov.tr.
7. Goldman Sachs Global Investment Research. *United States: Healthcare Services: CROs*; December 2007.
8. Akan H. Clinical research in Turkey. *Turkish Journal of Hematology* 2007;**24**:1–3.
9. Gündüz O. *Turkey: clinical trials in Turkey during the transition period*; 2010.
10. Turkish Clinical Research Association. http://www.klinikarastirmalar.org.tr/en
11. Lamb M, Setley D. *Clinical trial logistics: the trial of emerging markets*. Clinical Trial Services-ALMAC; 2005.

Regulatory Capacity

SECTION

Regulatory Capacity

Development of Regulatory Capacity in Monitoring, Oversight, Enforcement, and Approval of Clinical Trials

Taiwan's Experience as an Example

Herng-Der Chern
Center for Drug Evaluation, Taipei, Taiwan

129

DRUG REGULATION: AN INSTRUMENT FOR PUBLIC ASSURANCE OF DRUG SAFETY AND EFFICACY

The products of the biopharmaceutical industry, drugs, often have a profound impact on public health. To protect public health, every step in the development of a new drug is highly

Global Clinical Trials Playbook. DOI: 10.1016/B978-0-12-415787-3.00012-6

regulated based not only on best international practice, such as International Conference on Harmonisation (ICH) guidelines and good science, but also on special local regulatory requirements of national regulatory authorities (NRAs) so that they can be held accountable to their congress and citizens for their regulatory actions. However, most NRAs also recognize that early access to innovative medicinal products by patients can promote public health. To assure the general public of the safety and efficacy of the drugs at the same time supporting new drug development, such as H1N1 vaccine or therapies for acquired immunodeficiency syndrome (AIDS), the development of the capacity and capability of the NRA becomes a critical priority for many countries. Since all approved drugs are likely to be used globally, i.e. in a large human population, clinical trials have become indispensable and important steps in new drug development.

Conceptual Spheres of Investigational New Drug Regulations

Regulation for investigational new drugs (INDs) should be stated in the law, order, guidance, or points to consider. The review process should be transparent, efficient, and responsive, and run under standard operating procedures (SOPs) with a good quality assurance and control system in place. The review principles should be consistent and fair to all stakeholders. There should be no conflict of interest in regulatory evaluation and the information submitted to the NRA must be kept confidential. For the NRA to approve a specific indication carrying specific labeling, a large amount of clinical data needs to be submitted through a series of INDs during clinical development. As all INDs have different levels of built-in risk for trial subjects, the NRA has dual responsibilities to both protect public health and promote public health in the IND review. The first role of the NRA is to protect public health. All individual INDs should be carefully reviewed by the NRA based on sound study design with good risk/benefit ratio, preclinical data, ethical concerns, informed consent, and safety measures to decide whether it is safe to proceed. Good IND study design aiming for an NDA is mainly the responsibility of the sponsor. This is why the US Food and Drug Administration (FDA) does not use wording such as "this IND is approved by the FDA", to avoid any implication that the scientific merit of the sponsor's study design was endorsed by the FDA. The second role of the NRA is to promote public health. The sponsor is encouraged to seek early regulatory advice, such as through a pre-IND or an end of Phase II meeting with the FDA, or scientific advice from the European Medicines Agency (EMA) or Japanese Pharmaceuticals and Medical Devices Agency (PMDA), before making critical decisions for the drug development plan, to avoid potential regulatory surprises during the final NDA review.

Evolution of Clinical Research Regulations

The evolution of clinical research regulations can be briefly summarized in the following milestones:

- **1938**: Following the death of 107 people from sulfanilamide, the US Food, Drug and Cosmetic Act enforced the need for manufacturers to demonstrate safety.
- **1947**: Following inhumane experiments on prisoners of war in World War II, the Nuremberg Code was implemented, with the following key points:
  - The concept of informed consent was first proposed, so that informed consent of volunteers must be obtained without coercion in any form.
  - Human experiments should be based on prior animal experimentation.
  - Anticipated scientific results should justify the experiment.
  - Only qualified scientists should conduct medical research.
  - Physical, mental suffering, and injury should be avoided.
  - There should be no expectation of death or disabling injury from the experiment.
- **1962**: The USA passed the Kefauver-Harris Drug Amendment, meaning that proof of efficacy was required for NDA approval.

- **1964**: The Declaration of Helsinki was developed by the World Medical Association. These ethical codes provide principles for medical research involving human subjects.
- **1989**: Good Clinical Practice (GCP) of the European Community.
- **1996**: ICH-GCP was first accepted in the USA, the European Union (EU), and Japan. The ICH-GCP was followed by many non-ICH countries. GCP defines the basic principles used to protect trial subjects and data integrity in clinical trials.

Following the spirit of the FDA's IND process, the Center for Drug Evaluation (CDE) in Taiwan offers free regulatory consultations throughout the new drug development process. Of 600 consultations requested by sponsors in 2010, face-to-face meetings were granted in 20 percent. Taiwan FDA/CDE review INDs using the concept of "safe to proceed" and make regulatory recommendations for regulatory requirements for potential NDAs.

DIMENSIONS OF REGULATORY CAPACITY

Structure

The main components of regulatory capacity are a legal regulatory administrator, in-house full time technical staff, and an external advisory committee. Under the concept of risk-based evaluation, different review processes were set up with different levels of regulatory intensity, such as full review, abbreviated review, and clinical trial notification system. In Taiwan, the CDE/Taiwan Food and Drug Administration (TFDA) were set up as an innovative model for regulatory review.[1] The CDE was established in 1998 as a non-profit, non-governmental organization (NGO), fully sponsored and authorized by the Taiwan government to conduct regulatory consultation and evaluation for INDs, NDAs, guidance drafting, and international affairs. This special set-up has given the CDE the flexibility to recruit professionals in terms of increased headcount, competitive salary scales, and the ability to avoid many of the limitations applied to civil servants. The CDE/TFDA Integrated Medicinal Products Review Office (iMPRO) was established on June 1, 2011, with reviewers from both the CDE and the TFDA sharing an office and following the same SOPs for reviewing. The combination of legal authority and accountability with the capacity for in-house technical expertise under a streamlined process is the cornerstone in taking complicated regulatory action based on good regulatory science. In the early 2000s, when the capacity and capability of the CDE and TFDA were inadequately provided, the advisory committee played an important role in sharing the review work and serving as a quality check for the CDE's recommendations. Since the establishment of the iMPRO, the CDE/TFDA's in-house review team has been independently responsible for most IND and NDA reviews (Figure 12.1). The role of the advisory committee has been transformed into a real advisory one, to serve the NRA only on complicated regulatory challenges. The evolution of this regulatory structure has streamlined the review process significantly.

Human Resources

Regulatory science is both an art and a science involving many disciplines, such as biomedical science, ethics, law, management, and communication skills. The best way to learn it is through hands-on review experience supervised by experienced staff in a multidisciplinary review team. It takes time and a carefully planned training program to nurture good reviewers. To maintain qualified human resources, we need to create a learning organization, career path development, passion in their work in protecting and promoting public health, organizational prestige recognized by their peer groups and the general public, a good working environment, and competitive pay. Since 1998, the CDE has nurtured an experienced review team, with 170 full-time staff as of February 2012, working on step-by-step coverage of the review of INDs, NDAs, some new medical devices, and health technology assessment. The CDE has 25 full-time medical doctors, seven statisticians, 35 PhDs, and 48 with a master's degree (two of whom are lawyers), making it a major thinktank for the TFDA (Figure 12.2). A dedicated IND

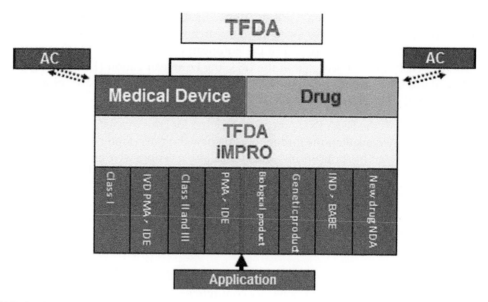

FIGURE 12.1

Excellence in regulatory science: in-house review capacity of the Center for Drug Evaluation/Taiwan Food and Drug Administration (CDE/TFDA). The Integrated Medicinal Product Review Office (iMPRO) has integrated reviewers and project managers from TFDA and CDE since June 1, 2011. AC: Advisory Committee; IVD: in vitro diagnostics; PMA: premarket approval; IDE: investigational device exemption; IND: investigational new drug; BABE: bioavailability and bioequivalence; NDA: new drug application. (Please refer to color plate section)

132

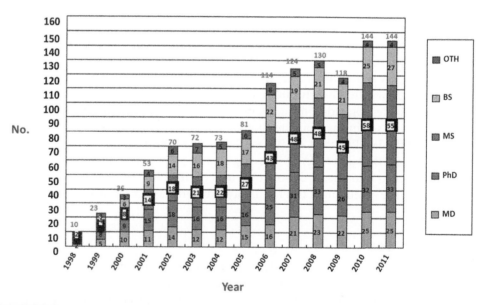

FIGURE 12.2

Full-time employees in the Center for Drug Evaluation (CDE), March 2011. (Please refer to color plate section)

review team is mainly composed of full-time medical doctors and statisticians, with preclinical review supported by the preclinical division, including chemistry, manufacturing, and control (CMC), pharmacology/toxicology, pharmacokinetics, and biological reviewers. The team leader of an IND review team will be the medical reviewer, so he or she can make a clinical judgment as to whether an IND is safe to proceed based on the clinical risk/benefit ratio. The

CDE has project managers serving as the main contact to manage the whole IND review according to SOPs.

Financial Resources

Stable and sufficient financial resources are a critical element in building and maintaining regulatory capacity. The financial resources can normally either be allocated a budget from the government or receive a user fee from the sponsors, mostly pharmaceutical companies. For example, NRAs such as the EMA, the Medicines and Healthcare Products Regulatory Agency (MHRA) in the UK, and the Therapeutic Goods Administration (TGA) in Australia are fully supported by the user fee, while the US FDA and Japanese PMDA are only partially supported by the user fee. The magnitude of NRAs' annual budget can vary even though they have similar responsibilities and regulatory challenges. However, almost all NRAs have problems of inadequate financial resources, from the well-resourced US FDA to the NRAs in most developing countries. Unfortunately, significant increases in resources usually only come after a safety disaster with a product under the NRA's jurisdiction, with the aim of fixing the system for better public health protection.

As NRAs also have a role in public health promotion, some NRAs have been relatively successful in justifying their budgets as investment expenditure, as a critical component of the infrastructure in the development of innovative medicinal products. As the CDE is a non-profit NGO, it was 100 percent supported by Taiwanese government funding under grants from different government sectors, including the Ministry of Economic Affairs, the National Translational Medicine Research Program, and the Ministry of Health, without any application fee for the products evaluated by the CDE. The nominal application fee goes to the TFDA, not the CDE. Over the years, the CDE has been relatively successful in securing financial support, about US $10 million in 2012, from different government sectors in Taiwan for the concept of public health promotion. Other than review work entrusted by the TFDA, the CDE provides regulatory consultations, grant reviews for clinical research, and regulatory training programs to serve stakeholders under different government projects. Although all projects need to be reviewed annually and there is some financial instability, this special working model links the CDE's performance and the satisfaction of all stakeholders via the annual budget review process. Since the CDE and TFDA have recently been functionally integrated under the iMPRO, the next step will be the formal establishment of an expanded iMPRO as an independent administrative agency, with both a legal basis for regulatory authority and flexibility in management, similar to the PMDA in Japan.

Planning, Monitoring, and Evaluating Implementation

To nurture the capacity and capability of a reputable NRA requires (1) careful stepwise planning based on the correct principles of regulatory science, (2) a good quality assurance and quality control system to monitor its performance by benchmarking other reputable NRAs, and (3) periodical evaluation of its overall implementation based on the vision, mission, goal, objectives, action plans, and roadmap, via a high-level advisory committee. In the following section, the CDE/TFDA model will be used as an experimental model of regulatory science in Asia to illustrate the importance of the approaches stated above.

PLANNING

In 1997, Taiwan chose the biopharmaceutical industry as one of its national priorities for economic development. As the biopharmaceutical industry is a regulation-intensive industry involving human health, many experts recommended upgrading the capacity of local NRAs to best international practice. The CDE was set up in 1998 (see Structure, above, for more details) to conduct regulatory consultation and evaluation of medicinal products with good regulatory science to support the final decision of the legal authority, now the TFDA.

From the beginning, the strategy of the CDE has been to follow the spirit of the FDA in regulatory science and the EMA format in reviews, to harmonize with the ICH guidance, and to network with reputable NRAs. Both the CDE and the TFDA have strived to be the leader in regulatory challenges related to Asia, by thinking globally but acting locally. Some highlights of its achievements are:

- the implementation of the ICH E5 in accepting foreign clinical data via Bridging Study Evaluation (BSE), since 2000
- setting up an IND process and providing free regulatory consultation
- initiating critical path projects for in-depth regulatory consultation for the index cases selected[2]
- setting up a Clinical Trial Notification (CTN) system following the spirit of TGA Australia, in which a qualifying IND (the same protocol has been approved by at least one of the 10 reference NRAs) can be approved within an average regulatory time of only 17.3 calendar days from submission to receipt of an approval letter
- leading international projects, e.g. the APEC Network of Regulatory Science since 2000 and APEC Good Regulatory Practice, including hosting the Good Pharmaceutical Review Practice workshop on drugs/devices and promoting the exchange of regulatory information among NRAs in 2011–2012.

MONITORING

Building quality into the decision-making process of the assessment requires good quality assurance and quality control systems to monitor the performance and improve consistency, transparency, timeliness, and competency in the review process. Good monitoring measures can improve stakeholder satisfaction and communication within the NRA, and serve as a guide for the allocation of regulatory resources.

The CDE/TFDA has a good internal quality assurance/quality control tracking system to monitor the IND review in terms of efficiency (regulatory time and sponsor time compared with the target time in SOPs), quantity (number of new protocols and clinical sites) and composition of INDs (number of Phase I, II, III, or multiregional trial), reasons for any delay in review, approval rate, and reasons for non-approval. External experts from different review disciplines (CMC, pharmacology and toxicology, statistics, medical, clinical pharmacology, etc.), many with US FDA review experience, periodically perform external quality audits on the CDE's assessment reports. Feedback from stakeholders is carefully reviewed through complaints, annual meetings, workshops, and surveys. Regulatory capacity and capability have been gradually improved since the establishment of the CDE in 1998. Progress is planned and monitored annually by the biotechnology committee at cabinet level, and by the TFDA on an almost daily basis.

Political Influence and Accountability

A clinical trial involves testing a new drug, with some unpredictable risks, in human subjects who volunteer not only for their own benefit but also to advance public health. If clinical trial conduct were treated lightly, without due respect and with no precautions regarding ethical trial conduct, the political repercussions from society may cause major setbacks to the future recruitment of subjects. Consumer groups and many politicians have been very active and concerned about the safe and ethical conduct of clinical trials. A lot of legislation relating to the conduct of clinical trials, informed consent, qualification of the principal investigators, accreditation of the hospitals, handling of genetic material, and guidance for cell and gene therapy has been stipulated. If there is major violation of a clinical trial protocol, the TFDA can take strong regulatory action, and even ban the whole hospital from submitting new INDs before a risk management plan is submitted. The principal investigator may face criminal charges for major misconduct in the clinical trial. Another kind of political pressure may come from lobbying of the sponsors. To avoid potential undue political influence in the independent evaluation of NRAs, the CDE/TFDA has set up an internal quality audit system with primary and secondary reviewers and supervisors from different disciplines to ensure consistent and impartial review. All reviewers' assessment reports will be signed and archived without any internal changes. The reviewers will be accountable for their own assessment reports only. If a higher manager wishes to overrule a recommendation from the primary reviewers, he or she will be accountable for the decision and his or her points documented. There is also an ombudsman system to investigate any significant issues efficiently and fairly.

Transparency

Transparency for an NRA refers to the ability and willingness of the agency to allocate time and resources, and to provide information on its activities to both the informed public (which includes health professionals) and industry. Transparency may provide assurance on safety safeguards to the public, and increase confidence in the system and predictability for the industry. Information provided may include the approval basis of a product, approval time, summary of approval for the product, advisory committee members, and meeting dates. The information may be made available through an official journal, a periodical publication, or an official website.

For the CDE/TFDA, any disapproval of an IND should give clear reasons to the sponsor. The sponsor can check the progress of their IND review on the Internet. If the sponsor has questions about the reasons for IND disapproval, they can request a free face-to-face consultation with the CDE to clarify any questions. The request for a meeting will normally be granted within one month. Periodically, the CDE/TFDA will invite stakeholders to discuss topics of concern and the performance index of the review efficiency, and conduct anonymous satisfaction surveys. The CDE's performance will be reviewed during the budget application process by many key opinion leaders in the country.

Inspections and Surveillance

The integrity of clinical trial data will be the presumption for all NDA approval. Thus, it is very important to ensure the integrity of clinical trial conduct and data management through GCP inspection. Since 1997, the TFDA has been conducting GCP inspection on at least one clinical site for all INDs in Taiwan. About 10 percent of the trials were disqualified for major GCP violation. The inspection team is composed of senior physicians and experienced statistical experts from the medical centers and TFDA staff. So far, no overseas GCP inspection has been conducted, but this aspect is being seriously considered. The CDE sent senior clinical reviewers to the EMA for GCP inspector training in 2010–2011. There are many accreditation schemes that can serve as a model of surveillance for personnel conducting clinical trials, e.g. the Association of Clinical Research Professionals (ACRP); for institutional review boards (IRBs), e.g. the Forum for Ethical Review Committee in the Asian and Western Pacific Region (FERCAP); and for clinical trial sites, e.g. the Association for the Accreditation of Human Research Protection Programs (AAHRPP).

Evaluating Regulatory Capacity and Performance

The capacity of an NRA can be evaluated by its annual budget, size, scope, and remit, the number and qualifications of its reviewers, and the type of the data assessment used (full review, abbreviated review, abridged review by reference to the approval of recognized NRAs, role of the external advisory committee).[3] The performance of an NRA can be evaluated by good review practice (GRP). GRP concerns the process and documentation of review procedures, and aims to standardize and improve the overall documentation, and ensure the timeliness, predictability, consistency, and high quality of the review and any reports. GRP also refers to whether the reviewers have good qualifications and on-the-job training programs, and perform the review based on good regulatory science. Another indicator for GRP is whether the regulatory action of the NRA is recognized by other NRAs. The CDE/TFDA is one of the few Asian NRAs to have an in-house review team that conducts a full review for a new molecular entity. For example, in 2009, the CDE/TFDA approved an H1N1 vaccine IND and NDA developed by a local company under a rolling review approach. Five million doses of vaccine were administered, which controlled the H1N1 epidemic successfully.

GLOBALIZATION OF CLINICAL RESEARCH AND INTERNATIONAL CONFERENCE ON HARMONISATION: SHARING EXPERTISE FOR CAPACITY BUILDING

The ICH has been relatively successful in harmonizing major scientific guidance for new drug development and common technical dossier (CTD) for global regulatory submission. The EMA has been known for creating a closed regulatory club that involved NRAs sharing their expertise and regulatory information among themselves. The dilemma of the inadequate capacity and capability of many small NRAs has been resolved by EMA's model of "compare and contrast" for GRP. Not only is the review process streamlined by coordinated collective regulatory effort, but the goal of protecting and promoting public health is also achieved. There are many regulatory harmonization initiatives with different levels of success ongoing worldwide. For example, the Association of Southeast Asian Nations (ASEAN), the Asia-Pacific Economic Cooperation (APEC), the Life Science Innovation Forum (LSIF), the Regulatory Harmonization Steering Committee (RHSC), the Korea–Japan–China Tripartite Clinical Trial Collaboration, the Cross Strait Agreement on Medicine and Public Health Affairs between China and Taiwan[4], and many other bilateral agreements in regulatory cooperation all indicate the future trend towards the globalization of clinical research and the sharing of regulatory expertise and information.

The TFDA/CDE has been routinely participating in the regulatory forum of ICH-GCG for several years. The TFDA/CDE is leading an APEC Best Regulatory Practice project in 2011–2012. Besides hosting the Good Review Practice (GRP) Workshop for Drugs and Medical Devices, another highlight is the Pharmaceutical Evaluation Report among APEC member economies (APEC PER Scheme). With help from the Center for Innovation in Regulatory Science (CIRS), Taiwan completed a survey for gap analysis of GRP among APEC NRAs in 2011.

REGULATION OF CLINICAL TRIALS IN DEVELOPING COUNTRIES

Six major essential elements of clinical trial infrastructure are required to attract global clinical trials to a particular country:

- quality of trial conduct up to ICH-GCP standard
- efficiency, including IND review of NRA and IRB
- efficiency of clinical trial conduct in hospitals
- regulatory requirements for local clinical trial or bridging study for NDAs
- cost of the trial, including whether there are any government incentives
- potential market size.

Using the evolving clinical trial status in Taiwan as an example for other developing countries,[5,6] it is obvious that the regulatory infrastructure is the driver for the rapid improvement in clinical trials in Taiwan in terms of both quantity and quality. Five phases of clinical trial regulatory infrastructure may be identified:

- **1993–1996**: There was an administrative requirement that all NDAs to be approved in Taiwan would need to conduct a clinical trial involving a minimum of 40 Taiwanese subjects. This regulatory requirement was simple and clear and brought some trials, mostly Phase IV trials of drugs already marketed in other countries, to Taiwan.

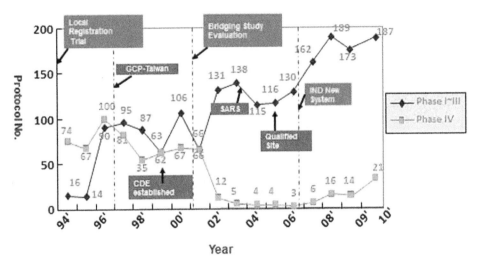

FIGURE 12.3

Built-up regulatory infrastructure: investigational new drugs (INDs) from 1994 to 2010 in Taiwan. GCP: good clinical practice; CDE: Center for Drug Evaluation. (Please refer to color plate section)

- **1997–2000**: Taiwan GCP was promulgated with GCP inspection and the CDE was set up for IND review. These measures guaranteed the quality of clinical trial conduct in Taiwan, so about 50 percent of the trials were Phase I–III trials conducted together with other countries.
- **2000–2006**: The 40 case regulatory requirement was gradually replaced by the BSE for potential ethnic sensitivity in accepting foreign clinical trial data.[7] Ninety-five percent of the trials were Phase I–III trials and Taiwan became the preferred site for multiregional clinical trials in Asia. This means that most companies decided to include Taiwan in their global clinical development so they could better determine whether the NDA was ethnically sensitive at the time of BSE, before NDA.
- **2006–2010**: The number of the clinical trials increased by 12–15 percent per year, which reflected the continuous improvement in the efficiency of regulatory IND review and clinical trial conduct in more qualified sites, including the five National Centers of Excellence for Clinical Trials and Research[8] and a dozen General Clinical Research Centers supported by government funding.
- **2011–present**: The CDE/TFDA announced the CTN scheme on August 18, 2010. The average regulatory review time was 17.3 calendar days for CTN cases (26 cases, about 19 percent of all INDs submitted) compared with 38.3 days for non-CTN cases (112 cases) (data from August 18, 2010 to March 31, 2011). Among these 26 CTN cases, 12 (46 percent) were Phase I and II trials, compared with only 25 percent of the non-CTN cases. This means that CTN schemes can attract early phase trials to Taiwan by improving the efficiency of the review time.

The regulatory infrastructure for INDs in Taiwan from 1994 to 2010 is shown in Figure 12.3.

ETHICS COMMITTEES AS CO-REGULATORS

Ethics committee or IRB approval is needed for the IND to be conducted at the site that bestows them with the role of co-regulators of INDs. Although the minimum requirements for IRB structure and operation are stipulated in the ICH-GCP, there are still many challenges in establishing a robust IRB. Many IRBs face the following challenges:

- Members may not have adequate training for ethical review and may insist on something that is "nice to know" and/or "scientifically interesting" but not necessarily needed for protocol modification.

137

- There may be a lack of administrative support and SOPs.
- For a multicenter trial, different IRBs may make different comments on the same IND protocol.
- There may be a lack of resources to monitor the progress of the INDs.

To target these challenges, in 1997 Taiwan established a Joint IRB, composed of members from five medical centers, the National Health Research Institute, and laypeople. At one time, the Joint IRB's decision was honored by two-thirds of medical centers in Taiwan for multicenter clinical trials. The Taiwan Association of IRBs was established in 2009 to serve as an open platform for all IRBs in terms of education, research, policy recommendations, and international interaction. More than 20 IRBs in Taiwan have passed the FERCAP IRB accreditation and the country has the highest number of accredited IRBs in Asia.

CONCLUSION

The past decade has witnessed the rapid development of the methodology of study design and related regulation, ethical principles for clinical trials as a critical component of new drug development, and marketing registration. During the trend towards simultaneous global drug development and regulatory convergence, there has been a focus on bringing the quality of the clinical trial conduct and its regulatory capacity up to best international practice, especially in many emerging countries. Taiwan has come a long way over the past 20 years, although there is room for improvement, considering all the new challenges to reach its current capacity and capability in regulatory science. This experience can serve as a good reference for other NRAs in developing a best fit regulatory system to protect and promote public health in their own jurisdiction.

References

1. Chern H-D, Gau Chen C-S, H-MH, Liao C-C. An experimental model of regulatory science in Asia: Center for Drug Evaluation in Taiwan. *Drug Information Journal* 2009;43:301–4.

2. Lin B-B, Lin C-H, Chern H-D. The Critical Path Program in Taiwan. *Drug Information Journal* 2009;43:311–7.

3. McAuslane N, Cone M, Collins J, Walker S. Emerging markets and emerging agencies: a comparative study of how key regulatory agencies in Asia, Latin America, the Middle East, and Africa are developing regulatory processes and review models for new medicinal products. *Drug Information Journal* 2009;43:349–59.

4. Cross Strait Cooperation Agreement on Medicine and Public Health Affairs. http://www.cde.org.tw/SubLink/CSCA/cross_strait_Cooperation_Agreement.pdf [accessed 25.01.12].

5. Wong ECK. Clinical trials in Southeast Asia: an update. *Drug Information Journal* 2009;43:57–61.

6. Liao J-J, Liao C-C, On A, Chern H-D, Lin M-S. Updates on IND process and clinical trials status in Taiwan. *Drug Information Journal* 2009;43:63–8.

7. Su L-L, Chern H-D, Ryan Lee I-L, Lin C-L, Lin M-S. An overview of bridging study evaluation in Taiwan. *Drug Information Journal* 2009;43:371–6.

8. Lin C-C, Yang C-H, Cheng A-L, Chan W-K, Ho H-N. National Center of Excellence for Clinical Trials and Research at National Taiwan University. *Drug Information Journal* 2009;43:361–3.

How to Build and Enhance Pharmacovigilance and Risk Management Capacity and Capability

CHAPTER 13

Pharmacovigilance and Risk Management

Suzanne Gagnon*, Peter Schueler**, James (Dachao) Fan†
*ICON Clinical Research, North Wales, Pennsylvania, USA
**ICON Clinical Research, Langen, Hessen, Germany
†ICON Clinical Research Pte Ltd/Asia Pacific, Singapore

Global Clinical Trials Playbook. DOI: 10.1016/B978-0-12-415787-3.00013-8

DEFINITION OF PHARMACOVIGILANCE AND RISK MANAGEMENT

The World Health Organization (WHO) defines pharmacovigilance as the science and activities relating to the detection, evaluation, understanding, and prevention of adverse reactions to medicines or any other medicine-related problems. The definition and scope of pharmacovigilance have evolved to recognize the importance of a systems approach for monitoring and improving the safe use of medicines.[1]

A simpler definition describes pharmacovigilance as the processes and science of monitoring the safety of medicines and taking action to reduce risk and increase benefit.[2] Therefore, the assessment of benefit versus risk must begin during the preclinical evaluation of a medicinal product and must extend throughout its full life cycle.

As a result, there is now added focus on safety and risk assessment after a product has received regulatory approval, when it is placed on the market and prescribed to large populations. Although there is no international standard that dictates the components of an adequate pharmacovigilance system or the processes to be engaged in risk management, there is consensus among the major regulators that pharmacovigilance is necessary and important in the development and commercialization of medicinal products.

Therefore it is essential in building capacity for clinical trials to understand the components, the functions, and the processes required for full and effective pharmacovigilance and risk management.

THE IMPORTANCE OF IMPLEMENTING A SYSTEMATIC PHARMACOVIGILANCE APPROACH IN GLOBAL CLINICAL TRIALS

The amount and variety of safety-relevant data gathered from different patient populations in global clinical trials are enormous; therefore it is crucial that a concise and systematic approach to pharmacovigilance be implemented. Systematic safety monitoring is needed to identify previously recognized and unrecognized adverse drug reactions and to evaluate the safety and efficacy of medicinal products during clinical trials and in the postmarketing period.

It is important that pharmacovigilance not be perceived as a burden put upon the pharmaceutical product development industry by the regulating bodies. Ongoing pharmacovigilance should be understood as essential to the only appropriate way to develop safe medicines, introduce them into the market, and have them survive in the market once approved. Not only does the failure to perform ongoing safety assessment activities increase the chances of placing subjects at risk unnecessarily, it also increases a company's risk of investing in the development of the wrong molecules.

The following example illustrates the value of ongoing systematic pharmacovigilance. Figure 13.1 displays aggregate alanine aminotransferase (ALT) data reported during a clinical trial performed to evaluate a new oncology compound. The product was dosed cyclically, administered intravenously every 21 days. Review of aggregate data from the initial eight patients suggested that the product caused a transient hepatitis, particularly apparent after the first dose, as shown by the spiking ALT levels. It was thus advisable to re-evaluate the initial dosing and the dosing intervals, and closely monitor liver function in all patients to avoid unacceptable toxicity and to better assess the benefit/risk value and the appropriate population for the drug. Because the review was part of ongoing pharmacovigilance during the clinical trial, the safety issue was identified and addressed early in clinical development. Such laboratory trend analysis yields maximum benefit when part of a systematic approach to safety monitoring.

Capacity building for pharmacovigilance and medicine safety should address all processes for developing individual and system capacity and enable achievement of sustainable ability to

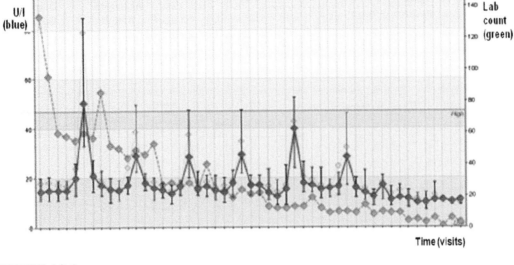

FIGURE 13.1
Ongoing surveillance and trend analysis of liver function tests showing potentially liver-toxic effects in a cyclic dosing scheme. *Source: IMRA—ICON Medical Review Application.* (Please refer to color plate section)

manage effectively the safety of patients and health products.[3] Performing systematic pharmacovigilance requires a full understanding of the scope of pharmacovigilance, which includes both active safety reporting and postmarketing surveillance. It involves the ongoing processes of risk identification, risk assessment, and risk mitigation. All of these processes are equally important to the pharmaceutical company, the regulatory authorities, the investigator, and the patient.

There are many ways of building pharmacovigilance capability, and many differences in how pharmacovigilance systems are created. Historically, companies created pharmacovigilance functionality as the need arose to assess their products under development. Since there are variations in the required sample size of studies, geographical site distribution, adjuvant or comparator products used, and in the definition of "standard treatment" in different countries, differences naturally evolved. Global pharmacovigilance is an ongoing process of harmonization. Currently, there are many national, cultural, and regulatory differences among countries in how pharmacovigilance is implemented. The goal is always the accurate assessment of the benefit versus the risk of a product in the populations who receive it, and mature pharmacovigilance systems are able reach accurate conclusions despite different types of data.

OPERATIONAL OVERVIEW OF PHARMACOVIGILANCE

An operational overview of pharmacovigilance begins with safety information coming from a variety of sources, including clinical trials data, safety call centers, spontaneous reports, and literature searches, each of which has the potential to create an individual case. Within the pharmacovigilance department each case is processed, assessed as to its relationship (causality) to the investigational product, and reported to the regulatory authorities and other stakeholders, either as an expedited report or as part of an aggregate report, based upon pharmacovigilance policies, regulations, and guidance documents. In addition, each case becomes part of the total safety dataset for that medicinal product.

Aggregate data are systematically analyzed for safety issues and assessed for benefit versus risk, and periodic safety update reports (PSURs) are submitted to the regulatory authorities as additional safety information is collected. This continues throughout the product's life cycle. Safety findings are addressed in order to mitigate risk. This may include modification to a clinical trial design, changes in proposed labeling, implementation of a risk mitigation plan,

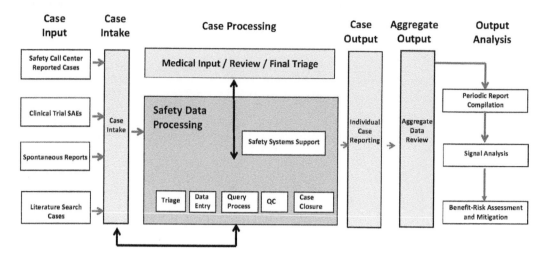

FIGURE 13.2

Summary of the major activities associated with pharmacovigilance. SAE: serious adverse event; QC: quality control.
(Please refer to color plate section)

or discontinuation of development or use of a marketed product. A flow diagram summarizing the major activities associated with pharmacovigilance is shown in Figure 13.2.

COMPONENTS AND CAPABILITIES OF A COMPLETE PHARMACOVIGILANCE SYSTEM

Based upon the intent and scope of pharmacovigilance, there are certain components and capabilities that are essential to a fully functioning pharmacovigilance system, regardless of how a company's safety department is constructed (Figure 13.3). These include:

- a qualified person for pharmacovigilance (QPPV) (Europe)
- safety systems (database) support.
- safety case processing and review
- medical writing and aggregate reporting
- a sound quality management system including standard operating procedures (SOPs), quality standards, metrics, and training
- signal detection and risk analysis
- global safety reporting

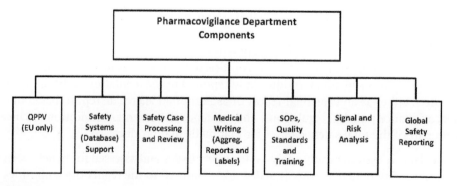

FIGURE 13.3

Components and capabilities of a fully functional pharmacovigilance system. QPPV: qualified person for pharmacovigilance; EU: European Union; SOP: standard operating procedure.

In some companies some activities may be performed by different departments, for example, safety regulatory reporting may be part of regulatory affairs, or aggregate report writing may be done within a company's medical writing department. Some activities may be outsourced to contract research organizations (CROs) or safety niche providers, while others are kept in-house, but all must be covered for complete pharmacovigilance capacity.

PHARMACOVIGILANCE POLICIES, REGULATIONS, AND GUIDANCE DOCUMENTS

In the major regions of the world where medicinal products are developed, pharmacovigilance is highly regulated. Structures, systems, and roles are determined by laws, regulations, guidances, and guidelines; it is within this context that the department's organizational structure is established, the individual roles and the systems required are defined, the skill sets necessary are determined, and the tools to perform pharmacovigilance effectively are created.

The major regulatory stakeholders driving the formation of global pharmacovigilance regulation are the US Food and Drug Administration (FDA), the European Medicines Agency (EMA), and Japan's Pharmaceuticals and Medical Devices Agency (PMDA). In the USA, the Code of Federal Regulations is legally binding, as are the European national laws and ordinances. Directives reflect current thinking on a topic and bind member states to common objectives, which must be implemented into national law within a given timeframe. Guidance documents, guidelines, and recommendations are not legally binding, but should be respected and play an important role in actual practice.

Global principles are harmonized through the International Conference on Harmonisation (ICH). ICH E1–E2F focus on clinical safety. Direction is provided in ICH E2A–C (Clinical Safety Data Management), E2D (Post-Approval Safety Data Management: Definitions and Standards for Expedited Reporting), E2E (Pharmacovigilance Planning), and E2F (Development Safety Update Report).

ICH E6 (Good Clinical Practice) describes the responsibilities and expectations of all stakeholders in the conduct of clinical trials.

However, even as efforts to harmonize pharmacovigilance processes continue, companies must still comply with national laws and local regulations. As in other areas of development, companies should have SOPs around pharmacovigilance processes in order to ensure consistency, compliance, and quality.

Adverse Event Reporting

DEFINITIONS

Reporting of adverse events is the cornerstone of pharmacovigilance, and therefore closely supervised by regulatory authorities. ICH E2A defines the following adverse events (AEs), adverse drug reactions (ADRs), and serious adverse events (SAEs) as follows:

Adverse event (or adverse experience)

Any untoward medical occurrence in a patient or clinical investigative subject administered a pharmaceutical product and which does not necessarily have to have a causal relationship with this treatment.

An adverse event (AE) can therefore be an unfavorable and unintended sign (including an abnormal laboratory finding, for example), symptom or disease temporally associated with the use of a medicinal product, whether or not considered related to the medicinal product.

Adverse drug reaction

In the pre-approval clinical experience with a new medicinal product or its new usages, particularly as the therapeutic dose(s) may not be established: all noxious and unintended responses to a medicinal product related to any dose should be considered adverse drug reactions.

The phrase "responses to a medicinal product" means that a causal relationship between a medicinal product and an adverse event is at least a reasonable possibility, i.e. the relationship cannot be ruled out.

Regarding marketed medicinal products, a well-accepted definition of an ADR in the post-marketing setting is found in WHO Technical Report 498 (1972) and reads as follows:

Unexpected adverse drug reaction

An adverse reaction the nature or severity of which is not consistent with the applicable product information (e.g. the Investigator Brochure for an unapproved investigational medical product).

Adverse events are defined as "serious" based upon patient event outcome or action criteria usually associated with events that pose a threat to a patient's life or functioning. Seriousness (not severity) serves as a guide for defining regulatory reporting obligations.

A serious adverse event (experience) or reaction is any untoward medical occurrence at any dose which:

- results in death,
- is life threatening,
- requires inpatient hospitalization or prolongation of existing hospitalization,
- results in persistent or significant disability/incapacity or
- is a congenital anomaly/birth defect.

Medical and scientific judgment should be exercised in deciding whether expedited reporting is appropriate in other situations, such as important medical events that may not be immediately life-threatening or result in death or hospitalization but may jeopardize the patient or may require intervention to prevent one of the other outcomes listed in the definition above. These should also usually be considered serious.

ADVERSE EVENT REPORTING TIMELINES

According to ICH E6, all SAEs should be reported to the sponsor immediately, except for those identified in the protocol or other document as not needing immediate reporting.

Fatal or unexpected ADRs occurring in clinical investigations should be reported to the regulatory authorities as soon as possible, but no later than seven calendar days after knowledge of the event by the sponsor, followed by as complete a report as possible within eight additional calendar days.

Serious unexpected reactions (ADRs) which are not fatal or life threatening must be filed as soon as possible but no later than 15 calendar days after first knowledge by the sponsor that the case meets the minimum criteria for expedited reporting.

Adverse events that do not meet the requirements for expedited reporting are reported at the end of the clinical trial as part of the marketing application or in PSURs.

EUROPEAN DIRECTIVE ON UNBLINDING

Volume 10 of the publication "The Rules Governing Medicinal Products in the European Union" provides guidance on unblinding the treatment allocation when suspected unexpected serious adverse reactions (SUSARs) occur. In the European Union (EU) SUSARs must be unblinded prior to submission to the regulatory authorities; this is not required by other regulatory authorities in Asia or the USA. Recently, the FDA acknowledged the potential need for unblinding some expedited safety reports, but recommends alternatives to unblinding be undertaken if possible; this rule came into effect on March 28, 2011.[4]

Procedures related to unblinding must ensure that only those who need to review unblinded data have access to them, and that everyone else involved in the trial remains blinded as to treatment assignment. This is required to preserve the integrity of the study.

Standard Operating Procedures, Study-Specific Procedures, and Safety Plans

The number of SOPs related to pharmacovigilance may vary from few in number to many, depending upon the length and complexity of the processes involved. Companies with few SOPs may write individual study-specific procedures (SSPs) consistent with their SOPs, but which provide more detail in relation to a specific product under development. Sometimes all of the pharmacovigilance procedures are combined into a safety plan, or pharmacovigilance plan, which becomes a summary of all of the processes to be followed by the assigned staff in conjunction with the clinical trial or across trials. In Europe, a detailed description of the pharmacovigilance system must be included in the marketing authorization application.

At a minimum, SOPs/SSPs should cover the following activities:

- serious adverse event reporting
- safety case handling (intake, process flow, assessment, documentation, archiving)
- safety database
- safety data conventions
- review of patient (clinical/laboratory) data
- aggregate data review
- signal detection
- unblinding
- regulatory reporting of safety information and 24 hour safety coverage.

Other SOPs/SSPs are developed as relevant to the specific product or therapeutic area. At the beginning of each trial safety reporting timelines should be reviewed, the timeframes for ongoing review and assessment of patient data should be agreed upon, and the assignment of any unblinded staff should be determined. Studies utilizing a drug safety monitoring board (DSMB) or clinical endpoint committee (CEC) will have additional SOPs/SSPs or charters created to clearly define the roles and processes to be performed by these groups.

In addition to written procedures, regular teleconferences and/or meetings should be held to ensure adequate communication of information, make modifications in best practices as needed during the study, and maintain compliance and audit readiness. Because processes may change during a clinical trial, training is an important part of pharmacovigilance and risk management.

Quality Management System

Pharmacovigilance departments should include a quality management system (QMS) for safety reporting processes, data review, and documentation. The purpose of a QMS is to ensure that all pharmacovigilance activities are performed to the highest ethical standards and conform to relevant regulatory requirements and contractual obligations to any licensing partners. Key elements include a quality policy, an approved documented library of SOPs, quality control procedures, key performance indicators (KPIs), job descriptions, and training plans.

A QMS is part of continuous process improvement. Within the QMS each process is reviewed through quality control steps within the process. The result of the quality control is measured against defined KPIs. Deviations from defined processes are identified, and those suggesting a quality issue are addressed through a root cause analysis followed by the creation of a corrective action and preventive action (CAPA) plan. Quality assurance can then check to ensure that quality is being managed within the pharmacovigilance department and that all quality issues are being addressed.

ORGANIZATIONAL STRUCTURE OF A PHARMACOVIGILANCE DEPARTMENT

Departmental Organization

The basic functional "unit" within the pharmacovigilance department is comprised of the drug safety physician (DSP), drug safety associate (DSA), and medical assistant. A "team" may consist of several DSAs, a single physician providing medical review, and one or two medical assistants for administrative support. Depending on the size of the company and the number of employees, pharmacovigilance teams may be organized by product or by therapeutic area, or may be separated into premarketing and postmarketing groups. Matrix structures are common. Global pharmacovigilance departments may exist in a limited number of regional hubs, with each hub having a senior pharmacovigilance member who provides oversight. An example of a pharmacovigilance organizational chart is depicted in Figure 13.4. Figure 13.5 shows an example of a matrix structure within pharmacovigilance.

Collaboration and Teamwork on Global Clinical Trials

Successful pharmacovigilance requires cross-functional, cross-regional, and cross-cultural collaboration. For example, within the pharmacovigilance department itself, safety case processing and assessment may occur in several locations, particularly if some steps in the

148

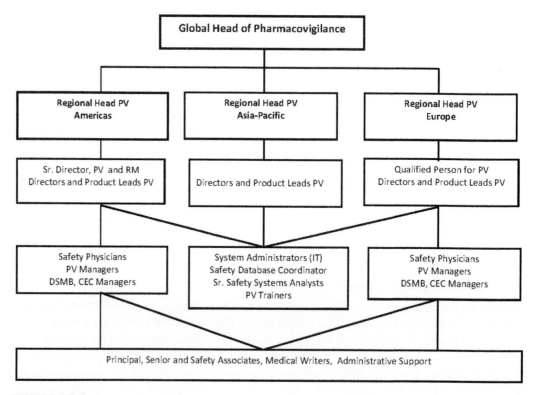

FIGURE 13.4

Sample organizational structure of a mid-sized pharmacovigilance (PV) department. RM: risk management; DSMB: drug safety monitoring board; CEC: clinical endpoint committee; IT: information technology.

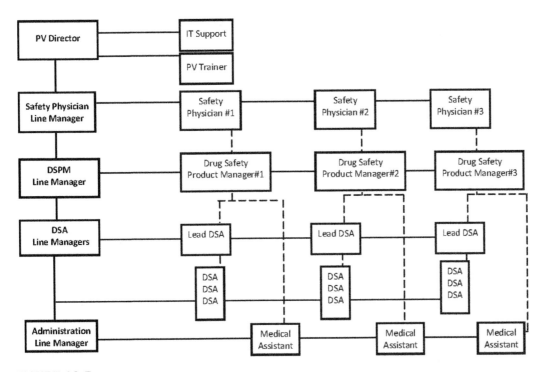

FIGURE 13.5
Sample matrix structure in pharmacovigilance (PV) by product. DSPM: drug safety product manager; DSA: drug safety associate; IT: information technology.

workflow are provided in low-cost centers. Global pharmacovigilance capacity can allow round-the-clock pharmacovigilance, but can only be successful with global systems, consistent processes and workflows, adequate and ongoing training, and excellent communication across regions.

As members of the clinical development team, pharmacovigilance staff also interact regularly with site investigators, clinical research associates (CRAs), clinical project managers (CPMs), clinical data managers (CDMs), biostatisticians, and medical writers. In addition, for projects using DSMBs or CECs, pharmacovigilance staff independent of the clinical team may work with the committee members to provide or clarify the safety information needed for clinical endpoint review or for periodic DSMB meetings.

ROLE OF THE MEDICAL MONITOR

ICH-GCP does not define or describe the responsibilities of a medical monitor. A practical definition might be "a physician or other qualified individual, separate from the principal investigator, who is responsible for medical and safety monitoring of research subjects for conditions that may arise during the conduct of a clinical trial".

The role of the medical monitor is to be the clinical team's advocate for subject safety and well-being. This extends beyond individual patient safety monitoring and may include medical assessment of the clinical study protocol for feasibility, upfront risk analysis, input into decisions on study design, treatment regimens, comparator selection, medical interpretation of data, and input into data analysis and report generation.

During the study the medical monitor is an important member of the clinical project team. Responsibilities include interaction with site investigators to provide them with known information on the product under study, ongoing assessment of the medical and safety aspects of the medicinal product, serving as the medical consultant to the project team by providing medical and therapeutic area expertise, participating in data review and interpretation, and helping to ensure overall project success. Despite regular interaction with clinical site personnel, the medical monitor should not interfere with the investigator's responsibility for medical assessment and treatment of individual subjects, but should provide the investigator with all medical information known by the company to ensure that the best assessment and treatment decisions may be made.

In essence, the medical monitor plays a unique role that bridges the site, the pharmacovigilance department, and the rest of the clinical development team.

ROLES AND RESPONSIBILITIES OF THE PHARMACOVIGILANCE TEAM

In different regions of the world, job titles vary for similar roles on the pharmacovigilance team. The titles drug, or product, safety associate or safety specialist may be used interchangeably with pharmacovigilance associate; the title drug safety physician is commonly used when referring to the physicians providing pharmacovigilance.

Head of Pharmacovigilance

The head of pharmacovigilance plays a critical role in the pharmacovigilance department, and is the person ultimately responsible for all of the safety and risk management activities performed within the department. Typically, he or she will have many years of experience in pharmacovigilance and be an authority on pharmacovigilance regulations and reporting requirements. In addition to providing leadership and oversight within the department, the head of pharmacovigilance acts as a senior resource throughout the company on matters such as safety strategy, regulatory and safety risk management, safety compliance, and safety quality assurance. The head of pharmacovigilance may be identical with the QPPV in smaller European companies. However, typically the role is separate from the QPPV to ensure the independence of the QPPV from the daily operational tasks.

Drug Safety Physician/Directors of Drug Safety

It is frequently necessary for the medical monitor to remain blinded as to the medicinal product causing an adverse reaction in a clinical trial. Knowledge of the treatment arm may bias the medical monitor in decisions affecting other aspects of the study. In such cases, a physician not otherwise associated with the study will be assigned to assess adverse events, possibly as an unblinded medical reviewer. In large, global pharmaceutical companies, these DSPs exist in the pharmacovigilance department completely separate from the medical monitors on the clinical team. In smaller companies where physicians may play multiple roles, it is important to firewall blinded and unblinded medical staff in order to protect the integrity of the clinical data.

Other responsibilities of the DSPs include medical review of aggregate data and reports. More experienced DSPs or directors of drug safety are involved in signal detection and analysis. Some may be responsible for creating and implementing development risk minimization plans (Europe) or risk evaluation and mitigation plans (USA), which are now required by many regulatory authorities.

Qualified Person for Pharmacovigilance in Europe

The QPPV is a required role for all pharmaceutical companies in Europe, but not yet required in other regions of the world. A named person is responsible for all aspects of pharmacovigilance for a medicinal product. The QPPV must be a physician or someone acting under the supervision of a qualified physician. He or she ensures the adequacy of the pharmacovigilance system and full compliance with meeting regulatory obligations and timelines for safety reporting. Therefore, the QPPV must be very experienced in clinical trial safety as well as safety regulations, compliance, and policy. The QPPV oversees the pharmacovigilance plan development and proactive risk minimization strategies. He or she is the single point of contact for safety with the regulatory authorities.

Pharmacovigilance/Drug Safety Product Manager

The pharmacovigilance or drug safety product manager (DSPM) is an experienced member of the pharmacovigilance department assigned to oversee specific safety products, usually when large numbers of safety staff are required. Examples of projects requiring a DSPM include studies with large numbers of SAEs, case reports, studies with clinical endpoints that are also SAEs, projects involving a number of different safety functions (e.g. case reporting and regulatory submission, literature review, and aggregate reporting), and other safety projects of special interest. A DSPM may also organize and coordinate DSMBs and CECs, utilizing key opinion leaders and medical and statistical experts.

Drug Safety Associate

The role of a DSA is to monitor and track SAEs, serious and non-serious ADRs, and other medically related product information. It is paramount to ensure the timely processing and reporting of such information in accordance with company and regulatory reporting timelines. The DSA usually has an educational background in one of the life sciences; it is also advantageous to have a working knowledge of medical terminology. Many DSAs are nurses, pharmacists, or other allied health professionals. The DSA works under the supervision of the DSPM, director of drug safety, QPPV, or medical monitor.

Some of the other functions performed by the DSA include, but are not limited to, developing safety plans and other SSPs; providing input to and reviewing study safety tracking reports for accuracy and quality; maintaining electronic and paper files; assisting the medical monitor with the documentation and processing of routine exceptions and rescreen approvals; performing safety review of clinical [case report forms (CRFs)] and patient laboratory data; liaising with sponsors, investigational sites, and/or reporters regarding safety issues; and participating in project team meetings and teleconferences.

Medical Assistant

The medical assistant plays an important role in maintaining efficient and accurate organization of documents and information within the department by providing administrative support to the pharmacovigilance team. Duties of the medical assistant include filing; faxing; assisting with the planning and organization of meetings, teleconferences, and training sessions; maintaining meeting minutes; handling mailing activities; answering SAE hotline and other departmental telephone lines; documenting contacts and submitting to appropriate personnel; maintaining office supplies and equipment; creating, maintaining and auditing work tracking systems; and ensuring accuracy and audit readiness of the departmental files and file room. In some cases, medical assistants may be trained as data entry personnel and can assist in the data entry of safety information into appropriate safety databases.

Safety Systems Specialists

Owing to the large amounts of data involved, numerous databases and technology systems are required to manage the daily workflow associated with pharmacovigilance, including individual case management and aggregate data analysis. This requires staff who have backgrounds in information technology (IT). In some cases, these staff are further specialized in the creation, validation, and maintenance specifically of safety systems. In smaller companies, the safety systems specialist may be part of the IT department, assigned as needed to support pharmacovigilance.

151

Pharmacovigilance Trainer

In the current dynamic environment surrounding pharmacovigilance and risk management, ongoing training for pharmacovigilance staff is essential to maintain awareness of current global and local regulations, policies, and guidelines. Pharmacovigilance training includes subject matter training on the therapeutic area of the product under development and specific training on the science related to the investigational product. Often the medical monitor or an expert in another therapeutic area supplies this training. Training related specifically to pharmacovigilance is continuous, with more senior staff reviewing and mentoring the junior staff. Beyond a certain size, however, staff specifically dedicated to performing pharmacovigilance training is usually necessary. All training should be documented and filed appropriately. Pharmacovigilance staff should be "audit ready" in terms of their knowledge of the rules, regulations, SOPs, and confidentiality requirements surrounding the specific protocol or project, as well as safety reporting requirements and general confidentiality requirements regarding clinical research subjects and their data.

APPROPRIATE FACILITIES FOR PHARMACOVIGILANCE

No specific requirements exist for the physical structure of a pharmacovigilance department. However, it is imperative that all subject data be kept confidential, and that there is adequate storage area with appropriate security, limited data access, and adequate disaster recovery. Infrastructure that enables documenting receipt and forwarding of time-sensitive safety information must be in place. It is crucial that unblinded safety information is not accessible to staff who must remain blinded during the clinical trial. This may be achieved through physical separation or through appropriate security measures for system and data access.

Although not required by regulation in most countries, many pharmacovigilance departments maintain a 24 hour emergency telephone system to allow prompt interaction with the investigative sites in fatal or life-threatening situations and to facilitate expedited case assessment and reporting. In the EU, a QPPV must be readily available at all times for any crisis situation.

SAFETY DATABASES

A safety database allows the pharmacovigilance department to monitor, assess, and report to the regulatory authorities serious safety information. The utilization of any specific safety system is not a direct legal requirement. However, under most circumstances, a more powerful database is needed, therefore the use of safety databases is currently standard. Specifically developed commercial safety databases are available. The database owner may maintain the system on their servers or install the full system on a company server and allow access through licenses. Alternatively, access to a safety database can be provided though a CRO or safety niche provider. This may be a more attractive solution financially for limited case volumes.

The database must be validated (e.g. CFR 21 compliant) and acceptable to all regulatory authorities on the global level. A recently established requirement is to have the capability for reporting expedited cases electronically. The specifications for electronic reporting are detailed in ICH E2B. Such an "E2B compliant" gateway allows direct export of such expedited cases to the authorities' databases such as EudraVigilance in Europe. For smaller companies not having their own safety database, expedited cases may be entered directly (manually) into any authority database. In the USA, electronic safety reporting is not yet mandatory.

SAFETY CASE PROCESSING AND REVIEW

Most commercial safety databases provide the functionality of a paperless workflow, allowing all case processing steps to be performed within the system. The company's process should be

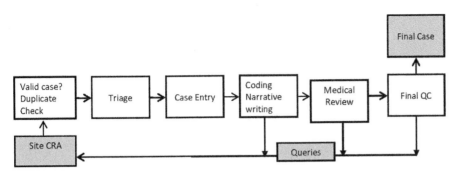

FIGURE 13.6

Example of a serious adverse event case processing workflow within a safety database. CRA: clinical research associate; QC: quality control.

described in an SOP available to auditors. Even if no safety database is used, the case processing workflow should always be detailed in an SOP, SSP, or safety plan to ensure clear assignment of roles and responsibilities. This is especially important when various steps in the workflow are distributed among different global locations. Updating cases as new information is obtained requires a clear audit trail to all prior information.

An example of such a workflow is depicted in Figure 13.6.

Steps in Serious Adverse Event Case Processing

1. When an investigator, healthcare provider, or clinical site monitor identifies a potential SAE, the event is reported to the sponsor immediately.
2. Upon receipt of an SAE at the pharmacovigilance department, the report is assessed as to whether it fulfills the minimum requirements for reporting.
3. A valid case is checked for duplication, i.e. whether the same case was previously reported, or whether this is follow-up information on a previously opened case.
4. If the case is identified as valid for initial data entry, it will undergo a triage step, being reviewed for expectedness, relatedness, and seriousness, with special attention as to whether the case is fatal or life threatening. This determines the appropriate timeline for processing and reporting to the regulatory authorities.
5. The case then undergoes data entry, a case narrative is created and the case undergoes medical review. Any missing or unclear information is queried and added to the case.
6. Once all of these activities are completed and quality checked, the case is finalized within the allotted timeframe and if expedited reporting is required the information is sent to the appropriate recipients.
7. The process is repeated as additional information becomes available until the event is resolved or no further information can be obtained.

GLOBAL SAFETY REPORTING

Since the main objective of pharmacovigilance is the identification of information that may affect the safety of patients, once a potential risk is noted, it must be communicated to all stakeholders. The distribution follows well-defined rules described in ICH E2A: Clinical Safety Data Management: Definitions and Standards for Expedited Reporting. According to ICH E2A,

All adverse drug reactions (ADRs) that are both serious and unexpected (SUSARs = Suspected Unexpected Serious Adverse Reactions) are subject to expedited reporting. This applies to reports from spontaneous sources and from any type of clinical or epidemiological investigation, independent of design or purpose.

Initial reports should be submitted within the prescribed timeframe providing the following minimum criteria are met:

- an identifiable patient
- a suspect medicinal product
- an identifiable reporting source, and
- an event or outcome that can be identified as serious and unexpected, and for which, in clinical investigation cases, there is a reasonable suspected causal relationship.

During global clinical trials, a SUSAR that occurs in one country may require expedited reporting to regulatory authorities, institutional review boards/ethics committees, and investigators in all participating countries. This must be done in accordance with each country's local laws and regulations. Unfortunately, countries vary in their requirements as to the format and timeframe for the reporting of cases. In addition, reporting requirements are frequently changing at the country level.

Keeping aware of the reporting requirements in various countries is a time-consuming task, which requires staff that fully understand the global pharmacovigilance reporting requirements. There are commercial databases available to provide up-to-date regulatory reporting intelligence. In some companies staff within the pharmacovigilance department perform safety regulatory reporting; this may be part of the electronic workflow. In other companies a team that is part of the regulatory department may perform this activity.

SAFETY DATA REVIEW AND ASSESSMENT

During a clinical trial, safety data will be collected from a number of different sources. These include the subject CRF, laboratory reports, SAE reports, and information specific to a particular study or therapeutic area such as electrocardiographic or radiographic imaging data. All safety data should be reviewed in an ongoing manner with the intent of minimizing risk to the participating and future subjects, and determining whether the benefit exceeds the risk if the product becomes commercially available (i.e. whether the product is safe enough for general use). This is done through the combined processes of individual subject data assessment and aggregate data review and assessment.

Individual Subject Data

The scope of individual data review begins with information on the subject CRFs. Screening and baseline information such as demographics, significant past medical history, concomitant diseases and medications, and prior treatment regimens are recorded and become part of the clinical database for the study. Laboratory and other ancillary information are also collected. Prior to the start of each study, alert triggers are determined in order to flag potential safety issues, and criteria for withholding or discontinuing treatment due to adverse events are written into the study protocol. When a subject experiences a serious adverse event or a safety alert is triggered, all available safety information on that subject should be reviewed in order to minimize harm to the subject under study.

Subject Profiles

Reviewing individual subject data effectively requires that either repetitive data cuts be reviewed or the pharmacovigilance staff must be able to look at cumulative data in real time. Commercial tools are available which enable cumulative data to be reviewed for each individual subject as well as in aggregate. Figure 13.7 shows an example of a subject profile depicting temporal information between an adverse event (vertigo), the receipt of medications, and selected laboratory results. An individual subject's safety parameters can be reviewed in context throughout his participation in the study. This helps to ensure maximum safety monitoring of individual subjects.

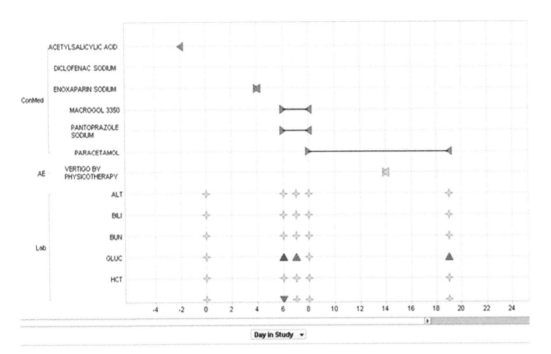

FIGURE 13.7

Subject profile. *Source: TIBCO Spotfire.* (Please refer to color plate section)

Review of Aggregate Data

The scope and timing of aggregate data review activities vary among clinical trials. These should be determined before the start of the study. Parameters to be determined include the objectives of the review; data fields to be reviewed; the frequency of the review; the process for raising, monitoring, and resolving queries generated; and how the review and any findings will be documented.

The main safety objective of ongoing review is the timely identification of potential safety issues. Other objectives may include identifying subjects included in a study inappropriately who may be placed at unintentional risk, or other systemic protocol violations that may be recurring. Aggregate data review may also identify training needed at sites or by the clinical study team in order to minimize subject risk, which may occur owing to unclear or misinterpreted direction in the protocol.

Review of aggregate data may be done in-house or by an external and independent team of experts such as a DSMB or data monitoring committee (DMC). If a DSMB or DMC is used, pharmacovigilance staff are often involved in the organization of the data along with an assigned (unblinded) statistician. Figure 13.8 shows an example of a decision tree for the use of a DSMB for a clinical trial.

Signal Detection and Analysis

The WHO defines a safety signal as reported information on a possible causal relationship between an adverse event and a drug, the relationship being unknown or incompletely documented previously.[1] When a signal is detected, further investigation is warranted to determine whether an actual causal relationship exists.

Signal detection uses data imports from the safety database or other clinical, laboratory, or epidemiological databases, as well as regulatory data sources. A compliant and suitable safety database should be able to process data related to signal detection. Signals can be suggested by alerts or trends in incoming data.

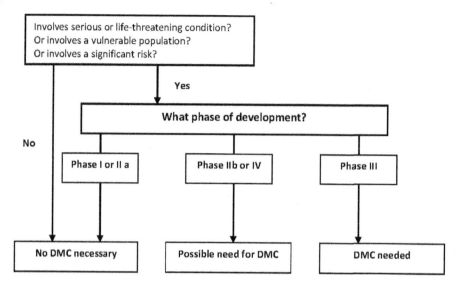

FIGURE 13.8

Decision tree for the use of a data safety monitoring board (DSMB, DMC) for a clinical trial. *Source: Day, S. (2010). Data monitoring committees — not for the faint-hearted. Pharmacovigilance Review 4(2), 9—12.*

Signals can also be identified by major statistical algorithms and advanced analysis in conjunction with biostatistics. Commercial tools are also available for data mining and signal detection and analysis. Signal detection consists of several activities:

- Signal detection tools:
  - single case evaluation, including literature surveillance
  - aggregate report creation
  - software tools for large case volumes and trend analysis
- Signal generation/detection procedure:
  - permanent monitoring of single case reports/report series
  - periodic report review
  - ad hoc analysis of reports from external sources, e.g. literature reports, requests from competent authorities (CAs) on report/reports
- Signal work-up and documentation:
  - quality of the information
  - other risk factors (e.g. natural history of the underlying disease/severity, specificity and outcome)
  - biological and pharmaceutical plausibility
  - class effect
  - epidemiological context
  - frequency
  - drug utilization/population exposure/age, gender and indication
- Signal assessment and documentation:
  - QPPV or other senior pharmacovigilance involvement/decision
    - signal not confirmed (no further actions, only documentation)
    - signal doubtful (special scrutiny for future cases)
    - signal confirmed.

Upon confirmation of a safety signal, the subsequent course will be variable but may involve action by company executives and/or the regulatory authorities, depending on the magnitude of risk. It is important that action is taken promptly in order to avoid any unnecessary harm; therefore, an ongoing and systematic approach is essential.

For safety findings that have low or minimal safety impact, these will be reported in the clinical study report (clinical trials), in updates to the investigator brochure, in the core data sheet, or in periodic safety update reports required by the regulatory authorities. The conclusion of any update report must comment on any new safety issue. Reports may be written within the pharmacovigilance department or by a medical writing team, with input from pharmacovigilance staff. In the case of marketed products, changes to labeling may be required. All of this is part of the communication of any safety risk to those who might use the product.

MANAGING RISK

Consequences of finding a significant safety issue may include any of the following activities:

- Amending the protocol
- Temporarily suspending enrollment
- Discontinuing the study
- Discontinuing development of the medicinal product
- Implementing a development risk management plan (RMP) or risk evaluation and mitigation strategy (REMS).

Risk management represents the top of the pharmacovigilance activity pyramid (Figure 13.9). These activities are the culmination of the processing and review of individual adverse events and other safety data, the review and assessment of aggregated data, and the identification, analysis, and interpretation of safety signals.

Risk Management Plans and Risk Evaluation and Mitigation Strategies

The RMP (EU) and the REMS (USA) are now a standard part of pharmacovigilance planning. ICH E2E (Pharmacovigilance Planning) was originally created to achieve consistency and harmonization, particularly during the early postmarketing period of medicinal products. Within the past few years, the US and European regulatory agencies have increased their guidance on benefit risk assessment and risk minimization.

157

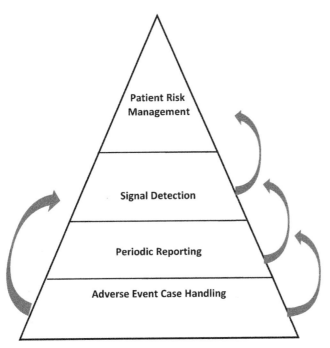

FIGURE 13.9
Pharmacovigilance activity pyramid. (Please refer to color plate section)

The intent of both the RMP and the REMS is to minimize risks related to a medicinal product through interventions and to communicate those risks to patients and healthcare providers. Elements may include medication guides or patient package inserts, a detailed communication plan about safety issues, specific elements to assure safe use of a product such as required laboratory testing or prescriber training, an implementation plan and a timetable for assessment.

Currently, the RMP or REMS may be created at any time during clinical development, but most often they are submitted as part of the marketing application. In the EU, RMPs are routinely required as part of the detailed description of the pharmacovigilance system. In the USA, the regulatory authorities can request a plan if there is a reason to suspect that one may be necessary, based upon non-clinical data, early use data, class data for the medicinal compound, or other factors.

If new safety information becomes available after regulatory approval, the regulatory authorities may request a REMS or an updated RMP. Additional pharmacovigilance such as active surveillance, other clinical or epidemiological trials, specialized training, or restricted access may be included in the plan. The activities must be sufficient to minimize the likelihood of harm so that benefits still outweigh risks, and to ensure that the risk reduction procedures are communicated and implemented.

OUTSOURCING WHILE BUILDING PHARMACOVIGILANCE CAPACITY

Large, global pharmaceutical companies usually have well-established pharmacovigilance systems. In countries where pharmacovigilance is not well established there may be a need to build pharmacovigilance capacity. For example, some companies only have medical affairs departments whose function is mainly to provide medical input to marketing strategy and ensure that product literature and marketing brochures meet legal and ethical requirements. They lack the capacity for complete, product life-cycle pharmacovigilance and risk management. To have a complete and systematic approach to pharmacovigilance requires the ability to perform all of the defined pharmacovigilance activities. Outsourcing some aspects of pharmacovigilance to a CRO or safety niche equivalent while building internal capacity may be an option.

Worldwide pharmacovigilance can be centralized in a few regions, or hubs, if the systems are global and there is good communication and process flow between regions. Some of the functions may be competently performed in low-cost regions. If outsourcing, sponsors must ensure that any vendors performing pharmacovigilance and risk management have the experience and capacity to perform those services, and that they are sufficiently knowledgeable in the regulations associated with pharmacovigilance.

Outsourcing those functions best performed by pharmacovigilance experts such as signal detection, aggregate data interpretation, and risk evaluation and mitigation, requires careful selection of vendors. Many CROs are able to provide complete safety services and resources, acting as a smaller company's pharmacovigilance department permanently or until such time as the company is able to manage the expense on its own. These services include performing safety audits; creation of SOPs and SSPs; medical and safety monitoring; individual case management; creating and maintaining pharmacovigilance databases; signal detection; trend analysis; organizing and managing DSMBs, DMCs, and CECs; and reporting of expedited and periodic safety reports to regulatory authorities, principal investigators, and institutional review boards.

GENERAL CONSIDERATIONS AND CONCLUSIONS

Pharmacovigilance and risk management are an essential part of pharmaceutical product development and commercialization, the activities of which are highly regulated in many parts of the world. Rare adverse events may not be identified until large numbers of patients receive the product, so pharmacovigilance and risk management must extend throughout the product's life cycle. Benefit and risk must be continually assessed as more is learned about the product through its use. Building pharmacovigilance and risk management capacity requires a systematic approach to ensure that all safety aspects are monitored and addressed properly. Since capacity building takes time and resources, outsourcing of certain activities may enable capacity building to proceed before all capabilities can be done in-house. The use of a limited number of safety centers is a viable and cost-effective option, provided there are good processes, good tools, and good communication of responsibilities and events.

References

1. World Health Organization. *The Importance of Pharmacovigilance: Safety Monitoring of Medicinal Products.* Geneva: WHO, http://apps.who.int/medicinedocs/pdf/s4893e/s4893e.pdf; 2002.

2. European Commission. *Assessment of the European Community System of Pharmacovigilance: Final Report — Final version, January 25. Submitted by Fraunhofer Institute Systems and Innovation Research, Karlsruhe, Germany, to the European Commission Enterprise and Industry Directorate-General, Unit F2, Pharmaceuticals,* http://ec.europa.eu/enterprise/pharmaceuticals/pharmacovigilance/docs/acs_consultation_final.pdf; 2006.

3. Nwokike J. *Technical Assistance for the Establishment of a Pharmacovigilance and Medicine Safety System in Rwanda. Submitted to the US Agency for International Development by the Strengthening Pharmaceutical Systems (SPS) Program.* Arlington, VA: Management Sciences for Health; 2009.

4. US Food and Drug Administration. 21 CFR Parts 312 and 320, Final Rule: Investigational New Drug Safety Reporting Requirements for Human Drug and Biological Products and Safety Reporting Requirements for Bioavailability and Bioequivalence Studies in Humans, http://www.fda.gov/Drugs/DevelopmentApprovalProcess/HowDrugsareDevelopedandApproved/ApprovalApplications/InvestigationalNewDrugINDApplication/ucm226358.htm.

Electronic Data Capture

CHAPTER 14

Setting Up Electronic Data Capture Capabilities

Yaw Asare-Aboagye
United Therapeutics, Durham, NC, USA

163

INTRODUCTION

Today's changing economic and political environments, coupled with the rising cost of clinical trials in the USA and Europe, are factors driving pharmaceutical companies to explore newer countries for research and development activities. Many pharmaceutical companies are looking beyond the traditional model of conducting studies in the USA, Japan, and Western Europe, and are increasingly taking advantage of the lower costs and the abundance of treatment-naïve populations in Eastern Europe, Asia, South America and, more recently, sub-Saharan Africa. In 2008, 80 percent of approved marketing applications for drugs and biologicals contained data from foreign clinical trials and more than half of the clinical trial subjects and sites were located outside the USA.[1] The US Food and Drug Administration (FDA) notes that based on the increase in foreign clinical investigators conducting trials on investigational new drugs (INDs) over the past 10 years and observations of FDA reviewers, sponsors' reliance on foreign clinical trials for FDA-regulated drugs and biologicals is likely to grow.[1] A review of the clinicaltrials.gov website, the global registry of clinical trials, in March 2011, showed about 241 clinical trials sponsored by pharmaceutical companies being conducted in Africa.[2] The European and Developing Countries Clinical Trials Partnership (EDCTP) announced in June 2008 its intention to inject over €80 million into African medical research,

Global Clinical Trials Playbook. DOI: 10.1016/B978-0-12-415787-3.00014-X with a goal of providing resources for joint clinical trials, capacity building, and networking activities, as well as empowering Africans to take ownership of projects.[3] In 2009, Quintiles, a global contract research organization (CRO), opened its third African office in Accra, Ghana, "to improve efficiency and expand capacity to monitor the growing number of clinical studies being conducted in Western sub-Saharan Africa".[4]

Despite such initiatives, conducting clinical trials in some of these emerging countries, particularly in sub-Saharan Africa, continues to be a daunting task, but with careful planning, proper information technology (IT) enablement, and adequate training of site and research personnel, sponsors can ensure success for their trials. Even though the abundance of naïve patient populations appears to be one of the major drivers for the increase in global trials, the future of clinical trials in these emerging countries will depend not only on recruitment efficiencies but also, and perhaps largely, on the provision of quality data. Efforts are currently underway at the FDA to inspect more clinical trials in more countries, especially in countries where good clinical practice standards have only recently been adopted.[1]

THE ROLE OF DATA MANAGEMENT IN CLINICAL TRIALS

Data management is an essential component of all clinical trials. The accuracy of the trial's results will ultimately be determined by the quality of the collected data, and how it conforms to 21 CFR Part 11 and other FDA and International Conference on Harmonisation (ICH) guidelines. The primary role of the data managers therefore is to ensure that data are of the highest possible integrity as well as ensuring that data collection methods and processes do not cause any delays to the availability of data for analysis. It is very important to solicit input from data management during the protocol development stage to avoid collection of duplicate data that may lead to numerous reconciliation issues.

Data managers have several responsibilities, including:

- design, validation, and release of the database for production work
- development of data capture tools, data entry procedures, data cleaning, and data review procedures
- development of procedures for ensuring data quality throughout the study
- management of dictionaries for coding adverse events
- integration of data from external sources, such as laboratories
- safety procedures, including reconciliation of serious adverse events
- locking of the database and production of datasets for statistical analysis
- training of staff and research personnel throughout the duration of the study.

In global trials involving many countries, the traditional "paper" method of data acquisition is too costly and inefficient for several reasons. Shipping and handling costs may become prohibitive, especially if there are several amendments to the protocol that necessitates the development of new case report forms (CRFs). To ensure quality data in global clinical trials, the use of electronic data capture (EDC) is highly recommended. This author has seen a steady decrease in EDC pricing compared to paper since 2002, yielding significant savings in overall study costs and the savings will continue to increase as the EDC systems evolve and costs drop. In addition, suites of EDC software now combine tools for protocol authoring, study budgeting and contracting, clinical trials management system (CTMS), remote data monitoring, and source data verification. The goal of these EDC tools is to replace the paper-based process of study design and data capture with electronic systems that are very well integrated, facilitate study builds, expedite the availability of accurate data, and enhance ability to manage investigator sites. This chapter will discuss EDC systems for data management only. These systems have revolutionized data management in the past decade.

The Biostatistics and Data Management Technical Group of the Pharmaceutical Research and Manufacturers of America, PhRMA, in its position paper on electronic data capture, defines EDC as "a technique for collecting clinical trial data in such a way that they are delivered to the sponsor in electronic form instead of on paper".[5] PhRMA's position paper also recognizes that EDC can take many different forms, including the electronic laboratory data that are not re-entered by the sponsor, electronic diaries or patient-reported outcomes (ePRO), interactive voice response systems (IVRS), patient data captured directly by instrumentation, and data that are captured in an electronic version of the case report form (eCRF) and delivered electronically to the sponsor or sponsor's representative (such as a CRO) without a handwritten CRF.

EDC systems offer several advantages over the traditional "paper" method for all personnel involved in the study. Data entry is performed by site personnel at the site, a process that eliminates data transcription errors as well as illegible data, and, if the site is properly trained, ensures that data are made available to the sponsors within days of the patients' visits. The sites have immediate access to queries and, with proper training, can resolve queries with minimum involvement of the data managers. Clinical research associates (CRAs) can monitor data remotely and concentrate their efforts on sites that need help, which could lead to potential cost savings. A built-in dictionary system can automatically code adverse events, and external data such as laboratory results can be loaded into the system by an automated process. Overall, there is almost real-time availability of data to all members of the team, especially if investigator reimbursement is tied to the availability of data in the system.

The following features of an EDC system are desirable. The system should:

- support role-based eLearning for all staff, and be an easy-to-use, self-paced, fully integrated web learning tool, and be able to provide certification at the end of the training; users must be able to return to the eLearning module at any time during the study to retake any modules without disabling their accounts
- be fully web based, support any of the popular browsers (Microsoft Internet Explorer, Google Chrome, Safari, etc.), and not require any plug-ins
- provide intuitive navigation
- be able to adopt standards such as CDISC and CDASH
- support a flexible workflow and allow flexible data entry
- be capable of displaying role-based task lists
- time out a configurable time interval if left unattended
- be capable of sending notification and alert systems that are triggered by activity in the EDC system
- be able to send time-sensitive messages via e-mail to selected roles, both internally (sponsor and CRO staff) and externally (investigator site staff)
- support protocol amendments and multiple versions of the eCRFs, and not have to be taken offline to make changes
- provide simple, intuitive, ad hoc reporting tools in addition to a set of standardized reports
- be able to provide data on demand in multiple formats.

OPPORTUNITIES AND CHALLENGES WHEN OUTSOURCING DATA MANAGEMENT

Most pharmaceutical companies outsource data management activities for global studies to their CRO partners either as a function or as part of a full outsourcing model. Many CROs have very good geographical coverage and can provide realistic timelines for development activities, based on their experience and knowledge obtained from years of managing trials in these countries, or by having local offices staffed with local experts in regulatory guidelines. Outsourcing to CROs allows sponsor companies to manage large numbers of trials without having to increase internal resources. For global trials, especially in the emerging countries, it is the opinion of this author that some of the medium or smaller sized CROs may be better choices because they are more responsive and more flexible to changing priorities. Regardless of whether sponsors choose a large CRO or use a medium-sized CRO to manage global studies, it is very important to adopt an EDC strategy that optimizes both internal and external resources.

At the start of the sponsor– CRO relationship, it is very important to decide who should be the EDC system owner. For larger sponsors, it may be more cost-effective for the sponsor to be the system owner as they may be able to negotiate better pricing from the EDC vendor based on their volume of studies. The advantages of using the sponsor's EDC system include the ability to reuse the sponsor's library of eCRFs, custom-written functions, and edit checks, as well as having all the data in one location. The disadvantages to the sponsor include the increased investment for the installation, including the extensive testing and validation of the system. Smaller biotech companies, with just a few studies per year, may prefer to use the CRO as system owner so that they are not tied to costly long-term contracts with the EDC vendor. Alternatively, some EDC vendors allow sponsors to use the system on a study-by-study basis and provide study builds as a service.

The next crucial step is to decide which company's EDC process would be used for the study. In general, if all data management activities are to be performed by the CRO then using the CRO's standard operating procedures (SOPs) is considered best practice as most CROs have very well-defined processes in which they perform extremely well, but may fail if they are forced to use a different process. In such instances, the CRO's SOP should be carefully reviewed by the sponsor to clearly understand the EDC workflow and any areas of ambiguity should be clarified upfront to avoid unnecessary conflicts during the study. The team should:

- document roles and responsibilities for each company as well as individuals on the team
- clarify and publish the processes to be used, defining all terms so that they are understood by all parties
- set up metrics for performance management
- define an issue escalation process to be followed during the course of the study
- set up an executive oversight committee made up of senior management staff from both companies who will manage the relationship between sponsor and CRO.

To ensure quality oversight of the CRO when data management activities are fully outsourced, the data management team should include an EDC system programmer, a lead data manager, a statistical programmer, and an IT support person from the sponsor side. The lead data manager's role would be to lead the review and approval of all parts of the data management plan. The EDC system programmer would be responsible for reviewing and signing off on all technical decisions made in the design of the eCRFs and the flow of the database. The programmer would also, together with the lead data manager, review all test scripts that would be used for the user acceptance testing of the database before going live. Having participants from the sponsor side ensures that all procedures included in the design of the database are relevant. The role of the statistical programmer would be to test that data transfers can occur at the appropriate time. The IT support person ensures that all systems are compatible between the sponsor and CRO systems, and facilitates the creation of secure connections for data transfers, if necessary.

SETTING UP ELECTRONIC DATA CAPTURE CAPABILITIES IN AN EMERGING COUNTRY

The first step towards setting up EDC and of clinical data management capability is to create a data center in each of the regions where the trial is to be conducted to allow for rapid interaction between clinical trial staff and the data managers. These centers would be staffed by data management personnel with specialized training in EDC system processes. Each regional center would then be responsible for a group of neighboring countries. For example, a data center in Accra, Ghana, could be responsible for managing centers in West Africa. Support for research staff, including system and protocol training, would be supplemented by staff from these centers.

The next step is to assess the capabilities for EDC at each of the selected sites in each country. This should ideally be part of the feasibility study so as to develop a strategy for technology deployment. The assessments include determining the number and types of computers at each site, what versions of browsers are being used and what version of Microsoft Office or equivalent software is available. In most of sub-Saharan Africa, there may be the need to provide laptops, software, and mobile Internet connections to avoid disruption due to instability in electricity supply. Fortunately, Internet services in sub-Saharan Africa have improved dramatically in the past few years. According to www.speedtest.net, a website that compares and ranks consumer Internet download speeds around the globe, most of the sub-Saharan countries have speeds that are either similar to, or better than, Russia, China, India, Brazil, Mexico, and Argentina.

The final step is to provide training to the data center staff. For a new data center, it may be necessary to hire new personnel if experienced data managers are not readily available. A typical data manager or data programmer would have a college degree in quantitative science, nursing, or health science. The first set of training programs, the system training, will consist of the following:

- "EDC train the trainer" training: This training is for staff who will eventually become the trainers for the center. This will be a comprehensive two-week training program that covers all aspects of the EDC system for all roles. At the end of the training period, the new trainer will be able to train other users including data managers, CRA, and site coordinators and investigators.
- "EDC database build" training: This is a comprehensive training program that teaches staff how to use the EDC system to build a study based on the protocol. It is typically a five-day training program, depending on the EDC system selected followed by at least one week of practising database builds. At the end of this training, the trainee would be able to understand how the EDC system works, how to build an eCRF, how to develop an edit check, and how to manage a study.
- Becoming familiar with the SOPs: A list of recommended SOPs is provided at the end of this chapter (Appendix 1).
- How to get support from the EDC vendor.

Because the EDC system allows for direct entry of data by the investigator site staff, each member should be trained and given a separate user account. Study coordinators or other designated staff at the site will log into the system directly to enter data. The principal investigator also logs into the system to review patient data and to sign eCRFs to confirm that the data are correct. All users should be educated on the need to not share their usernames and passwords, as required in 21 CFR Part 11.

GOOD CLINICAL DATA MANAGEMENT PRACTICES

Good data management practices begin with the development of a good data management plan. The plan, which should be version controlled and signed by at least one member of the clinical operations team as well as data management, should include plans for developing the eCRF, the edit checks specifications, data specifications and plans for collecting external data, plans for locking the database, and specifications for the delivery of data to biostatistics for analysis. The plan should be started at the beginning of the study and updated throughout the study if the plans change. eCRFs must be developed to collect data specified in the protocol only and care must be taken to avoid collecting duplicate information as this invariably leads to reconciliation issues. Whenever possible, data must be collected in coded form by providing a pick list in the eCRFs and care must be taken to avoid excessive use of free text fields. Care must be taken when using some of the "fancy" functionality of the EDC systems, such as the "dynamic" fields in form design, as these usually confuse the sites. If dynamic fields are used, this should be emphasized during training so that the sites truly understand it. Form designers must be aware of data privacy laws in each of the jurisdictions where the study will be conducted and must adopt a policy that meets the strictest guidelines in any of the regions represented. A good rule is to design data collection forms with the minimum subject identifiers and to educate all study personnel who handle personally identifiable data on company procedures.

APPENDIX 1
Selected Standard Operating Procedures for Electronic Data Capture Systems

The following SOPs have been recommended by PhRMA:[5]

- EDC preparation of investigator site
- EDC set-up process
- EDC set-up testing
- EDC installation procedures
- EDC help-desk process
- EDC training process
- EDC user access
- EDC data migration
- EDC site monitoring
- EDC change control
- EDC disaster recovery
- EDC records retention
- EDC study/server closedown
- EDC postclosure changes.

APPENDIX 2
Sample Job Description: Systems Associate

CDM Systems Associate
This position supports Clinical Data Management systems and provides custom data listings and reports to the study team.

Qualifications:
Bachelor's degree or equivalent in life science, computer science or related discipline, or equivalent combination of education and experience.

Responsibilities/Key activities
Responsible for one or more of the following activities:
- Configuring and supporting EDC systems for all CDM activities
- Defining studies in clinical databases
- Defining standards for external datasets/loading electronic datasets into EDC system
- Providing programming support for CDM activities
- Maintaining case report form standards
- Supporting data management systems activities for electronic submissions to regulatory agencies
- Developing/providing EDC system and study training for end users

- Executing formal testing of all purchased or developed software for data management
- Maintaining library of all objects used in database builds in a global library
- Managing third party vendors such as CROs, EDC vendors, and local/central laboratories on defined data standards, content specifications, and timelines for deliverables
- Participating in DM system selection, evaluation, and implementation

Experience
Minimum of 4 years' experience in data management and programming, with knowledge in:
- Drug development and clinical trial processes
- Data management processes
- Good clinical practices
- Programming in SAS, SQL, etc.
- Project management

Key Competencies:
- Effective communication and collaboration skills
- Problem-solving skills
- Attention to detail

APPENDIX 3
Sample Job Description: Manager, Clinical Data Management

Manager, Clinical Data Management
This position is responsible for the day-to-day data management activities supporting clinical trials, including working with external vendors and external business partners.

Qualifications:
Bachelor's degree or equivalent in natural/life science or related discipline, or equivalent combination of education and experience.

Responsibilities/Key activities
- Responsible for data management deliverables for all clinical studies to ensure timely delivery and high data quality
- Participates in developing standards, SOPs, and working practice
- Participates in DM system selection, evaluation, and implementation
- Participates in DM vendor selection
- Oversees development of data management plans including eCRF specifications, edit specifications, and plans for the flow and management of external data
- Oversees data management activities of external business partners, such as CROs
- Management of internal and external staff; identifies resources needed to meet new project demands
- Maintains awareness of global regulatory developments relevant to data management of clinical trials and ensures that staff and colleagues are kept informed
- Direct responsibility for providing budgetary input on projects and managing budgets

Experience
- Minimum of 8 years' experience in data management
- Hands-on experience with an EDC system
- Knowledge of regulatory requirements related to clinical data management and systems

Key Competencies:
- Excellent project management skills
- Ability to work in a fast-paced, team-oriented environment

169

- Excellent verbal and written communication skills
- Attention to detail
- Knowledge of clinical study design, basic statistics, and SAS programming a plus

APPENDIX 4
Sample Data Capture Standard Operating Procedure

SOP Number: CDM-0001	Version 00	Title Design, Review and Approval of Electronic Case Report Forms (eCRF)		
Status Approved	Supersedes XX	Effective Date		Page X of Y

APPROVALS

Author	Title	Print Name	Signature	Date
Approver	CDM Systems Associate			
Approver	Clinical Data Manager			
Approver				
Approver				

1.0 Purpose

    1.1 This standard operating procedure (SOP) outlines the process for the review and approval of electronic case report forms (eCRFs) used to capture clinical trial data. The eCRF review and approval process establishes procedures to ensure eCRFs accurately represent the clinical trial data collection objectives of the associated protocol.

2.0 Scope

    2.1 This SOP applies to all clinical studies conducted by, or on behalf of (Company Name) on either investigational or marketed products for which the results may be submitted to regulatory agencies.

3.0 Definitions

    3.1 Electronic Case Report Form (eCRF): Electronic document designed to record all protocol-required information to be reported to the sponsor on each trial subject.

    3.2 eCRF Designer: Clinical data management system associate or any member of the data management team designated to design or review the eCRF for a study.

    3.3 eCRF Reviewer(s): Study team members or designees who are assigned the responsibilities of reviewing the draft eCRF. The reviewers include the Study Manager, Clinical Data Manager, and Statistical Programmer.

4.0 Responsibilities

    4.1 The Clinical Data manager is responsible for

        4.1.1 Initiating, reviewing and approving eCRF specifications

    4.2 The eCRF Developer is responsible for

        4.2.1 Developing, reviewing and approving eCRF specifications

        4.2.2 Developing (and/or revising) the eCRFs using approved eCRF specifications and existing library of eCRFs

        4.2.3 Obtaining approval and signing off on the draft eCRF

4.3 The eCRF Reviewers are responsible for

    4.3.1 Reviewing and approving eCRF specifications

    4.3.2 Reviewing and approving final eCRFs.

5.0 Procedure

  5.1 The Clinical Data Manager initiates the eCRF development specifications upon the availability of the schedule of assessments. This process can run concurrently with the protocol development.

  5.2 The eCRF Designer develops the eCRF specifications for review and approval by the study team. The final schedule of events must be available before the eCRF specifications can be signed off.

  5.3 The Clinical Data Manager reviews the eCRF specifications to ensure that they accurately support the following:

    5.3.1 Protocol objectives

    5.3.2 Capture of all applicable data points.

  5.4 The Clinical Data Manager works with the eCRF designer to ensure the accuracy of the specification document and signs off on the document for database build to begin.

  5.5 Using the approved specifications document, the eCRF Designer develops the eCRFs.

  5.6 Once the final protocol is approved, the Data Manager and the eCRF Designer perform a final review of the eCRF specifications document and the final protocol to determine if any changes are needed.

    5.6.1 If changes are needed, the specification document is updated and communicated to the study team, as necessary.

  5.7 Once the final eCRF specification document is approved, the eCRF Designer completes the eCRF development and notifies the Clinical Data Manager.

  5.8 The Clinical Data Manager either schedules a meeting for a group review and approval of the eCRFs or notifies the eCRF Reviewers to review the eCRFs online.

  5.9 The eCRF Reviewers review the eCRFs (either separately or together) and provide feedback to the Clinical Data Manager and the eCRF Designer.

    5.9.1 If changes need to be made to the eCRFs, the Data Manager updates and signs the eCRF specifications document and the eCRF Designer makes the necessary changes to the eCRF. This step will continue until no further changes are needed.

    5.9.2 If there are no changes, the eCRF reviewers, the Clinical Data Manager and the eCRF Designer sign the eCRF Approval Form.

6.0 Revisions to an eCRF

  6.1 Once the eCRF is finalized, the eCRF version is saved in the EDC system and released into the production.

  6.2 If further changes to the eCRF are needed during the course of the study (e.g. due to a protocol amendment), the procedure described from Section 5.0 should be followed.

7.0 Attachments and forms

Attachment Number	Attachment Title

Form Number	Form Title
xxx.yyy.1	Sample eCRF Approval Form
xxx.yyy.2	Sample eCRF Specification Document

8.0 Revision history

Change Number	Description

References

1. Department of Health and Human Services. (June 2010). *Challenges to FDA's ability to monitor and inspect foreign clinical trials.* http://oig.hhs.gov/oei/reports/oei-01-08-00510.pdf [accessed 03.11]

2. http://www.clinicaltrials.gov [accessed 03.11]

3. Clinical trials in Africa receive funding boost. http://www.scidev.net/en/news/clinical-trials-in-africa-receive-funding-boost.html [accessed 03.11]

4. Quintiles increases capacity to manage clinical studies for diseases including malaria, HIV and tuberculosis. http://www.medicalnewstoday.com/releases/154314.php [accessed 03.11].

5. Clinical Trial EDC Task Group of PhRMA Biostatistics & Data Management Technical Group. Electronic Clinical Data Capture. (May 1, 2005). *Position Paper, Revision, 1.*

Ethics, Human Resources, and Intellectual Property

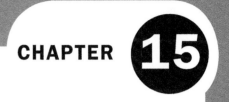

CHAPTER 15

Ethics and Institutional Review Board Capacity Building

Richard Chin
Institute for OneWorld Health and UCSF School of Medicine, San Francisco,
California, USA

175

Some of the material in this chapter is based on or excepted with permission from Chin and Lee's Principles and Practice of Clinical Trial Medicine[4] and Chin and Bairu's Global Clinical Trials.[5]

BACKGROUND

Conducting clinical trials is an inherently risky endeavor. Patients are treated with drugs of unknown efficacy and safety. In some cases, they are treated with drugs of unknown efficacy or with placebo when efficacious treatments are available. Enrollment in a clinical trial involves the risks of additional procedures in most cases. In addition, patients in a clinical trial are treated not with the intent of improving their own individual health or welfare but for the benefit of other patients who may receive therapies that are developed on the basis of the clinical trials.

The above important facets of clinical research, combined with ethics disasters in the past involving human research, including the Nazi war experiments, the Tuskegee experiment, and Japanese Unit 731 war experiments, have led to a host of guidelines, declarations, and laws being developed to protect patients' safety and rights. These are specified by the Declaration of Helsinki, the Council for International Organizations of Medical Sciences (CIOMS) international ethical

Global Clinical Trials Playbook. DOI: 10.1016/B978-0-12-415787-3.00015-1

guidelines for biomedical research involving human subjects, the Belmont Report, International Conference on Harmonisation (ICH) guidelines, the Nuremberg Code, and others.[1,2]

ETHICAL GUIDELINES

NUREMBERG CODE

1. The voluntary consent of the human subject is absolutely essential. This means that the person involved should have legal capacity to give consent; should be so situated as to be able to exercise free power of choice, without the intervention of any element of force, fraud, deceit, duress, over-reaching, or other ulterior form of constraint or coercion; and should have sufficient knowledge and comprehension of the elements of the subject matter involved as to enable him to make an understanding and enlightened decision. This latter element requires that before the acceptance of an affirmative decision by the experimental subject there should be made known to him the nature, duration, and purpose of the experiment; the method and means by which it is to be conducted; all inconveniences and hazards reasonable to be expected; and the effects upon his health or person which may possibly come from his participation in the experiment.
   The duty and responsibility for ascertaining the quality of the consent rests upon each individual who initiates, directs or engages in the experiment. It is a personal duty and responsibility which may not be delegated to another with impunity.
2. The experiment should be such as to yield fruitful results for the good of society, unprocurable by other methods or means of study, and not random and unnecessary in nature.
3. The experiment should be so designed and based on the results of animal experimentation and knowledge of the natural history of the disease or other problem under study that the anticipated results will justify the performance of the experiment.
4. The experiment should be so conducted as to avoid all unnecessary physical and mental suffering and injury.
5. No experiment should be conducted where there is an a priori reason to believe that death or disabling injury will occur; except, perhaps, in those experiments where the experimental physicians also serve as subjects.
6. The degree of risk to be taken should never exceed that determined by the humanitarian importance of the problem to be solved by the experiment.
7. Proper preparations should be made and adequate facilities provided to protect the experimental subject against even remote possibilities of injury, disability, or death.
8. The experiment should be conducted only by scientifically qualified persons. The highest degree of skill and care should be required through all stages of the experiment of those who conduct or engage in the experiment.
9. During the course of the experiment the human subject should be at liberty to bring the experiment to an end if he has reached the physical or mental state where continuation of the experiment seems to him to be impossible.
10. During the course of the experiment the scientist in charge must be prepared to terminate the experiment at any stage, if he has probable cause to believe, in the exercise of the good faith, superior skill and careful judgment required of him that a continuation of the experiment is likely to result in injury, disability, or death to the experimental subject.

From the National Institutes of Health.

DECLARATION OF HELSINKI

Adopted by the 18th World Medical Association (WMA) General Assembly, Helsinki, Finland, June 1964, and amended by the:

29th WMA General Assembly, Tokyo, Japan, October 1975
35th WMA General Assembly, Venice, Italy, October 1983
41st WMA General Assembly, Hong Kong, September 1989
48th WMA General Assembly, Somerset West, South Africa, October 1996
52nd WMA General Assembly, Edinburgh, Scotland, October 2000

53rd WMA General Assembly, Washington, DC, USA, October 2002
(Note of Clarification on paragraph 29 added)
55th WMA General Assembly, Tokyo, Japan, October 2004
(Note of Clarification on Paragraph 30 added)
59th WMA General Assembly, Seoul, Korea, October 2008

A. Introduction

1. The World Medical Association (WMA) has developed the Declaration of Helsinki as a statement of ethical principles for medical research involving human subjects, including research on identifiable human material and data.
   The Declaration is intended to be read as a whole and each of its constituent paragraphs should not be applied without consideration of all other relevant paragraphs.
2. Although the Declaration is addressed primarily to physicians, the WMA encourages other participants in medical research involving human subjects to adopt these principles.
3. It is the duty of the physician to promote and safeguard the health of patients, including those who are involved in medical research. The physician's knowledge and conscience are dedicated to the fulfillment of this duty.
4. The Declaration of Geneva of the WMA binds the physician with the words, "The health of my patient will be my first consideration", and the International Code of Medical Ethics declares that, "A physician shall act in the patient's best interest when providing medical care".
5. Medical progress is based on research that ultimately must include studies involving human subjects. Populations that are underrepresented in medical research should be provided appropriate access to participation in research.
6. In medical research involving human subjects, the well-being of the individual research subject must take precedence over all other interests.
7. The primary purpose of medical research involving human subjects is to understand the causes, development and effects of diseases and improve preventive, diagnostic and therapeutic interventions (methods, procedures and treatments). Even the best current interventions must be evaluated continually through research for their safety, effectiveness, efficiency, accessibility and quality.
8. In medical practice and in medical research, most interventions involve risks and burdens.
9. Medical research is subject to ethical standards that promote respect for all human subjects and protect their health and rights. Some research populations are particularly vulnerable and need special protection. These include those who cannot give or refuse consent for themselves and those who may be vulnerable to coercion or undue influence.
10. Physicians should consider the ethical, legal and regulatory norms and standards for research involving human subjects in their own countries as well as applicable international norms and standards. No national or international ethical, legal or regulatory requirement should reduce or eliminate any of the protections for research subjects set forth in this Declaration.

B. Principles for All Medical Research

11. It is the duty of physicians who participate in medical research to protect the life, health, dignity, integrity, right to self-determination, privacy, and confidentiality of personal information of research subjects.
12. Medical research involving human subjects must conform to generally accepted scientific principles, be based on a thorough knowledge of the scientific literature, other relevant sources of information, and adequate laboratory and, as appropriate, animal experimentation. The welfare of animals used for research must be respected.
13. Appropriate caution must be exercised in the conduct of medical research that may harm the environment.
14. The design and performance of each research study involving human subjects must be clearly described in a research protocol. The protocol should contain a statement of the ethical considerations involved and should indicate how the principles in this Declaration have been addressed. The protocol should include information regarding funding, sponsors, institutional affiliations, other potential conflicts of interest, incentives for subjects and provisions for treating and/or compensating subjects who are harmed as a consequence of participation in the research study. The protocol should describe arrangements for post-study access by study subjects to interventions identified as beneficial in the study or access to other appropriate care or benefits.

15. The research protocol must be submitted for consideration, comment, guidance and approval to a research ethics committee before the study begins. This committee must be independent of the researcher, the sponsor and any other undue influence. It must take into consideration the laws and regulations of the country or countries in which the research is to be performed as well as applicable international norms and standards but these must not be allowed to reduce or eliminate any of the protections for research subjects set forth in this Declaration. The committee must have the right to monitor ongoing studies. The researcher must provide monitoring information to the committee, especially information about any serious adverse events. No change to the protocol may be made without consideration and approval by the committee.

16. Medical research involving human subjects must be conducted only by individuals with the appropriate scientific training and qualifications. Research on patients or healthy volunteers requires the supervision of a competent and appropriately qualified physician or other health care professional. The responsibility for the protection of research subjects must always rest with the physician or other health care professional and never the research subjects, even though they have given consent.

17. Medical research involving a disadvantaged or vulnerable population or community is only justified if the research is responsive to the health needs and priorities of this population or community and if there is a reasonable likelihood that this population or community stands to benefit from the results of the research.

18. Every medical research study involving human subjects must be preceded by careful assessment of predictable risks and burdens to the individuals and communities involved in the research in comparison with foreseeable benefits to them and to other individuals or communities affected by the condition under investigation.

19. Every clinical trial must be registered in a publicly accessible database before recruitment of the first subject.

20. Physicians may not participate in a research study involving human subjects unless they are confident that the risks involved have been adequately assessed and can be satisfactorily managed. Physicians must immediately stop a study when the risks are found to outweigh the potential benefits or when there is conclusive proof of positive and beneficial results.

21. Medical research involving human subjects may only be conducted if the importance of the objective outweighs the inherent risks and burdens to the research subjects.

22. Participation by competent individuals as subjects in medical research must be voluntary. Although it may be appropriate to consult family members or community leaders, no competent individual may be enrolled in a research study unless he or she freely agrees.

23. Every precaution must be taken to protect the privacy of research subjects and the confidentiality of their personal information and to minimize the impact of the study on their physical, mental and social integrity.

24. In medical research involving competent human subjects, each potential subject must be adequately informed of the aims, methods, sources of funding, any possible conflicts of interest, institutional affiliations of the researcher, the anticipated benefits and potential risks of the study and the discomfort it may entail, and any other relevant aspects of the study. The potential subject must be informed of the right to refuse to participate in the study or to withdraw consent to participate at any time without reprisal. Special attention should be given to the specific information needs of individual potential subjects as well as to the methods used to deliver the information. After ensuring that the potential subject has understood the information, the physician or another appropriately qualified individual must then seek the potential subject's freely-given informed consent, preferably in writing. If the consent cannot be expressed in writing, the non-written consent must be formally documented and witnessed.

25. For medical research using identifiable human material or data, physicians must normally seek consent for the collection, analysis, storage and/or reuse. There may be situations where consent would be impossible or impractical to obtain for such research or would pose a threat to the validity of the research. In such situations the research may be done only after consideration and approval of a research ethics committee.

26. When seeking informed consent for participation in a research study the physician should be particularly cautious if the potential subject is in a dependent relationship with the physician or

may consent under duress. In such situations the informed consent should be sought by an appropriately qualified individual who is completely independent of this relationship.

27. For a potential research subject who is incompetent, the physician must seek informed consent from the legally authorized representative. These individuals must not be included in a research study that has no likelihood of benefit for them unless it is intended to promote the health of the population represented by the potential subject, the research cannot instead be performed with competent persons, and the research entails only minimal risk and minimal burden.

28. When a potential research subject who is deemed incompetent is able to give assent to decisions about participation in research, the physician must seek that assent in addition to the consent of the legally authorized representative. The potential subject's dissent should be respected.

29. Research involving subjects who are physically or mentally incapable of giving consent, for example, unconscious patients, may be done only if the physical or mental condition that prevents giving informed consent is a necessary characteristic of the research population. In such circumstances the physician should seek informed consent from the legally authorized representative. If no such representative is available and if the research cannot be delayed, the study may proceed without informed consent provided that the specific reasons for involving subjects with a condition that renders them unable to give informed consent have been stated in the research protocol and the study has been approved by a research ethics committee. Consent to remain in the research should be obtained as soon as possible from the subject or a legally authorized representative.

30. Authors, editors and publishers all have ethical obligations with regard to the publication of the results of research. Authors have a duty to make publicly available the results of their research on human subjects and are accountable for the completeness and accuracy of their reports. They should adhere to accepted guidelines for ethical reporting. Negative and inconclusive as well as positive results should be published or otherwise made publicly available. Sources of funding, institutional affiliations and conflicts of interest should be declared in the publication. Reports of research not in accordance with the principles of this Declaration should not be accepted for publication.

C. Additional Principles for Medical Research Combined with Medical Care

31. The physician may combine medical research with medical care only to the extent that the research is justified by its potential preventive, diagnostic or therapeutic value and if the physician has good reason to believe that participation in the research study will not adversely affect the health of the patients who serve as research subjects.

32. The benefits, risks, burdens and effectiveness of a new intervention must be tested against those of the best current proven intervention, except in the following circumstances:
   - The use of placebo, or no treatment, is acceptable in studies where no current proven intervention exists; or
   - Where for compelling and scientifically sound methodological reasons the use of placebo is necessary to determine the efficacy or safety of an intervention and the patients who receive placebo or no treatment will not be subject to any risk of serious or irreversible harm. Extreme care must be taken to avoid abuse of this option.

33. At the conclusion of the study, patients entered into the study are entitled to be informed about the outcome of the study and to share any benefits that result from it, for example, access to interventions identified as beneficial in the study or to other appropriate care or benefits.

34. The physician must fully inform the patient which aspects of the care are related to the research. The refusal of a patient to participate in a study or the patient's decision to withdraw from the study must never interfere with the patient–physician relationship.

35. In the treatment of a patient, where proven interventions do not exist or have been ineffective, the physician, after seeking expert advice, with informed consent from the patient or a legally authorized representative, may use an unproven intervention if in the physician's judgment it offers hope of saving life, re-establishing health or alleviating suffering. Where possible, this intervention should be made the object of research, designed to evaluate its safety and efficacy. In all cases, new information should be recorded and, where appropriate, made publicly available.

The Tuskegee Experiment

The Tuskegee experiment is one of the most notorious cases of ethics violations in clinical research. Commencing in the 1930s, the experiment continued until 1970 when the details of the experiment were uncovered, causing an uproar. Researchers followed 400 African American men with syphilis and kept them from receiving treatment so that they could observe the natural course of the disease. This experiment had two major problems. First, the researchers denied the subjects available treatment for a major disease for so long. Second, the researchers were Caucasian and the subjects were African Americans. There was no scientific reason why all the subjects had to be African Americans. The experiment appeared to be a case of one race experimenting on another.

These developments prompted action from the major governing bodies in the USA. For the first time, clinical researchers were no longer allowed to regulate themselves. The violations had demonstrated that oversight was needed. The National Institutes of Health (NIH) began requiring that each institution conducting clinical research have an institutional review board (IRB) to review and approve clinical study protocols. The Food and Drug Administration (FDA) followed suit by strengthening its drug and medical device rules and regulations. In 1973, the US Congress assembled the 11-member National Commission for the Protection of Human Subjects of Biomedical and Behavioral Research, which issued the Belmont Report in 1979.[3] This report clearly defined three major principles of ethical clinical research: respect for persons, beneficence and justice. It included guidelines on weighing the risks and benefits of a study and subject selection.

THE BELMONT REPORT

Ethical Principles and Guidelines for the Protection of Human Subjects of Research
The National Commission for the Protection of Human Subjects of Biomedical and Behavioral Research

April 18, 1979

AGENCY: Department of Health, Education, and Welfare.

ACTION: Notice of Report for Public Comment.

SUMMARY: On July 12, 1974, the National Research Act (Pub. L. 93-348) was signed into law, thereby creating the National Commission for the Protection of Human Subjects of Biomedical and Behavioral Research. One of the charges to the Commission was to identify the basic ethical principles that should underlie the conduct of biomedical and behavioral research involving human subjects and to develop guidelines which should be followed to assure that such research is conducted in accordance with those principles. In carrying out the above, the Commission was directed to consider: (i) the boundaries between biomedical and behavioral research and the accepted and routine practice of medicine, (ii) the role of assessment of risk—benefit criteria in the determination of the appropriateness of research involving human subjects, (iii) appropriate guidelines for the selection of human subjects for participation in such research, and (iv) the nature and definition of informed consent in various research settings.

The Belmont Report attempts to summarize the basic ethical principles identified by the Commission in the course of its deliberations. It is the outgrowth of an intensive four-day period of discussions that were held in February 1976 at the Smithsonian Institution's Belmont Conference Center supplemented by the monthly deliberations of the Commission that were held over a period of nearly four years. It is a statement of basic ethical principles and guidelines that should assist in resolving the ethical problems that surround the conduct of research with human subjects. By publishing the Report in the Federal Register, and providing reprints upon request, the Secretary intends that it may be made readily available to scientists, members of Institutional Review Boards, and Federal employees. The two-volume Appendix, containing the lengthy reports of experts and specialists who assisted the Commission in fulfilling this part of its charge, is available as DHEW Publication No. (OS) 78-0013 and No. (OS) 78-0014, for sale by the Superintendent of Documents, US Government Printing Office, Washington, DC 20402.

Unlike most other reports of the Commission, the Belmont Report does not make specific recommendations for administrative action by the Secretary of Health, Education, and Welfare. Rather, the Commission recommended that the Belmont Report be adopted in its entirety, as a statement of the Department's policy. The Department requests public comment on this recommendation.

National Commission for the Protection of Human Subjects of Biomedical and Behavioral Research

Members of the Commission

Kenneth John Ryan, MD, Chairman, Chief of Staff, Boston Hospital for Women.
Joseph V. Brady, PhD, Professor of Behavioral Biology, Johns Hopkins University.
Robert E. Cooke, MD, President, Medical College of Pennsylvania.
Dorothy I. Height, President, National Council of Negro Women, Inc.
Albert R. Jonsen, PhD, Associate Professor of Bioethics, University of California at San Francisco.
Patricia King, JD, Associate Professor of Law, Georgetown University Law Center.
Karen Lebacqz, PhD, Associate Professor of Christian Ethics, Pacific School of Religion.
*** David W. Louisell, JD, Professor of Law, University of California at Berkeley.
Donald W. Seldin, MD, Professor and Chairman, Department of Internal Medicine, University of Texas at Dallas.
Eliot Stellar, PhD, Provost of the University and Professor of Physiological Psychology, University of Pennsylvania.
*** Robert H. Turtle, LLB, Attorney, VomBaur, Coburn, Simmons & Turtle, Washington, DC.
*** Deceased.

Ethical Principles and Guidelines for Research Involving Human Subjects

Scientific research has produced substantial social benefits. It has also posed some troubling ethical questions. Public attention was drawn to these questions by reported abuses of human subjects in biomedical experiments, especially during the Second World War. During the Nuremberg War Crime Trials, the Nuremberg code was drafted as a set of standards for judging physicians and scientists who had conducted biomedical experiments on concentration camp prisoners. This code became the prototype of many later codes intended to assure that research involving human subjects would be carried out in an ethical manner.

The codes consist of rules, some general, others specific, that guide the investigators or the reviewers of research in their work. Such rules often are inadequate to cover complex situations; at times they come into conflict, and they are frequently difficult to interpret or apply. Broader ethical principles will provide a basis on which specific rules may be formulated, criticized and interpreted.

Three principles, or general prescriptive judgments, that are relevant to research involving human subjects are identified in this statement. Other principles may also be relevant. These three are comprehensive, however, and are stated at a level of generalization that should assist scientists, subjects, reviewers and interested citizens to understand the ethical issues inherent in research involving human subjects. These principles cannot always be applied so as to resolve beyond dispute particular ethical problems. The objective is to provide an analytical framework that will guide the resolution of ethical problems arising from research involving human subjects.

This statement consists of a distinction between research and practice, a discussion of the three basic ethical principles, and remarks about the application of these principles.

Part A: Boundaries Between Practice and Research

It is important to distinguish between biomedical and behavioral research, on the one hand, and the practice of accepted therapy on the other, in order to know what activities ought to undergo review for the protection of human subjects of research. The distinction between research and practice is blurred partly because both often occur together (as in research designed to evaluate a therapy) and partly because notable departures from standard practice are often called "experimental" when the terms "experimental" and "research" are not carefully defined.

For the most part, the term "practice" refers to interventions that are designed solely to enhance the well-being of an individual patient or client and that have a reasonable expectation of success. The purpose of medical or behavioral practice is to provide diagnosis, preventive treatment or therapy to particular individuals.*(2)* By contrast, the term "research" designates an activity designed to test a hypothesis, permit conclusions to be drawn, and thereby to develop or contribute to generalizable knowledge (expressed, for example, in theories, principles, and statements of relationships). Research is usually described in a formal protocol that sets forth an objective and a set of procedures designed to reach that objective.

When a clinician departs in a significant way from standard or accepted practice, the innovation does not, in and of itself, constitute research. The fact that a procedure is "experimental", in the sense of new, untested or different, does not automatically place it in the category of research. Radically new procedures of this description should, however, be made the object of formal research at an early stage in order to determine whether they are safe and effective. Thus, it is the responsibility of medical practice committees, for example, to insist that a major innovation be incorporated into a formal research project.*(3)*

Research and practice may be carried on together when research is designed to evaluate the safety and efficacy of a therapy. This need not cause any confusion regarding whether or not the activity requires review; the general rule is that if there is any element of research in an activity, that activity should undergo review for the protection of human subjects.

Part B: Basic Ethical Principles

The expression "basic ethical principles" refers to those general judgments that serve as a basic justification for the many particular ethical prescriptions and evaluations of human actions. Three basic principles, among those generally accepted in our cultural tradition, are particularly relevant to the ethics of research involving human subjects: the principles of respect of persons, beneficence and justice.

1. Respect for Persons – Respect for persons incorporates at least two ethical convictions: first, that individuals should be treated as autonomous agents, and second, that persons with diminished autonomy are entitled to protection. The principle of respect for persons thus divides into two separate moral requirements: the requirement to acknowledge autonomy and the requirement to protect those with diminished autonomy.

An autonomous person is an individual capable of deliberation about personal goals and of acting under the direction of such deliberation. To respect autonomy is to give weight to autonomous persons' considered opinions and choices while refraining from obstructing their actions unless they are clearly detrimental to others. To show lack of respect for an autonomous agent is to repudiate that person's considered judgments, to deny an individual the freedom to act on those considered judgments, or to withhold information necessary to make a considered judgment, when there are no compelling reasons to do so.

However, not every human being is capable of self-determination. The capacity for self-determination matures during an individual's life, and some individuals lose this capacity wholly or in part because of illness, mental disability, or circumstances that severely restrict liberty. Respect for the immature and the incapacitated may require protecting them as they mature or while they are incapacitated.

Some persons are in need of extensive protection, even to the point of excluding them from activities which may harm them; other persons require little protection beyond making sure they undertake activities freely and with awareness of possible adverse consequence. The extent of protection afforded should depend upon the risk of harm and the likelihood of benefit. The judgment that any individual lacks autonomy should be periodically reevaluated and will vary in different situations.

In most cases of research involving human subjects, respect for persons demands that subjects enter into the research voluntarily and with adequate information. In some situations, however, application of the principle is not obvious. The involvement of prisoners as subjects of research provides an instructive example. On the one hand, it would seem that the principle of respect for persons requires that prisoners not be deprived of the opportunity to volunteer for research. On the other hand, under prison conditions they may be subtly coerced or unduly influenced to engage in research activities for which they would not otherwise volunteer. Respect for persons would then dictate that prisoners be protected. Whether to allow prisoners to "volunteer" or to "protect" them presents a dilemma. Respecting persons, in most hard cases, is often a matter of balancing competing claims urged by the principle of respect itself.

2. Beneficence – Persons are treated in an ethical manner not only by respecting their decisions and protecting them from harm, but also by making efforts to secure their well-being. Such treatment falls under the principle of beneficence. The term "beneficence" is often understood to cover acts of kindness or charity that go beyond strict obligation. In this document, beneficence is understood in a stronger sense, as an obligation. Two general rules have been formulated as complementary expressions of beneficent actions in this sense: (1) do not harm and (2) maximize possible benefits and minimize possible harms.

The Hippocratic maxim "do no harm" has long been a fundamental principle of medical ethics. Claude Bernard extended it to the realm of research, saying that one should not injure one person regardless of the benefits that might come to others. However, even avoiding harm requires learning what is harmful; and, in the process of obtaining this information, persons may be exposed to risk of harm. Further, the Hippocratic Oath requires physicians to benefit their patients "according to their best judgment". Learning what will in fact benefit may require exposing persons to risk. The problem posed by these imperatives is to decide when it is justifiable to seek certain benefits despite the risks involved, and when the benefits should be foregone because of the risks.

The obligations of beneficence affect both individual investigators and society at large, because they extend both to particular research projects and to the entire enterprise of research. In the case of particular projects, investigators and members of their institutions are obliged to give forethought to the maximization of benefits and the reduction of risk that might occur from the research investigation. In the case of scientific research in general, members of the larger society are obliged to recognize the longer term benefits and risks that may result from the improvement of knowledge and from the development of novel medical, psychotherapeutic, and social procedures.

The principle of beneficence often occupies a well-defined justifying role in many areas of research involving human subjects. An example is found in research involving children. Effective ways of treating childhood diseases and fostering healthy development are benefits that serve to justify research involving children – even when individual research subjects are not direct beneficiaries. Research also makes it possible to avoid the harm that may result from the application of previously accepted routine practices that on closer investigation turn out to be dangerous. But the role of the principle of beneficence is not always so unambiguous. A difficult ethical problem remains, for example, about research that presents more than minimal risk without immediate prospect of direct benefit to the children involved. Some have argued that such research is inadmissible, while others have pointed out that this limit would rule out much research promising great benefit to children in the future. Here again, as with all hard cases, the different claims covered by the principle of beneficence may come into conflict and force difficult choices.

3. Justice – Who ought to receive the benefits of research and bear its burdens? This is a question of justice, in the sense of "fairness in distribution" or "what is deserved". An injustice occurs when some benefit to which a person is entitled is denied without good reason or when some burden is imposed unduly. Another way of conceiving the principle of justice is that equals ought to be treated equally. However, this statement requires explication. Who is equal and who is unequal? What considerations justify departure from equal distribution? Almost all commentators allow that distinctions based on experience, age, deprivation, competence, merit and position do sometimes constitute criteria justi-fying differential treatment for certain purposes. It is necessary, then, to explain in what respects people should be treated equally. There are several widely accepted formulations of just ways to distribute burdens and benefits. Each formulation mentions some relevant property on the basis of which burdens and benefits should be distributed. These formulations are (1) to each person an equal share, (2) to each person according to individual need, (3) to each person according to individual effort, (4) to each person according to societal contribution, and (5) to each person according to merit.

Questions of justice have long been associated with social practices such as punishment, taxation and political representation. Until recently these questions have not generally been associated with scientific research. However, they are foreshadowed even in the earliest reflections on the ethics of research involving human subjects. For example, during the 19th and early 20th centuries the burdens of serving as research subjects fell largely upon poor ward patients, while the benefits of improved medical care flowed primarily to private patients. Subsequently, the exploitation of unwilling prisoners as research subjects in Nazi concentration camps was condemned as a particularly flagrant injustice. In this country

183

[the USA], in the 1940s, the Tuskegee syphilis study used disadvantaged, rural black men to study the untreated course of a disease that is by no means confined to that population. These subjects were deprived of demonstrably effective treatment in order not to interrupt the project, long after such treatment became generally available.

Against this historical background, it can be seen how conceptions of justice are relevant to research involving human subjects. For example, the selection of research subjects needs to be scrutinized in order to determine whether some classes (e.g. welfare patients, particular racial and ethnic minorities, or persons confined to institutions) are being systematically selected simply because of their easy availability, their compromised position, or their manipulability, rather than for reasons directly related to the problem being studied. Finally, whenever research supported by public funds leads to the development of therapeutic devices and procedures, justice demands both that these not provide advantages only to those who can afford them and that such research should not unduly involve persons from groups unlikely to be among the beneficiaries of subsequent applications of the research.

Part C: Applications

Application of the general principles to the conduct of research leads to consideration of the following requirements: informed consent, risk/benefit assessment, and the selection of subjects of research.

1. Informed Consent – Respect for persons requires that subjects, to the degree that they are capable, be given the opportunity to choose what shall or shall not happen to them. This opportunity is provided when adequate standards for informed consent are satisfied.

While the importance of informed consent is unquestioned, controversy prevails over the nature and possibility of an informed consent. Nonetheless, there is widespread agreement that the consent process can be analyzed as containing three elements: information, comprehension and voluntariness.

Information. Most codes of research establish specific items for disclosure intended to assure that subjects are given sufficient information. These items generally include: the research procedure, their purposes, risks and anticipated benefits, alternative procedures (where therapy is involved), and a statement offering the subject the opportunity to ask questions and to withdraw at any time from the research. Additional items have been proposed, including how subjects are selected, the person responsible for the research, etc.

However, a simple listing of items does not answer the question of what the standard should be for judging how much and what sort of information should be provided. One standard frequently invoked in medical practice, namely the information commonly provided by practitioners in the field or in the locale, is inadequate since research takes place precisely when a common understanding does not exist. Another standard, currently popular in malpractice law, requires the practitioner to reveal the information that reasonable persons would wish to know in order to make a decision regarding their care. This, too, seems insufficient since the research subject, being in essence a volunteer, may wish to know considerably more about risks gratuitously undertaken than do patients who deliver themselves into the hands of a clinician for needed care. It may be that a standard of "the reasonable volunteer" should be proposed: the extent and nature of information should be such that persons, knowing that the procedure is neither necessary for their care nor perhaps fully understood, can decide whether they wish to participate in the furthering of knowledge. Even when some direct benefit to them is anticipated, the subjects should understand clearly the range of risk and the voluntary nature of participation.

A special problem of consent arises where informing subjects of some pertinent aspect of the research is likely to impair the validity of the research. In many cases, it is sufficient to indicate to subjects that they are being invited to participate in research of which some features will not be revealed until the research is concluded. In all cases of research involving incomplete disclosure, such research is justified only if it is clear that (1) incomplete disclosure is truly necessary to accomplish the goals of the research, (2) there are no undisclosed risks to subjects that are more than minimal, and (3) there is an adequate plan for debriefing subjects, when appropriate, and for dissemination of research results to them. Information about risks should never be withheld for the purpose of eliciting the cooperation of subjects, and truthful answers should always be given to direct questions about the research. Care should be taken to distinguish cases in which disclosure would destroy or invalidate the research from cases in which disclosure would simply inconvenience the investigator.

Comprehension. The manner and context in which information is conveyed is as important as the information itself. For example, presenting information in a disorganized and rapid fashion, allowing too little time for consideration or curtailing opportunities for questioning, all may adversely affect a subject's ability to make an informed choice.

Because the subject's ability to understand is a function of intelligence, rationality, maturity and language, it is necessary to adapt the presentation of the information to the subject's capacities. Investigators are responsible for ascertaining that the subject has comprehended the information. While there is always an obligation to ascertain that the information about risk to subjects is complete and adequately comprehended, when the risks are more serious, that obligation increases. On occasion, it may be suitable to give some oral or written tests of comprehension.

Special provision may need to be made when comprehension is severely limited — for example, by conditions of immaturity or mental disability. Each class of subjects that one might consider as incompetent (e.g. infants and young children, mentally disabled patients, the terminally ill and the comatose) should be considered on its own terms. Even for these persons, however, respect requires giving them the opportunity to choose to the extent they are able, whether or not to participate in research. The objections of these subjects to involvement should be honored, unless the research entails providing them a therapy unavailable elsewhere. Respect for persons also requires seeking the permission of other parties in order to protect the subjects from harm. Such persons are thus respected both by acknowledging their own wishes and by the use of third parties to protect them from harm.

The third parties chosen should be those who are most likely to understand the incompetent subject's situation and to act in that person's best interest. The person authorized to act on behalf of the subject should be given an opportunity to observe the research as it proceeds in order to be able to withdraw the subject from the research, if such action appears in the subject's best interest.

Voluntariness. An agreement to participate in research constitutes a valid consent only if voluntarily given. This element of informed consent requires conditions free of coercion and undue influence. Coercion occurs when an overt threat of harm is intentionally presented by one person to another in order to obtain compliance. Undue influence, by contrast, occurs through an offer of an excessive, unwarranted, inappropriate or improper reward or other overture in order to obtain compliance. Also, inducements that would ordinarily be acceptable may become undue influences if the subject is especially vulnerable.

Unjustifiable pressures usually occur when persons in positions of authority or commanding influence — especially where possible sanctions are involved — urge a course of action for a subject. A continuum of such influencing factors exists, however, and it is impossible to state precisely where justifiable persuasion ends and undue influence begins. But undue influence would include actions such as manipulating a person's choice through the controlling influence of a close relative and threatening to withdraw health services to which an individual would otherwise be entitled.

2. Assessment of Risks and Benefits — The assessment of risks and benefits requires a careful arrayal of relevant data, including, in some cases, alternative ways of obtaining the benefits sought in the research. Thus, the assessment presents both an opportunity and a responsibility to gather systematic and comprehensive information about proposed research. For the investigator, it is a means to examine whether the proposed research is properly designed. For a review committee, it is a method for determining whether the risks that will be presented to subjects are justified. For prospective subjects, the assessment will assist the determination whether or not to participate.

The nature and scope of risks and benefits. The requirement that research be justified on the basis of a favorable risk/benefit assessment bears a close relation to the principle of beneficence, just as the moral requirement that informed consent be obtained is derived primarily from the principle of respect for persons. The term "risk" refers to a possibility that harm may occur. However, when expressions such as "small risk" or "high risk" are used, they usually refer (often ambiguously) both to the chance (probability) of experiencing a harm and the severity (magnitude) of the envisioned harm.

The term "benefit" is used in the research context to refer to something of positive value related to health or welfare. Unlike, "risk", "benefit" is not a term that expresses probabilities. Risk is properly contrasted to probability of benefits, and benefits are properly contrasted with harms rather than risks of harm. Accordingly, so-called risk/benefit assessments are concerned with the probabilities and magnitudes of possible harm and anticipated benefits. Many kinds of possible harms and benefits need to be taken into account. There are, for example, risks of psychological harm, physical harm, legal harm, social harm and economic harm and the corresponding benefits. While the most likely types of harms to research subjects are those of psychological or physical pain or injury, other possible kinds should not be overlooked.

Risks and benefits of research may affect the individual subjects, the families of the individual subjects, and society at large (or special groups of subjects in society). Previous codes and Federal regulations have required that risks to subjects be outweighed by the sum of both the anticipated benefit to the subject, if any, and the anticipated benefit to society in the form of knowledge to be gained from the research. In balancing these different elements, the risks and benefits affecting the immediate research subject will normally carry special weight. On the other hand, interests other than those of the subject may on some occasions be sufficient by themselves to justify the risks involved in the research, so long as the subjects' rights have been protected. Beneficence thus requires that we protect against risk of harm to subjects and also that we be concerned about the loss of the substantial benefits that might be gained from research.

The systematic assessment of risks and benefits. It is commonly said that benefits and risks must be "balanced" and shown to be "in a favorable ratio". The metaphorical character of these terms draws attention to the difficulty of making precise judgments. Only on rare occasions will quantitative techniques be available for the scrutiny of research protocols. However, the idea of systematic, non-arbitrary analysis of risks and benefits should be emulated insofar as possible. This ideal requires those making decisions about the justifiability of research to be thorough in the accumulation and assessment of information about all aspects of the research, and to consider alternatives systematically. This procedure renders the assessment of research more rigorous and precise, while making communication between review board members and investigators less subject to misinterpretation, misinformation and conflicting judgments. Thus, there should first be a determination of the validity of the presuppositions of the research; then the nature, probability and magnitude of risk should be distinguished with as much clarity as possible. The method of ascertaining risks should be explicit, especially where there is no alternative to the use of such vague categories as small or slight risk. It should also be determined whether an investigator's estimates of the probability of harm or benefits are reasonable, as judged by known facts or other available studies.

Finally, assessment of the justifiability of research should reflect at least the following considerations: (i) Brutal or inhumane treatment of human subjects is never morally justified. (ii) Risks should be reduced to those necessary to achieve the research objective. It should be determined whether it is in fact necessary to use human subjects at all. Risk can perhaps never be entirely eliminated, but it can often be reduced by careful attention to alternative procedures. (iii) When research involves significant risk of serious impairment, review committees should be extraordinarily insistent on the justification of the risk (looking usually to the likelihood of benefit to the subject — or, in some rare cases, to the manifest voluntariness of the participation). (iv) When vulnerable populations are involved in research, the appropriateness of involving them should itself be demonstrated. A number of variables go into such judgments, including the nature and degree of risk, the condition of the particular population involved, and the nature and level of the anticipated benefits. (v) Relevant risks and benefits must be thoroughly arrayed in documents and procedures used in the informed consent process.

3. Selection of Subjects — Just as the principle of respect for persons finds expression in the requirements for consent, and the principle of beneficence in risk/benefit assessment, the principle of justice gives rise to moral requirements that there be fair procedures and outcomes in the selection of research subjects.

Justice is relevant to the selection of subjects of research at two levels: the social and the individual. Individual justice in the selection of subjects would require that researchers exhibit fairness: thus, they should not offer potentially beneficial research only to some patients who are in their favor or select only "undesirable" persons for risky research. Social justice requires that distinction be drawn between classes of subjects that ought, and ought not, to participate in any particular kind of research, based on the ability of members of that class to bear burdens and on the appropriateness of placing further burdens on already burdened persons. Thus, it can be considered a matter of social justice that there is an order of preference in the selection of classes of subjects (e.g. adults before children) and that some classes of potential subjects (e.g. the institutionalized mentally infirm or prisoners) may be involved as research subjects, if at all, only on certain conditions.

Injustice may appear in the selection of subjects, even if individual subjects are selected fairly by investigators and treated fairly in the course of research. Thus injustice arises from social, racial, sexual and cultural biases institutionalized in society. Thus, even if individual researchers are treating their research subjects fairly, and even if IRBs are taking care to assure that subjects are selected fairly within a particular institution, unjust social patterns may nevertheless appear in the overall distribution of the burdens and benefits of research. Although individual institutions or investigators may not be able to resolve a problem that is pervasive in their social setting, they can consider distributive justice in selecting research subjects.

Some populations, especially institutionalized ones, are already burdened in many ways by their infirmities and environments. When research is proposed that involves risks and does not include a therapeutic component, other less burdened classes of persons should be called upon first to accept these risks of research, except where the research is directly related to the specific conditions of the class involved. Also, even though public funds for research may often flow in the same directions as public funds for health care, it seems unfair that populations dependent on public health care constitute a pool of preferred research subjects if more advantaged populations are likely to be the recipients of the benefits.

One special instance of injustice results from the involvement of vulnerable subjects. Certain groups, such as racial minorities, the economically disadvantaged, the very sick, and the institutionalized may continually be sought as research subjects, owing to their ready availability in settings where research is conducted. Given their dependent status and their frequently compromised capacity for free consent, they should be protected against the danger of being involved in research solely for administrative convenience, or because they are easy to manipulate as a result of their illness or socioeconomic condition.

(1) Since 1945, various codes for the proper and responsible conduct of human experimentation in medical research have been adopted by different organizations. The best known of these codes are the Nuremberg Code of 1947, the Helsinki Declaration of 1964 (revised in 1975), and the 1971 Guidelines (codified into Federal Regulations in 1974) issued by the US Department of Health, Education, and Welfare. Codes for the conduct of social and behavioral research have also been adopted, the best known being that of the American Psychological Association, published in 1973.

(2) Although practice usually involves interventions designed solely to enhance the well-being of a particular individual, interventions are sometimes applied to one individual for the enhancement of the well-being of another (e.g. blood donation, skin grafts, organ transplants) or an intervention may have the dual purpose of enhancing the well-being of a particular individual, and, at the same time, providing some benefit to others (e.g. vaccination, which protects both the person who is vaccinated and society generally). The fact that some forms of practice have elements other than immediate benefit to the individual receiving an intervention, however, should not confuse the general distinction between research and practice. Even when a procedure applied in practice may benefit some other person, it remains an intervention designed to enhance the well-being of a particular individual or groups of individuals; thus, it is practice and need not be reviewed as research.

(3) Because the problems related to social experimentation may differ substantially from those of biomedical and behavioral research, the Commission specifically declines to make any policy determination regarding such research at this time. Rather, the Commission believes that the problem ought to be addressed by one of its successor bodies.

These and other ethical guidelines depend on mostly Western humanist and ethical philosophies built around individual rights and autonomy, beneficence, and justice. These concepts are discussed briefly below, and in detail in other books, including Chin and Lee's Principles and Practice of Clinical Trial Medicine and Chin and Bairu's Global Clinical Trials.[4,5]

These ethical principles must be followed both in substance and in form. In other words, the rights must not be violated, and in addition proper documentation and procedures must be followed. Even if the patients do not come to harm and are not put at risk, it is unethical to conduct a study without their consent, for example.

Each trial must be framed in a research protocol incorporating a statement of ethical considerations that includes information regarding funding, sponsorship, institutional affiliations, potential conflicts of interest, incentives, provisions for treatment or compensation to subjects harmed as a consequence of participation. The protocol must state the subjects' right to post-study interventions, including compassionate usage, identified as beneficial. The study must be scientifically well designed, address a significant medical question, and have equipoise.

Globalization of clinical research and drug development has exacerbated or highlighted ethical issues. By some estimates, over a third of all clinical trials are conducted outside the USA and Western Europe, a number that may double in the next decade.[6] According to the US Department of Health and Human Services' Office of Inspector General (OIG), 80 percent of the applications for drugs and biologicals approved for the USA in 2008 relied on data from overseas clinical trials. More than 50 percent of clinical trial participants and sites were located outside the USA.

Because many of the studies are performed in developing countries, there are some important ethical issues and practical challenges that must be resolved. While there is broad consensus over the acceptable ethical principles for research in developed countries, there are several highly contentious issues regarding clinical trials in developing countries.

FUNDAMENTAL ISSUES

One of the most important issues is the recognition of different cultural, ethical, religious, and political frameworks that exist in different countries. Whether ethics and morality should be viewed from a relativist viewpoint or not is a philosophical question that is beyond the scope of this book. What is clear, however, is that in general, it is necessary to satisfy the ethical requirements of both the originating and the receiving countries and not to violate ethical prohibitions of both countries. In cases where this is not possible, a study may not be feasible. Specific examples are provided later in this chapter.

Another important issue is the differing concepts of disease from one country or culture to the next. While differing concepts of disease can exist even in a Western country, such as homeopathy, Christian Scientist tradition, and others, concept of disease in a developing country may be dramatically different from the Western scientific concept. This may make informed consent particularly difficult. For example, it may be difficult to explain the possibility of anaphylactic shock to someone whose understanding of disease has no reference to cells or allergies. As another example, injection of a drug into an acupuncture meridian that may cause a particular side-effect as per Chinese acupuncture tradition may need to be disclosed in the informed consent form if the study is being conducted in Asia.

Originating and Destination Countries

Some ethicists make a distinction between a study sponsored by a party in a developed country that is conducted in a developing country from a study sponsored and conducted all within a developing country. They argue that standards in the former case must conform to the standards used in the developed country. They would accept different standards for the latter case. For example, if a sponsor in developing country wanted to utilize a placebo arm in a study because that was the standard of care in that country, these ethicists would accept that, but not if the sponsor came from another country where an expensive drug was the standard of care. Other ethicists make no such distinction.

Other ethicists draw a distinction not on the basis of where the sponsor is but rather whether the objective of the study is to improve patient care in a developing country or the developed country. They may find it problematic not to use the expensive standard of care in the control arm if the results of the study are intended to benefit mostly patients in the developed country, but not if the study is conducted to benefit mostly patients in the developing country in which the study is performed.

Many ethicists, however, assert that there can be only one standard, to which all clinical trials must adhere.

Placebo Controls

One of the most contentious issues is the use of placebo controls or controls other than the best standard of care available. In many impoverished countries, patients do not have access to expensive and effective therapies available in developed countries. In many clinical trials, patients in the control arm may receive the local standard of care. Often the local standard of care is no treatment, and therefore the patients receive placebo.

As an example, in 1997, the Centers for Disease Control and Prevention (CDC) and NIH published a study of randomized, placebo-controlled trials to test the effectiveness of short-course zidovudine (AZT) treatment in preventing perinatal transmission of the human immunodeficiency virus (HIV). The trials were conducted in sub-Saharan Africa and Thailand.[7] An intensive zidovudine regimen had already been proven effective and has been adopted as the standard of care in developed countries.

The use of placebos in these studies when there was a proven treatment available (albeit only in rich countries) triggered an firestorm. Hundreds of infants "needlessly contracted HIV infection", charged Drs Peter Laurie and Sidney Wolfe in the New England Journal of Medicine.[8] Comparing the trials to the Tuskegee syphilis study, Marcia Angell, NEJM editor-in-chief, condemned the "widespread exploitation of vulnerable Third World populations for research programs that could not be carried out in the sponsoring country".[9]

Lost in the clamor were findings demonstrating that the short-course (less costly) zidovudine regimen had shown a 51 percent reduction in perinatal HIV transmission. The use of placebo controls, CDC officials argued, had provided "the most rapid, accurate, and reliable answer to the question of the value of the intervention being studied compared to the local standard of care".

In the developing world, "local standard of care" may be an ethical slippery slope. "It is an unfortunate fact", the CDC noted, "that the current standard of perinatal care for the HIV-infected pregnant women in the sites of the studies does not include any HIV prophylactic intervention at all".[10]

An important distinction between the Tuskegee experiments and modern clinical trials that use placebo arms is informed consent. The patients in the Tuskegee studies were never informed that penicillin was available. In fact, they were not even informed that they had syphilis.

There is no consensus on the use of "local standard of care" as the control arm in developing countries. Those who argue that this practice is acceptable are arguing, in effect, that a patient can waive his right (if he has that right to begin with) to receive the developed countries' expensive standard of care. Those who argue that the practice is unacceptable are arguing, in effect, that the patient does not have the right to waive that right even with informed consent. They are arguing that the right to the most advanced standard of care within a clinical trial is an inalienable right that cannot be waived.

Some guidelines, such as the CIOMS guideline, specify that placebo is acceptable if the placebo is scientifically necessary and would not result in serious or permanent harm to the patient or put him at increased risk. On the other hand, the Declaration of Helsinki mandates that the best available therapy be given to the patients in the control arm:

> The benefits, risks, burdens and effectiveness of a new intervention must be tested against those of the best current proven intervention, except in the following circumstances:

- The use of placebo, or no treatment, is acceptable in studies where no current proven intervention exists; or
- Where for compelling and scientifically sound methodological reasons the use of placebo is necessary to determine the efficacy or safety of an intervention and the patients who receive placebo or no treatment will not be subject to any risk of serious or irreversible harm. Extreme care must be taken to avoid abuse of this option.

The use of placebo or less than the best standard of care is not an issue restricted to developing countries. The position of the FDA is that placebo-controlled studies can be ethical in some or many cases, and that is the reason why the FDA no longer subscribes to the Declaration of Helsinki, which mandates that the best available therapy be given to the patients in the control arm. In fact, many studies within the USA deny patients the best available therapy. One example is trials where osteoarthritis patients may receive placebo rather than a non-steroidal anti-inflammatory drug (NSAID) for a limited period.

The position of the European Medicines Agency (EMA) and most European countries is that placebo-controlled studies or studies using anything less than the best standard of care available in the world are always or nearly always unethical.

The controversy about placebo controls is part of a larger debate about whether a study that is unethical in a developed country could be ethical in a developing country. Laurie and Wolfe argue that it is never possible. Others argue that just as there are studies that are unethical in one developed country yet ethical in another developed country, there may be instances where a study may be ethical in one developing country without being ethical in another developing country or a developed country. One example might be a study of a rotavirus vaccine that causes a fatal side-effect in one in 5000 patients. In a developed country where mortality from childhood diarrhea is nearly zero, the study may not be ethical. In a developing country where childhood mortality from diarrhea is 10 percent, the same study may be ethical.

In any case, if the study uses a control group or a design different from what would be considered ethical in the originating developed country, it is imperative to justify the design clearly.

Intent to Market Within the Country

Conducting trials in a country or a region without any intent to make the drug available to the patients in that country is generally considered unethical. Conducting trials in a country or a region without any intent to make the drug available at an affordable price to the patients in that country is considered unethical by most ethicists.

Patients in clinical studies volunteer to put themselves at risk so that other patients may benefit. If those very patients and the patients from their communities will not have a chance to benefit from the results of the study, then most ethicists would agree that they are clearly being exploited. There is little or no debate about this issue.

Availability of Medical Care After the Study

Many ethicists and guidelines assert that the patients are entitled to the best proven therapy. Some assert that sponsors are obligated to continue to provide drug or other therapy to the patients in a study after the study has terminated. Others assert that the government is responsible for ensuring the care.

The most recent version of the Declaration of Helsinki states:

> At the conclusion of the study, patients entered into the study are entitled to be informed about the outcome of the study and to share any benefits that result from it, for example, access to interventions identified as beneficial in the study or to other appropriate care or benefits.

For both studies in developed and developing countries, some sponsors continue to make the study drug available to the patients after the study if the disease is life threatening and there are no alternative therapies; most do not make the drug available in other instances. Rarely do they provide the comparator drug or therapy after the conclusion of the study.

It is important, however, to make it clear to the patients at the informed consent stage what the availability of the therapies will be after the conclusion of the study.

Undue Inducement and Site Compensation

Undue inducement to a patient to participate in a study is always a potential issue in a clinical study. It is particularly important when the study involves vulnerable populations. In studies conducted in developing countries, the extreme poverty, lack of access to medical care, and other factors often make the population a vulnerable population.

The principles against undue influence are the same as for other studies, although the probability is higher in studies conducted in developing countries. The benefit or perceived benefit that the patient receives may be at a much lower level than the level that would trigger concerns of undue influence in a developed country. For example, even a $5 payment may be considered to be coercive.

In addition, ICH regulations and other laws and regulations typically prohibit paying investigators more than the value of their work, and they also prohibit donation of equipment and supplies beyond what is necessary for the study. In some cases, it is not practical to collect all study equipment after the study, especially if the equipment is bulky or specialized. In those cases, specific provisions should be made before the study, and the equipment to be left behind should be considered part of the study compensation.

Informed Consent

For any clinical research, informed consent must be obtained. US regulation 45 CFR 46.116(b) sets out the basic requirements for informed consent, and most other countries follow the same or similar requirements:

1. A statement that the study involves research, an explanation of the purposes of the research and the expected duration of the subject's participation, a description of the procedures to be followed, and identification of any procedures which are experimental.
2. A description of any reasonably foreseeable risks or discomforts to the subject.
3. A description of any benefits to the subject or to others which may reasonably be expected from the research.
4. A disclosure of appropriate alternative procedures or courses of treatment, if any, that might be advantageous to the subject.
5. A statement describing the extent, if any, to which confidentiality of records identifying the subject will be maintained and that notes the possibility that the FDA may inspect the records.
6. For research involving more than minimal risk, an explanation as to whether any compensation and an explanation as to whether any medical treatments are available if injury occurs and, if so, what they consist of, or where further information may be obtained.

7. An explanation of whom to contact for answers to pertinent questions about the research and research subjects' rights, and whom to contact in the event of a research-related injury to the subject.

8. A statement that participation is voluntary, that refusal to participate will involve no penalty or loss of benefits to which the subject is otherwise entitled, and that the subject may discontinue participation at any time without penalty or loss of benefits to which the subject is otherwise entitled.

When appropriate, one or more of the following elements of information shall also be provided to each subject:

1. A statement that the particular treatment or procedure may involve risks to the subject (or to the embryo or fetus, if the subject is or may become pregnant) which are currently unforeseeable.

2. Anticipated circumstances under which the subject's participation may be terminated by the investigator without regard to the subject's consent.

3. Any additional costs to the subject that may result from participation in the research.

4. The consequences of a subject's decision to withdraw from the research and procedures for orderly termination of participation by the subject.

5. A statement that significant new findings developed during the course of the research which may relate to the subject's willingness to continue participation will be provided to the subject.

6. The approximate number of subjects involved in the study.

The informed consent requirements in these regulations are not intended to pre-empt any applicable federal, state, or local laws which require additional information to be disclosed for informed consent to be legally effective.

Nothing in these regulations is intended to limit the authority of a physician to provide emergency medical care to the extent the physician is permitted to do so under applicable federal, state, or local law.

In addition, most modern ethicists recommend that any conflict of interest be disclosed to the patient.

Informed consent can be a challenge in developing countries for several reasons.

First, communication can be an issue. The patient's understanding of the disease and the disease or body framework may be different. Translations can be difficult. Standard practice is to translate the informed consent into the local language and then to back-translate it using another translator. The original and the back-translated versions are compared and any discrepancies corrected. The patients may not be literate.

In particular, the investigators must be careful to avoid therapeutic misconception, or belief that the study is designed to help the patients in the trial. This is a common misconception in developed countries and even more common in developing countries.

Second, the power relationship between the physician and the patient may be extremely wide. In many cultures, it may be almost impossible for the patient to refuse a request from the physician. In that case, a study may not be feasible.

Third, the patient may need permission from a family member (a wife from a husband for example) legally and/or culturally before they consent to the study. The patient may need permission from the elder of the village or family, or the village council before entering into the study. In general, in order to satisfy both local and international ethical requirements, the consent must be obtained from all appropriate parties. In cases where the elder or others may exert undue pressure on the patient to enroll in the study, it is important to ensure that this does not happen. If it is impossible to rule out such an influence, then the study may not be feasible.

It may be counterintuitive from a Western perspective, but respect for community and family rights in developing countries is often just as important as respect for individual rights. Whereas in a Western country, legal permission from a supercommunity (the state or federal government) and personal permission from an individual are generally necessary and sufficient, that is not always the case in communities where the family or the village still hold responsibilities and authority that had been devolved or evolved to the legal and individual level. Even in a Western community, however, there are traces of community authority and rights in certain circumstances. For example, for a study of defibrillation in patients undergoing sudden death, where neither the individual nor his kin may be available to give consent, community informed consent such as consent obtained via public meetings can substitute for individual consent.

In cases where the patient is not literate or is otherwise unable to sign the consent form, an independent witness must witness the consenting process and document it.

As mentioned above, many patients in developing countries may be considered a vulnerable population and great care must be taken in obtaining informed consent. Vulnerable research populations — those who cannot give or refuse consent for themselves and those vulnerable to coercion or undue influence — must be afforded special protection; the physician/researcher must make every effort to determine whether a potential subject is in a dependent relationship or under duress.

For incompetent, unconscious or incapacitated individuals, informed consent must be obtained from a legally authorized representative. If a potential subject deemed incompetent is able to give consent, the physician/researcher must procure his or her consent *in addition* to that of a legal representative.

Involvement of incompetent or incapacitated individuals in clinical trials can be justified only if their physical or mental condition is *a necessary characteristic* of the research population. Such individuals must be excluded from research that: can be undertaken with competent persons; entails significant risk or burden; and has no likelihood of benefit for them, except when the research may promote the health of the population they represent.

In some countries, certain diagnoses, such as cancer, are not divulged to patients. There is controversy about whether informed consent is possible in those circumstances, and most ethicists believe that it is not.

Although informed consent may be difficult to obtain, it is critical that a genuine informed consent be obtained and documented before the patient is enrolled in a clinical trial.

Institutional Review Board/Ethics Review Board

As per FDA and other regulatory body requirements, and as per international guidelines and standards, all studies must be approved by one or more institutional review board or ethics committee (EC). An EC has scientific, legal, and regulatory responsibilities. It reviews the design of the study to ensure that the study is scientifically sound, protects patient rights, and does not expose the patients to undue risk, that investigators are free from commercial or other bias, and that proper ethical safeguards are in place. In some cases, there is a separate scientific review board and the EC may not need to review the scientific merits of the study in as much detail. A scientific review board is charged with reviewing a study before the EC to determine its scientific validity and value.

An EC or an IRB must be properly constituted and must operate under certain requirements. US regulations as set forth in 21 CFR 56.107 mandate the following:

1. The IRB must have at least five members.
2. The members must have enough experience, expertise, and diversity to make an informed decision on whether the research is ethical, informed consent is sufficient, and appropriate safeguards have been put in place.

3. If the IRB works with studies that include vulnerable populations, the IRB should have members who are familiar with these groups. It is common for an IRB to include an advocate for prisoners when considering research that involves them.
4. The IRB should include both men and women, as long as they are not chosen specifically for their gender.
5. The members of the IRB must not be all of the same profession.
6. The IRB must include at least one scientist and at least one non-scientist. These terms are not defined in the regulations.
7. The IRB must include at least one person who is not affiliated with the institution or in the immediate family of a person affiliated with the institution. These are commonly called "community members".
8. IRB members may not vote on their own projects.
9. The IRB may include consultants in their discussions to meet requirements for expertise or diversity, but only actual IRB members may vote.
10. In order to vote on a proposal, more than half of the members of the board must be present and there must be a non-scientist present.
11. There are exceptions for expedited review, where only the chair of the committee or a designee reviews research, but these are relatively narrow.

In many cases, ECs in other countries follow the same or similar guidelines.

The EC must operate with a written charter, and must fully document its meetings and decisions. The investigator must submit protocols, informed consent forms, protocol amendments, serious adverse event reports/updates, and revised informed consent forms to the EC.

It is often difficult to properly constitute and operate an EC in a developing country. In one recent study, 44 percent of nearly 700 researchers conducting trials in lesser developed countries reported that their protocols had not been reviewed by local ECs or government ministries.[11] According to a 2005 survey, only 150 of India's approximately 14,000 general hospitals are adequately equipped to host clinical trials. Of these, only half have IRBs, many without the expertise to evaluate protocols.[12] Of published clinical trials conducted in China in 2004, 90 percent proceeded without a prior ethical review of protocols. Eighteen percent satisfied the requirements for obtaining subjects' informed consent.[13] Another survey of 200 health researchers found that a quarter of clinical trials in developing countries were not reviewed by an EC.[14]

In 1991, the US Department of Health and Human Services issued a set of guidelines (Federal Policy for the Protection of Human Subjects), referred to as the "Common Rule", incorporating standards for IRB membership, function, operations, review, and record keeping in trials funded or regulated by federal agencies and the FDA.

The sheer number, size, and complexity of research trials in the developing world create inordinate demands on sponsors, researchers, and host countries. Centralized IRBs — independently staffed and accredited oversight committees — can help to enforce best practices and standards, share non-proprietary information, and reduce redundancy. One model for the approach is the National Cancer Institute's Central Institutional Review Board Initiative. In some European countries, a single national EC serves to review studies for all clinical research in the country.

In many cases, there may be a need for two ECs for a study. One EC based in the originating developed country may review the study from the viewpoint of the originating country, while another EC based locally may review the study from the perspective of the developing country. The standards for where the EC review must occur are evolving, but in many cases, having double review of the protocol ensures that all ethical considerations have been met. For research sponsored by most US agencies, a US IRB must review the study.

The CIOMS guidelines call for both the originating (sponsor) and local (host) countries' ECs to review studies, whereas the Declaration of Helsinki suggests that the local EC is best suited. In some cases, approval by the originating country may unduly influence the local review because the local EC may be reluctant to overrule the more experienced EC in the originating country.

If only one EC can review the study, the local EC is preferred.

Capacity Building

In order to develop EC capacity in a developing country, several things must be accomplished. First, personnel with the requisite background must be recruited. In general, academic centers, government organizations, and personnel with experience in the World Health Organization or other international organizations make good candidates. Second, the personnel must be trained. There are multiple courses, publications, and other resources available for training. In some cases, some of the initial members for the EC might be personnel from developed countries who have previous experience on ECs. Third, the infrastructure must be established, with support personnel who can ensure smooth functioning of the EC. Fourth, proper documentation of the meetings must be maintained, with necessary documentation of quorums, votes, minutes, etc.

It is important that the EC operate in an environment of good clinical practice (GCP) compliance, and in the context of well-conducted and well-trained clinical investigators and studies. Otherwise, the beneficial effects of a well-functioning EC may be compromised. For example, if the investigator fails to provide the EC with timely reports of serious adverse events, then the EC cannot properly do its job.

Data Safety and Monitoring Board

A data safety monitoring board (DSMB) monitors a study during its course to ensure that patient safety is not being compromised. DSMBs are often used in clinical trials in developed countries, and can be very useful in developing countries because they add another layer of protection for the patient. A properly constituted DSMB has physicians, statistician(s), and other experts, and usually has access to the unblinded data upon which to base their decisions. A full explanation of a DSMB can be found in Chin and Lee.[4] A high functioning DSMB requires many of the same requirements as an EC, including expertise, training, and resources.

Early Phase Studies

CIOMS guidelines states that Phase I drug studies and Phase I and II vaccine studies should not be performed in a developing country. While there is no theoretical reason why Phase I studies should not be conducted in a developing country, there are practical reasons why such studies may be of particular concern in these countries. Primarily, the concern is that drugs or vaccines that may not be approved for testing in a developed country may be sent to a developing country for early phase studies. Many countries, including India and China, prohibit Phase I studies unless the drug and the sponsor are local. In addition, some countries frown upon studies that are only conducted locally without any sites in developed countries.

Responsibility to Maintain Privacy/Confidentiality

Every subject's right to privacy must be respected. The physician/researcher's responsibility is to assure that subjects' personal information is kept confidential. There are multiple guidelines on privacy/confidentiality in clinical research, including the US Health Insurance Portability and Accountability Act's Standards for Privacy of Individually Identifiable Health Information[14] and the European Commission's privacy guidelines, as well as local requirements.

Publication

The Declaration of Helsinki obligates authors and publishers to publish well-documented and accurate accounts of clinical trials — including negative data — and to reject "reports of experimentation not in accordance" with its principles. The International Committee of Medical Journal Editors has issued a set of standards covering trial design, access to data, control over the publication of results, and other issues. As noted elsewhere, information regarding funding, institutional affiliations, and potential conflicts of interest must be made public.

CONCLUSIONS

As clinical trials become more globalized, it is important to keep in mind and adhere to the highest levels of ethics. In addition to the typical issues surrounding clinical trials conducted in developed countries, studies in developing countries pose additional important issues, outlined above, that must be addressed carefully to ensure that patient rights are being protected and that the study is being conducted in an ethical manner.

Some of the material in this chapter is based on or excerpted with permission from Chin and Lee's Principles and Practice of Clinical Trial Medicine[4] and Chin and Bairu's Global Clinical Trials.[5]

References

1. World Medical Association. Declaration of Helsinki: ethical principles for medical research involving human subjects, http://www.wma.net/en/30publications/10policies/b3/index.html [accessed 30.07.10].

2. Council for International Organizations of Medical Sciences (CIOMS). International ethical guidelines for biomedical research involving human subjects, http://www.cioms.ch/publications/layout_guide2002.pdf [accessed 31.07.10].

3. The Belmont Report. http://www.nmmu.ac.za/documents/rcd/The%20Belmont%20Report.pdf

4. Chin R, Lee BY. Principles and Practice of Clinical Trial Medicine. 1st ed. New York: Academic Press; 2008.

5. Chin R, Bairu M. Global Clinical Trials: Effective Implementation and Management. 1st ed. New York: Academic Press; 2011.

6. Lamberti MJ, Space S, Gammbrill S. Going global. Applied Clinical Trials 2004;**13**:84–92.

7. Centers for Disease Control. Update on CDC Collaborative research studies on perinatal HIV prevention in the developing world: preliminary results find short-course AZT effective, http://www.cdc.gov/nchstp/od/Perinatal; 1998.

8. Lurie P, Wolfe SM. Unethical trials of interventions to reduce perinatal transmission of the human immunodeficiency virus in developing countries. New England Journal of Medicine 1997;**337**:853–6.

9. Angell M. The ethics of clinical research in the third world. New England Journal of Medicine 1997;**337**:847–9.

10. Varmus H, Satcher D. Ethical complexities of conducting research in developing countries. New England Journal of Medicine 1997;**337**:1003–5.

11. Glickman SW, McHutchison JG, Peterson ED, Cairns CB, Harrington RA, et al. Ethical and scientific implications of the globalization of clinical research. New England Journal of Medicine 2009;**360**:2793.

12. Nundy S, Gulhati CM. A new colonialism? Conducting clinical trials in India. New England Journal of Medicine 2005;**352**:1633–6.

13. Zhang D, Yin P, Freemantle N, Jordan R, Zhong N, Cheng KK. An assessment of the quality of randomized controlled trials conducted in China. Trials 2008;**9**:22.

14. Hyder A. Ethical review of health research: a perspective from developing country researchers. Journal of Medical Ethics 2004;**30**:68–72.

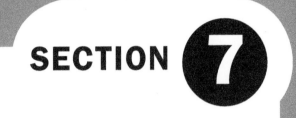

SECTION 7

Quality Assurance and Data Management

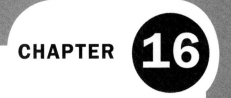
Clinical Quality Assurance and Data Management

Janice B. Wilson
Wilson Quality & Compliance Consulting, Antioch, California, USA

199

INTRODUCTION

The reasons for carefully managing the quality of data generated during drug development and clinical trials can be summed up quite simply: good clinical trial data are the only way a sponsor can ensure that the information submitted for review during a drug application process is accurate and meets the expectations of regulators, subjects and their families, and caregivers. Bad or questionable data can cause an ongoing study to be put on hold or suspended, a regulatory submission to be denied, or months or years of work and large sums of money and human resources to be wasted when an application is denied approval. Sponsors must ensure that data integrity is maintained throughout a clinical trial and that studies proceed according to development plans, protocols, and regulatory requirements. Changes to the original plan must be properly thought through, and documented in amended protocols, institutional review board (IRB) submissions, and study brochures. A system must be in place that can ensure that all activities are compliant with applicable regulations. Thus, there is the need for a quality system appropriately designed to address the various stages of product development.

Global Clinical Trials Playbook. DOI: 10.1016/B978-0-12-415787-3.00016-3

CLARIFYING THE TERMINOLOGY

Since it is important to understand the terminology specific to the topic of discussion, a list is provided of the most common quality-related terms along with a definition intended to provide clarification on how the term is applied in, or during clinical studies. The list is not intended to be inclusive of all quality-related terms, but does include those terms that are required to understand the structure and activities of an effective quality system that oversees all aspects of clinical trials according to good clinical practice (GCP).

- **Audit**: A form of review that provides confidence to the sponsor concerning the validity and accuracy of clinical study data that must be submitted to support a new drug application (NDA), biologicals license application (BLA), or premarket approval (PMA) application. Audits usually are conducted throughout the course of the study while problems are still "correctable".
- **Bioresearch monitoring**: The regulatory inspection programs related to clinical research designed to ensure the protection of research subjects and the integrity of data submitted in support of a marketing application. The FDA's Bioresearch Monitoring Program (BIMO) is an example.
- **Clinical quality assurance (CQA)**: An independent function whose primary responsibilities are to perform systematic and independent examinations/audits of all trial-related activities and documents to assure that the evaluated activities have been appropriately conducted and that the data have been generated, recorded, analyzed, and accurately reported according to protocol, standard operating procedures (SOPs), and GCPs.[1]
- **Compliance**: Adherence to the study protocol, relevant SOPs, GCP, and all other applicable regulatory requirements.
- **Corrective action and preventive action (CAPA)**: Actions taken to correct and prevent reoccurrence and occurrence of an incident or event that was found to be out of compliance, not according to procedures, or not within validated parameters.
- **Quality control (QC)**: The operational techniques and activities undertaken within the quality assurance (QA) system to verify that the requirements for quality of the study-related activities have been fulfilled.
- **Quality plan**: The plan that describes how the quality control and quality assurance processes will be applied throughout the clinical trial. It definitively defines the various quality-related tasks in the study. A quality plan documents specific quality practices, resources, and activities relevant to a specific project. This includes both operational QC and QA activities.
- **Quality system**: The organizational structure, responsibilities, procedures, processes, and resources for implementing quality management.
- **Quality system element (QSE)**: an individual/unique component of a quality management system designed to ensure that all internal policies, government regulations, and guidance requirements related to the element are met. Examples of QSEs are materials management, complaint handling, deviations and non-compliance, CAPA management, and computer validation.
- **Raw data**: Any original worksheets, calibration data, records, memoranda and notes of first-hand observations and activities of a study that are necessary for the reconstruction and evaluation of the study. Raw data may include, but are not limited to, photographic materials, magnetic, electronic or optical media, information recorded from automated instruments, and hand-recorded datasheets. Transcribed data are not considered raw data.
- **Regulatory inspection**: The act by a relevant regulatory authority of conducting, in accordance with its legal authority, an official review of study documentation, facilities, equipment, finished and unfinished materials (and associated documentation), labeling, and any other resources related to the registration of an investigational product and that may be located at any site related to the study. Regulatory inspections are performed by

regulatory agencies such as the US Food and Drug Administration (FDA) or a member state of the European Medicines Agency (EMA), and are intended to determine compliance with applicable regulations, adherence to appropriate guidelines, and the validity and integrity of clinical data submitted in applications for approval, and to assure that the rights and welfare of subjects participating in clinical studies have been protected.

BASIC QUALITY REQUIREMENTS

International Requirements

The quality requirements are spelled out quite clearly in the International Conference on Harmonisation (ICH) GCP guidelines.[2] The essence of what is written as the initial requirement in ICH E6 (R1), Part 5, clearly states that a system of quality must be employed and implemented by the sponsor (Table 16.1).

US Requirements

The US FDA has accepted the ICH GCP guidance, ICH E6, and does not have a consolidated guidance document for GCP as it does for good manufacturing practice (GMP). However, there are several other "Guidance to Industry" publications relative to GCP requirements. In the 2001 publication,[3] the responsibility for quality was clearly identified as being that of the sponsor.

- Section 4.2.16. Ensure the quality and integrity of data from clinical studies by implementing quality audit procedures that are consistent with well-recognized and accepted principles of quality assurance.
- Section 4.3.1. A sponsor may delegate any or all of the sponsor's study-related duties and functions to a contract research organization (CRO), but the ultimate responsibility for the quality and integrity of the study data always resides with the sponsor.

Having made the case for quality, required by the regulations, the next sections of this chapter present some best practices that ensure that the essence of these requirements is met. Throughout the following section, observations from documented bioresearch monitoring inspections will be interjected in an effort to support the position that a strong, well-defined quality management system is beneficial.

THE CASE FOR A GOOD CLINICAL PRACTICE QUALITY SYSTEM

There are no clearly defined requirements for a GCP quality management system equivalent to the one recommended by the Center for Devices and Radiological Health (CDRH) for

TABLE 16.1 ICH E6 (R1) Guidelines for Good Clinical Practices — Section 5.1
5.1.1 The sponsor is responsible for implementing and maintaining quality assurance and quality control systems with written SOPs to ensure that clinical studies are conducted and data are generated, documented (recorded), and reported in compliance with the protocol, GCP, and other applicable regulatory requirement(s).
5.1.2 The sponsor is responsible for securing agreement from all involved parties to ensure direct access (see 1.21) to all trial related sites, source data/documents, and reports for the purpose of monitoring and auditing by the sponsor, and inspection by domestic and foreign regulatory authorities.
5.1.3 Quality control should be applied to each stage of data handling to ensure that all data are reliable and have been processed correctly.
5.1.4 Agreements, made by the sponsor with the investigator/institution and any other parties involved with the clinical study, should be in writing, as part of the protocol or in a separate agreement.

ICH: International Conference on Harmonisation; SOP: standard operating procedure; GCP: good clinical practice.

TABLE 16.2 Common Inspection Findings (Deficiencies)

Sponsors/monitors	Study Investigators	IRBs/ECs
Inadequate monitoring	Failure to follow the investigational plan	Inadequate initial and/or continuing review
Failure to bring investigators into compliance	Protocol deviations	Inadequate SOPs
Inadequate accountability for the investigational product	Inadequate recordkeeping	Inadequate membership rosters
	Inadequate accountability for the investigational product	Inadequate meeting minutes
	Inadequate subject protection, including informed consent issues	
	Underreporting of safety issues	

IRB: independent review board; EC: ethics committee; SOP: standard operating procedure.

GMP activities related to medical devices. The sheer number of separate guidance documents related to GCP, beginning with the Helsinki Accord, would suggest that such a system would be massive, difficult to define, and/or not required. Of course, none of these is true. All one has to do is look at the number of inspections carried out by agencies such as the FDA and the EMA and observe the common issues found, some of which are listed in Table 16.2.

Even though the requirements as outlined in Table 16.1 leave little room for creative interpretation, quality systems do vary across the GxP disciplines. For GCP, a successful quality system would require QSEs that, at a minimum, address all of the subjects of concern during regulatory inspections or bioresearch monitoring. Since the FDA acceptance/endorsement of ICH E6 and the success of a joint inspection pilot by the FDA and the EMA in 2010, setting up a quality system that would meet global requirements is essential. In Part II of Chapter 48 of the FDA's Compliance Program Guidance Manual[4] the FDA provides clear guidance to its agents/inspectors on what to look for during inspections of sponsors, CROs, and monitors. Table 16.3 contains the major headings in this section of the guidance manual and is fairly representative of the subject areas that should be addressed in a GCP quality system.

In the FDA's compliance guidance manual, each of the components in Table 16.3 is expanded on to show how ensuring patient safety is the primary focus of the inspection. The purpose of this chapter is not to define the complete programs for all these subjects but rather to show how having an adequate quality system ensures that all are in place and in compliance with internal as well as applicable regulatory requirements.

The remainder of this chapter describes a quality assurance program that, when properly implemented, will ensure that clinical studies are conducted and data are generated, documented (recorded), and reported in compliance with the protocol, GCP, and other applicable regulatory requirements.

CLINICAL QUALITY ASSURANCE

Sponsors, CROs, and clinical investigators must have SOPs in place. These SOPs define the quality system. The degree to which the quality program has been thought out and planned determines the strength and cohesiveness of the quality system. There should be SOPs that govern all clinical activities and responsibilities initiated and carried out by sponsors, clinical

TABLE 16.3 Components of the FDA's Bioresearch Monitoring Program for Sponsors, Contract Research Organizations, and Monitors

Personnel qualification and training
Registration of clinical trial studies
Selection and monitoring of clinical investigators
Selection of monitors
Monitoring procedures and activities
Quality assurance activities
Safety/adverse event reporting
Data collection and handling
Record retention
Financial disclosure
Electronic records and electronic signatures
Test article management and control
Non-clinical laboratory studies

investigators, monitors, and ethics committees (ECs), and IRBs. It is important to address what CQA should do to ensure that the SOPs are adequate and complied with and to make sure that when deviations from SOPs or protocols occur they are properly investigated and resolved. Effective CQA cannot exist without a well-defined quality system. Since the primary role of CQA is to ensure compliance with internal and external requirements, the internal requirements must be as well defined as the regional and international regulatory requirements. The quality system for a CRO should cover all the activities of all the departments or functions; the quality system for a clinical site should relate to the specific clinical research activities involved.

Complexity must be avoided when developing a quality system. The well-known KIS principle (keep it simple) should be paramount. Recalling that the components of a quality system can be referred to as the QSEs of that system, one can use the list to determine the elements of the quality system. The subjects can be combined such that a separate QSE is not needed for each subject. For example, all those related to personnel and training can be combined into one QSE consisting of the subcomponents that address the overarching training program, personnel qualification requirements, training plans for various functions or departments, and training records. Similarly, subcomponents related to ensuring regulatory compliance such as vendor qualification, internal and external auditing, hosting, and responding to regulatory inspections could compile another QSE. Table 16.4 provides examples of the key QSEs and QSE topics related to the responsibilities and activities of the CQA function, i.e., the areas that the CQA group must monitor and audit to ensure compliance with in-house and regulatory requirements. It is the responsibility of CQA to ensure that the content of the quality system is fit for purpose. This requires a joint effort between CQA and all other stakeholders such as clinical development, regulatory affairs, biometrics, and medical affairs, to name a few.

Table 16.4 contains QSEs for which CQA should assure compliance. They are not all QSEs that CQA should own. Those items marked with an asterisk (*) are activities that are usually overseen by a GMP QA function. However, in many small companies or virtue companies, the CQA organization is a combination of individuals performing all GxP oversight.

The CQA or any quality assurance group must have their own SOPs in addition to reviewing and approving all SOPs. The SOPs that CQA own should clearly define how quality assurance activities should be carried out, while setting the standard for SOPs owned by other areas, departments, and functions in the company. Table 16.5 contains a list of SOPs typically owned by CQA. The list is not intended to be all inclusive and it may contain SOPs owned by other functions within an organization. The ownership and accountability for all SOPs must be carefully thought out, with the development, implementation, and maintenance of the SOPs in mind when assigning SOPs.

TABLE 16.4 Examples of Quality System Elements of a Good Clinical Practice (GCP) Quality System	
QSE title	**QSE subjects/subelements**
Personnel/organization	Training program
	Training plans
	Training records
	Quality organization
	Qualification of personnel
	Job descriptions
	Delegation and responsibilities
Documentation practices	Document control
	Standard operating procedures
	Document change control
	Development reports
	Data recording and management
	Study protocols
	Essential documents (GCP)
	Document and record retention
	Archiving
Materials control*	CTM manufacturing*
	Clinical trial API manufacturing*
	Review and release of CTM*
	CTM specifications*
	CTM shipping and storage*
	CTM distribution
	CTM accountability
Facilities and equipment	Investigation sites (suitability for study)
	Equipment (validation and calibration if applicable)*
	Facility, utilities, and equipment controls*
	Maintenance*
Regulatory compliance	Adverse event reporting
	Annual product review
	Audit programs (plans/schedules)
	Audit/inspection results
	Deviation investigation and reporting
	Test substance complaints
	Corrective and preventive actions
	Trend analysis
Validation	Cleaning validation and verification*
	Computerized systems validation and risk management*
	Test method validation*
	Shipping validation*
	Manufacturing process validation and verification*

QSE: quality system element; CTM: clinical trial material; API: Active Pharmaceutical Ingredient.
*Oversight of these activities is normally the responsibility of good manufacturing practice quality assurance (GMP QA) functions. For small or virtual companies these may be combined in the clinical quality assurance (CQA) function with the GMP QA specialist.

A huge part of CQA's responsibilities is to ensure that there are systems in place for managing all data and activities associated with a clinical trial or, more clearly stated, to ensure that a state of control is maintained throughout a trial. Data integrity and patient safety cannot be assured with a fine list of well-written SOPs. Today, with concepts and practices such as quality by design and quality risk management, the expectation is to have a quality management system in place that runs in parallel with well-established data management systems. The following section explains how CQA can demonstrate a state of control throughout and beyond the duration of a clinical study by utilizing the different types of quality assessments and audits that should be carried out.

TABLE 16.5 Examples of Clinical Quality Assurance (CQA) Standard Operating Procedure Titles
Preparation, use and maintenance of standard operating procedures
Training program (when training is owned by QA)
Training of CQA personnel
Qualification of third party vendors and service providers
Contract employees and consultants
Document change control process
Qualification/monitoring of contractors for manufacturing, packaging, distribution, and/or testing of clinical products (auditing program)
Investigation and deviation reporting procedure
Annual product review for INDs
Internal audit procedure
Procedure for regulatory agency inspections
Handling clinical product complaints
Contents of quality documentation central files
Expiration dating procedure
Recall/withdrawal of policy and procedure for clinical trial materials
Organization and responsibilities of quality and compliance
Quality assurance (GCP/GLP) audits of CROs
Distribution and management of notebooks
Archiving procedure for quality documentation
Controlled copy distribution
QA release of clinical supplies for Phase I–IV studies
Retained samples management program
Quality assurance review of documents
Preparation and distribution of audit reports
Handling and maintenance of regulatory agencies inspection records
CGMP requirements for manufacturing of CTM to support NDAs
Internal document processing procedure
Clinical quality assurance preapproval inspection process
Audit of clinical study report
CQA audit of clinical site
Contract manufacturer assessment program
Management of a CQA program of a CRO
Detecting and reporting misconduct or possible fraud in clinical studies
Clinical data processing audits
Clinical trial master file audit
Investigator brochure audit
QA procedure for CTM diversions

QA: quality assurance; CQA: clinical quality assurance; IND: investigational new drug; GCP: good clinical practice; GLP: good laboratory practice; CRO: contract research organization; CGMP: current good manufacturing practice; CTM: clinical trial material; NDA: new drug application.

GOOD CLINICAL PRACTICE QUALITY AUDITS

There are no well-defined regulatory requirements for performing QA audits during clinical studies. However, section 5.1 of ICH E6 — GCP clearly states:

> 5.1 Quality Assurance and Quality Control
>
> 5.1.1 The sponsor is responsible for implementing and maintaining quality assurance and quality control systems with written SOPs to ensure that trials are conducted and data are generated, documented (recorded), and reported in compliance with the protocol, GCP, and the applicable regulatory requirement(s).

Inadequate sponsor oversight of clinical studies is a common problem, according to information published in the annual Bioresearch Monitoring Reports[5] of the FDA as well as in warning letters that are also published by the FDA on its website.[6] Therefore, companies must periodically assess and audit studies to determine that all activities are being carried out and recorded according to protocols. This is done in addition to the clinical monitoring that occurs on a more frequent basis. How often to audit and what stage(s) of a study to audit become natural questions for CQA. This is where the GCP or clinical study quality plan comes into play.

The clinical study quality plan must be study specific, and developed and implemented by the company's CQA function. The most effective clinical study quality plan goes beyond the development of an audit schedule and includes ensuring CQA's involvement from study design to study end. This means that CQA should be involved in study execution team meetings, review of protocols, and protocol amendments, as well as performing scheduled audits at investigator sites, CROs, and other common GCP service providers such as IRBs and pharmacies. The audit schedule and subsequent audit plans are components of a well-defined quality plan. Quality plans must be developed with the ability to make modifications as the clinical study or schedule changes throughout the life cycle of the study. A quality plan may include the following components:

- clinical study oversight
- audits of clinical investigator sites
- audits of clinical study report
- database audits
- audits of clinical service providers.

Clinical Study Oversight

The quality plan should indicate the quality representative assigned to the study. This individual should be the regulatory compliance "go to subject matter expert" who attends study execution meetings on a regular basis, as well as special meetings called to discuss protocol amendments, study diversions/deviations, ongoing activities with vendors providing study-related services, etc.

Audits of Clinical Sites

Clinical investigator site audits are performed to ensure that the conduct of study is proceeding according to the protocol and in compliance with GCP. These audits must be scheduled in order to effect changes as close to the point when needed as possible. With an adequate schedule, when problems exist, they are detected, acted upon, and corrected in a timely fashion, with preventive measures put in place to avoid similar issues at other sites. These audits assure data integrity and subject protection. During site assessment planning, the parameters used to determine which sites are audited should include:

- projected site enrollment
- trial management arrangements
- site regulatory history
- site personnel issues
  - turnover of site personnel
  - consistency of site monitors or contracted monitoring organizations
  - use of subinvestigators
- participation in other studies (specifically other company-sponsored studies)
- screening trends.

For Phase I studies, a site assessment should occur before enrollment and possibly at the end of the study, based upon the length of the study and whether any issues arose during the study. For Phase II and III studies, which are larger and longer, auditing should begin when 25–50 percent of study enrollment has occurred at a site. When determining how many sites should be audited during a study, industry standards are that quality plans should ensure that 10–20 percent of the sites are audited. However, this number could increase dramatically during the course of a study; for example, if protocols are changed such that study arms are dropped or added, or if drug accountability becomes a problem during the study. In addition, the following parameters can lead to a site being selected for an audit or a reaudit:

- actual subject enrollment at a site
- issues reported from other areas in the organization, such as
  - drug safety: subject safety or safety trends
  - clinical operations: protocol or regulatory non-compliance
  - biostatistics: site data trends or inaccuracies
- changes in study monitors or monitoring organizations
- concerns raised by a monitor or another responsible person
- notification of regulatory inspection(s).

The primary purpose of the site audit is to ensure that the site has followed the protocol and study-related SOPs, and complied with all applicable regulations. To this end, some information to be reviewed during an investigator site audit is listed in Table 16.6. The list is not intended to be all inclusive. Other information, such as the records associated with the management of remote sites managed by an investigator, should also be reviewed during a site audit.

The results of the investigator site audit should be discussed with the investigator and all other key site study personnel at the close of the audit. Effort should be made to ensure that all findings are understood and agreed upon in the audit close-out meeting. The audit report should be issued on a "need to know" basis and should include a summary of the findings with a request for a formal response from the investigator within a set amount of time. Industry standards are that these responses, complete with root cause analyses and CAPAs, are submitted within 30 days of the close of the audit. However, there is nothing that precludes a shorter response time. Corrective and preventive actions will be expanded on at the end of this section.

Audits of Clinical Study Reports

The audit of the clinical study report (CSR) should occur when the report is considered finalized but before final approval and publication. The audit of this report is extremely important and should be done very thoroughly. The amount of report information/data to audit is often a question of "how much or how little is enough"? The percentage of data audited should be predetermined and justified or statistically and scientifically valid. Too large a sample size can be time consuming and equivalent to rewriting the entire report, while too

TABLE 16.6 Information to be Reviewed During an Investigator Site Audit

Investigator's and subinvestigators'/pharmacist's curriculum vitae
Training records of study personnel
Signature pages for protocol including amends if applicable
Form 1572 or other documentation of investigator's agreement
IRB initial approval of protocol and consent form
IRB ongoing or annual review
IRB approval of items such as amended protocols, revised consent forms, and study advertisements
IRB final review if study is completed
Subjects' records/case report forms (including individual consent forms)
Laboratory certifications and records
Study material records (shipments, usage, and returns)
Correspondence
Financial records related to the study

IRB: institutional review board.

TABLE 16.7 Points to Consider During Audits of Clinical Research Reports
Consistency of text, tables and figures with data reported
Adverse event reports — ensuring that what is reported is accurate and reflects the study history
Properly prepared and signed reports from specialists or subinvestigators
Verification of selected data points from case report forms — these can be specifically chosen based on observations or randomly selected
Verification of protocol compliance — including compliance to standard operating procedures identified in the protocol
Results, summaries, and study conclusions should be consistent with recorded data
Clinical study report should contain no typographical errors
Verification of signatures of all responsible persons — compliant with good documentation practices

small a sample can lead to missed detection of errors. Industry standards appear to be to randomly select data from a percentage of the total data points, with about 50 percent of the data being reviewed. In addition, the CSR audit should confirm that the table of contents is aligned with the actual text of the document, tables, and appendices. The most egregious errors that should be avoided are mislabeled or incorrectly numbered tables and appendices, since one numbering error may cause all subsequent numbering to be incorrect. Table 16.7 provides a list of areas to audit within the CSR and information that should be included in the audit report.

The results of the CSR audit should be documented in an audit report and all items that need correcting or were questionable should be sent to those responsible, with a request for corrections to be made. A medical writer or someone who can review the corrections and make sure that they are aligned with the data should make the actual corrections to the report with verification by CQA before final approval.

Database Audits

Database audits should occur before hard lock of the database. This is after the study ends and all data have been entered. Such audits are more common after Phase II and III clinical studies, where 10–15 percent of randomly selected subject cases are audited. Subject cases are defined as the case report forms for the subjects, any addendum pages, laboratory results pages, and data queries regarding the subject. The CQA audit should include an assessment of compliance with the protocol and applicable SOPs and a review of quality control documentation. Any corrective actions are also performed before database hard lock.

Audits of Essential Documents

Essential documents are those documents that individually and collectively permit evaluation of the conduct of a trial and the quality of the data produced. The accumulation of these documents is often referred to as the trial master file (TMF). While the TMF should contain all essential documents, it contains more than the essential documents listed in ICH E6 Section 8. For example, both the EMA and the FDA require that records of audits of study activities be included in the TMF.

Essential documents or TMFs can be audited at any time during a study and the audit can occur at the investigator or sponsor site. The files should always be readily available, complete, and compiled in chronological order aligned with the timing of or sequence of study activities. The CQA auditor should ensure that the documents comply with GCP requirements as well as SOPs relative to the study. A simple acronym that defines compliant documents is ALCOA: attributable, legible, contemporaneous, original, and accurate. Table 16.8 contains a list of generic audit findings when ALCOA is not apparent. During planning for these audits, CQA

TABLE 16.8 Common Frequent Findings Observed During Audits of Essential Documents

Documents are missing
Documents are stored elsewhere
Documents are incomplete
Documents are not signed and dated
Documents are not current (incorrect version)
Documents are absent
- Laboratory certification
- Audit certification
- Safety reports
- IRB/EC statement of compliance
- IRB/EC membership
- Product accountability documentation
- Monitoring visit reports
- Expected correspondence (IRB, sponsor, CRO)

Subject safety (consent forms)
- Signatures not dated
- Versions not current
- Patient privacy not assured
- Dating discrepancies
- Inadequate investigator oversight in consenting process

Study personnel
- Missing CVs
- No evidence of GCP training
- No record of study training (protocol, investigator brochure)
- Current position not listed
- Incomplete or missing signature log

Clinical trial material (IND, IMP)
- Shipping records
- Storage monitoring records
- Accountability inadequate

Contracts and agreements
- Missing contracts
- Responsibilities not clearly defined
- Contracts out of date

IRB: institutional review board; EC: ethics committee; CRO: contract research organization; CV: curriculum vitae; GCP: good clinical practice; IND: investigational new drug; IMP: investigational medicinal product.

should ensure that these problems do not exist, by looking for them. If problems are found, corrective and preventive actions should be implemented immediately.

One of the most important essential documents of a study is the informed consent form (ICF). ICFs should be audited specifically for compliance to the requirements of the protocol. In addition, the auditor should ensure that the language of the consent form is clear and written at a level that subjects and caregivers can understand. While this may be appear to be subjective, a very technically written ICF that the auditor finds difficult to map to the protocol is generally a clue that the protocol is not written at a level that can be easily comprehended. CQA's SOP related to auditing GCP activities should have a well-defined escalation process that allows issues related to consent forms to be addressed immediately. It should also require an assessment beyond the site where the problem was found, to ensure that the issues are not systemic. Such a problem can run the risk of endangering subjects or negating an entire clinical study. Table 16.9 provides a checklist that is typical of one used when reviewing or auditing the ICF for compliance to GCP. These are the minimum number of factors that should be assessed during the audit of the ICF.

TABLE 16.9 Informed Consent Form Checklist			
	Yes	No	Comments

Does the informed consent form contain:
1. Statement that the study involves research?
2. Explanation of purpose of research?
3. Expected duration of subjects' participation?
4. Description of procedures to be followed?
5. Identification of any procedures that are experimental?
6. Description of any reasonably foreseeable risks or discomforts to subjects?
7. Description of any benefits to subjects or to others, which reasonably may be expected from research?
8. Disclosure of appropriate alternative procedures or courses of treatment, if any that might be advantageous to subjects?
9. Statement regarding confidentiality of records and indicating possibility of regulatory agencies and sponsor reviewing records?
10. Explanation of any compensation or medical treatments available if injury occurs and where further information can be obtained?
11. Explanation of whom to contact for answers to pertinent questions about the research and research subjects' rights?
12. Statement regarding whom to contact in the event of research-related injury to the subjects?
13. Statement that participation is voluntary?
14. Statement that refusal to participate will involve no penalty or loss of benefits to which subject is otherwise entitled?
15. Statement that subject may discontinue participation at any time without penalty or loss of benefits to which subject is otherwise entitled?

There are times when the nature of the study will require that other statements be included, such as statements that a particular drug or treatment may involve risks. When this is the case, the ICF must spell out in clear and simple language what these risks are. If protocols are amended, the CQA auditor must verify during the audit of the ICFs that the forms were appropriately changed and that IRB/EC approval for the changed ICF occurred in a timely fashion.

Audits of Clinical Study Service Providers

Today, very few companies run clinical trial studies without contracting services from a third party vendor. CQA must have procedures in place to allow verification that these service providers are compliant with GCP, SOPs, and other appropriate regulations and guidelines. A list of service providers that also need auditing includes, but is not limited to:

- IRBs/ECs
- interactive voice response system providers
- pharmacies
- Active Pharmaceutical Ingredient (API) and clinical trial material contractors
- contract testing laboratories
- statisticians or firms providing such services.

Audit Closure and Corrective Action and Preventive Action

Audits almost always result in findings that need to be rectified or the discovery of gaps that must be remediated. At the close of the audit, the auditing SOP should require that the CQA auditor discuss all findings with personnel involved in the audit and that a reasonable effort is made to resolve issues before the audit report is finished or audit fieldwork is considered completed. It can also be beneficial for the auditor to notify the monitors of findings, because often the monitor can clarify issues and prevent misunderstandings from being recorded in the audit report. Audit reports should be issued within 14 days of the completion of the audit fieldwork. Responses to audit findings should be issued within 30 days of the written report.

A well-developed and implemented GCP quality management program must have root cause analyses and continuous improvement as part of their quality assessment component. The investigation of audit or inspection findings must be conducted systematically, identifying the most probable cause for a deficiency and developing corrective and preventative actions to address the system. A holistic CAPA program should include all such actions from all types of audits or inspections. The CAPA program should be governed by an SOP that requires association of the CAPA with a specific finding while also requiring assurance that an issue does not spread across different areas of the program. For example, if it is determined during an audit that a particular site has made an error during recruitment associated with exclusion/inclusion criteria, CQA should review a number of sites to make sure that the problem is localized, and not the result of poorly written instructions in the study protocol. In addition, a robust CAPA program allows for trending that may lead to an improvement in processes that result in better-run clinical studies in the future. Table 16.10 lists the eight commonly recognized elements that a sound CAPA SOP should require and Figure 16.1 illustrates some of the areas where deficiencies may lead to the development of corrective or preventive actions.

An audit should not close completely until satisfactory responses are received, including CAPAs that have been completed or will be completed. Such commitments must have a targeted due date as well as an individual who is responsible for developing and implementing the CAPA. Final closure of the audit occurs only after verification of the responses. Both FDA GCP (CFR 314.50.b.ix) and ICH E6 require audit certificates to be included in TMFs for all audits that become part of a regulatory submission. However, neither is clear about which audits require certificates. As with many other non-specific guidelines, industry has developed standards or common practices that are recognized as standards by the agencies by way of deficiencies noted in inspection reports or FDA Form 483s. Certificates are commonly issued for audits of clinical study reports regardless of the phase of the study (Phase I, II, or III), while certificates are issued for reviews and audits of TMFs, investigator sites, and databases associated with Phases II and III only. Certificates may be required for internal audits or audits

TABLE 16.10 Corrective and Preventive Action (CAPA) Steps[7]
1. Analyzing processes, work operations, concessions, quality audit reports, quality records, service records, complaints, returned product, and other sources of quality data to identify existing and potential causes of non-conforming product, or other quality problems. Appropriate statistical methodology shall be employed where necessary to detect recurring quality problems.
2. Investigating the cause of non-conformities relating to product, processes, and the quality system.
3. Identifying the action(s) needed to correct and prevent recurrence of non-conforming product and other quality problems.
4. Verifying or validating the corrective and preventive action to ensure that such action is effective and does not adversely affect the finished device.
5. Implementing and recording changes in methods and procedures needed to correct and prevent identified quality problems.
6. Ensuring that information related to quality problems or non-conforming product is disseminated to those directly responsible for ensuring the quality of such product or the prevention of such problems.
7. Submitting relevant information on identified quality problems, as well as corrective and preventive actions, for management review.
8. Documenting all CAPA activities.

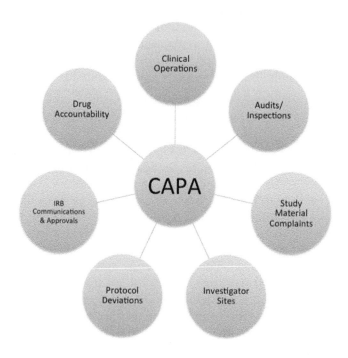

FIGURE 16.1
Sources for deficiencies that could lead to the need for corrective or preventive actions. CAPA: corrective action and preventive action; IRB: institutional review board. (Please refer to color plate section)

at CROs or other third party service providers, such as those manufacturing or testing clinical trial material, and such audits must be well documented with findings reported appropriately. These reports should also include a summary statement that allows stakeholders to assess the overall compliance of those audited.

GOOD CLINICAL PRACTICE QUALITY ORGANIZATION

In some larger organizations, CQA is part of a larger quality assurance unit or organization. The size of the quality assurance organization is dependent on the size of the organization. Regardless of size, the responsibilities of the CQA are the same. What will differ is who performs the duties: full- or part-time employees, consultants working for the organization, or contractors such as CROs. Regardless, all sponsors must have SOPs in place that ensure data integrity and subject safety. Either the SOPs will be written for employees or contractors to execute on behalf of the sponsor, or they are written to ensure that CROs have adequate SOPs in place.

The most effective quality assurance units are those whose leaders are equivalent in status or reporting order to the leaders of the departments that they support. For GCP, this means that the head of the CQA should be equivalent to medical directors, clinical research directors, and heads of regulatory affairs or drug safety. In addition to having the proper status and authority, the quality assurance unit/organization should have independence reflected in its reporting line. In some organizations this translates to the head of CQA reporting to the chairperson, president, chief medical officer, or head of research and development. In organizations where the quality assurance operations are provided by contractors or consultants, these individuals should also report as high up in the organization as possible. This ensures that CQA maintains the independence that is needed to ensure that reporting of issues goes through as few individuals as possible.

During inspections, regulatory agencies will look at organization charts to evaluate the independence and authority of its quality organization as well as the qualifications and training of the individuals. Table 16.11 provides a typical job description for the head of clinical quality assurance.

TABLE 16.11 Components of Job Description for Head of Clinical Quality Assurance

Position Summary:
The head of clinical quality assurance (CQA) will implement and maintain an effective clinical quality assurance function. This position will direct and manage the activities required to assure compliance with applicable regulations and industry accepted standards that govern clinical studies. CQA will provide oversight in all activities leading to or potentially leading to a regulatory filing [e.g. premarket approval (PMA), investigational device exemption (IDE), investigational new drug application (IND), biologic license application (BLA), new drug application (NDA), preapproval inspection (PAI), FDA-mandated post market studies (PMS), and market-driven PMS]. The CQA function is responsible throughout the clinical development process and post-launch clinical studies, from design of the protocol to the final clinical study report, to ensure compliance with applicable governmental regulations as well as company policies and procedures.

ESSENTIAL DUTIES AND RESPONSIBILITIES include the following. Other duties may be assigned.
- Develop and maintain quality management system documentation, including documents specific to regulatory and compliance processes and procedures
- Oversee internal training, including regulatory and compliance training of study personnel
- Ensure audits of internal processes and procedures to ensure staff compliance
- Ensure quality audits of external vendors and partners to evaluate prospective groups and review ongoing work under contract
- Perform audits of project procedures, training, documentation, and records
- Develop and implement quality programs including training personnel to ensure compliance with practices and procedures in support of quality programs such as ISO certification
- Ensure compliance of procedures with applicable regulations
- Manage the CAPA process to address findings, issues and non-compliances from both internal and client audits, working with other groups as applicable
- Develop, maintain and report on quality metrics related to compliance, training effectiveness, and resolution of issues including CAPAs and audit findings
- Host client audits of and regulatory inspections, including presentation of the company's QMS and responding to questions
- Deliver trainings as required on QMS processes and procedures
- Maintain internal training records and ensure timely compliance with company and job specific training requirements
- Provide in-house guidance on the application of national, regional, and local laws and regulations (e.g. privacy, data protection, ethics) to project-specific requirements and ensure compliance
- Ensure clinical compliance with respect to the development of and process for all clinical protocols and risk assessment for clinical trial execution
- Ensure that QA audits of clinical trial data are conducted effectively in order to assure compliance with SOPs, study protocols, good clinical practice guidelines, and relevant regulations including the CFR, ICH, and ISO 9000 requirements as applicable
- Ensure audits of CROs, central laboratories, and other vendor facilities
- Plan and coordinate specific projects related to the development and improvement of the QA clinical auditing program
- Ensure that audit results are formally and consistently recorded and reported and that corrective/preventive actions have been requested and documented effectively
- Ensure that regulatory inspections are effectively executed and provide support and direction during the hosting of such inspections
- Provide support to investigator sites for regulatory inspections related to company/sponsor-related clinical studies
- Prepare the local department budget and ensure effective cost control
- Liaise with all affected departments on quality aspects of studies, including attendance at marketing meetings, project meetings, oral presentations, and audits

Continued

213

TABLE 16.11	Components of Job Description for Head of Clinical Quality Assurance—continued

Required Skills and Experience

- Requires a bachelor's degree in a scientific discipline. A master's or PhD degree in life science, medicine, or related field would be a plus
- A minimum of 7 years' experience in quality and/or clinical practice within the pharmaceutical industry
- Strong knowledge and understanding of product development and the clinical trial process
- Auditing experience preferred
- Knowledge of relevant healthcare regulatory environment standards and regulations, e.g. GCP, FDA, ICH, other organizations
- Experience working in a structured but fast-paced environment
- Experience performing process and documentation audits
- Experience developing process documentation
- Proven ability to address and resolve non-compliances
- Ability to develop training programs and successfully train personnel
- Ability to prioritize and schedule time for various activities such as audits considering business needs
- Ability to organize and track documentation and records
- Excellent verbal and written communication skills
- Excellent communicator with demonstrated track record in fostering collaboration and building consensus to achieve collective objectives
- Travel required up to 75%
- Budget planning and expenditure management experience a plus

CAPA: corrective action and preventive action; QMS: quality management system; QA: quality assurance; SOP: standard operating procedure; CFR: Code of Federal Register; ICH: International Conference on Harmonisation; ISO: International Organization for Standardization; CRO: contract research organization; GCP: good clinical practice; FDA: Food and Drug Administration.

214

GOOD CLINICAL PRACTICE INSPECTION READINESS

Being ready for regulatory inspections should be part of the job of everyone involved in clinical trials. However, as with all other activities not owned by one department, sponsors and investigators can be woefully unprepared when the regulatory inspectors show up at the door or send notice that a clinical site will be inspected on a specific date. GCP inspection readiness should also be owned by CQA. Being prepared is much easier if the systems and processes previously discussed in this chapter have been adequately developed and implemented. In addition, because regulatory agencies need to know that their inspections are carried out consistently and in a manner that will ensure that their job of protecting the consumer is being done properly, all have their own guidance documents on performing such inspections. These are available to the public. The FDA has many guidance documents related to GCP inspections. Program 7348.8.10 in Chapter 48 of the FDA's Compliance Program Guidance Manual, as stated in section 15.4, addresses inspections of sponsors, CROs, and monitors. In that same chapter, Program 7348.8.11 is related to the inspection of investigators.[8] The EMA has a large number of guidance documents related to EMA inspections which can be found on their website as well.[9] Many emerging countries such as India have fashioned their GCP program after the ICH efficacy guidelines and have developed similar inspection process documents for their inspectors. India's inspection guidelines for inspectors are also available on their website.[10]

In addition to reading the above-referenced literature, the author recommends that CQA develop a short inspection readiness training module that addresses such things as:

- inspection notification telephone log
- inspection hosting areas

TABLE 16.12 Some Inspection Dos and Don'ts	
Dos	**Don'ts**
Know your procedures and processes	Do not make casual conversation
Have an SOP that covers inspection responsibilities of key functions	Do not assume the investigator is your "buddy"
Be prepared, organized, professional, and confident	Do not guess or make up an answer
Make sure that all anticipated documentation is readily available during the inspection	Do not lie
Have a scribe present at all times during the interview	Do not volunteer more information than necessary to completely answer the question
Listen carefully and repeat the question or ask it to be repeated, if necessary	Do not make the inspector wait for the information; explain legitimate delays
Answer completely, directly, and honestly	Do not speculate
Speak only for your area of expertise and be able to verify everything you say	Do not assume you know what the investigator means
Effectively guide questions posed by the inspector to SMEs with both the knowledge and the verbal skills to answer them	Ask for clarification, examples, or specifics
Communicate inspection results on a continuing basis	Never question the investigator's authority
Escalate serious issues as soon as they appear to be valid	Never argue or raise your voice
Summarize the results more formally after the inspection is complete	Do not allow photographs
Keep a record of all documentation reviewed by the inspector and a copy of any records taken by the inspector	Do not allow uncontrolled interchanges between personnel and the inspector; have a well-rehearsed signal that calls a discussion to an end when appropriate
Follow up to see that all written comments (e.g. 483s) and verbal comments have been addressed and resolved	
Ensure that responses are submitted to the agency in a timely fashion (14 days)	

SOP: standard operating procedure; SME: subject matter expert.

- need for various groups to identify their subject matter expert(s)
- inspection dos and don'ts such as those listed in Table 16.12.

The above list is also applicable to regulatory inspections at investigator sites.

When CQA is notified that an investigator site for a study is going to be inspected, the company should offer to assist the site in preparing for the inspector. Someone should be available to the site during the inspection. In the USA, this is usually done via telephone and e-mail; very seldom is the sponsor present during an inspection of a study site. However, it is expected that the sponsor will have a representative at the site during FDA inspections outside the USA.

SUMMARY

In summary, being ready for inspections allows a company to shine in the eyes of the inspector. The most successful inspections are those that run without hitches in logistics. It is important to know from where the inspection will be based, and to ensure that all departments have subject matter experts available throughout the inspection and that everyone is prepared by having a thorough training program that has been implemented and properly documented. Attention to details, such as ensuring that copiers and office supplies are available at the inspection, makes a positive impression. Before all of this, there must be CQA SOPs and a specific training program that has resulted in effective audits of all GCP activities. There must be complete follow-up for all audits, which includes verification of the effectiveness of implemented CAPAs. Finally, but not at all least, there must be a CQA organization staffed with well-trained personnel, with CVs in place that document their qualifications for the positions that they occupy.

References

1. ICH/GCP Good Clinical Practices Guidelines, E6. www.wilsonqcc.com [accessed 23.02.12]

2. ICH/GCP Good Clinical Practices Guidelines, E6, Section 5.1. www.wilsonqcc.com [accessed 23.02.12]

3. FDA. Guidance for Industry, Good Clinical Practice, 085. www.wilsonqcc.com [accessed 23.02.12]

4. FDA Compliance Program Guidance Manual, Program 7348.810. Chapter 48. Bioresearch monitoring – sponsors, contract research organizations and monitors. Implemented March 2011. www.wilsonqcc.com [accessed 23.02.12]

5. http://www.fda.gov/ScienceResearch/SpecialTopics/RunningClinicalTrials/ucm261409.htm [accessed 23.02.12]

6. http://www.fda.gov/ICECI/EnforcementActions/WarningLetters/2010/default.htm [accessed 23.02.12]

7. 21 CFR §820.100.

8. FDA Compliance Program Guidance Manual, Program 7348.811. Chapter 48. Bioresearch monitoring: clinical investigators. Implemented December 2008. www.wilsonqcc.com [accessed 23.02.12]

9. http://www.ema.europa.eu/ema/index.jsp?curl=pages/regulation/landing/human_medicines_regulatory.jsp&murl=menus/regulations/regulations.jsp&mid=WC0b01ac058001ff89 [accessed 23.02.12]

10. http://cdsco.nic.in/clinical_trial.htm [accessed 23.02.12]

Appendices

Sample Protocol Template

DCP CONSORTIA CHEMOPREVENTION PROTOCOL TEMPLATE

From National Cancer Institute - http://prevention.cancer.gov/clinicaltrials/management/pio/instructions

INSTRUCTIONS

The protocol template is a tool to facilitate rapid protocol development. It is not intended to supersede the role of the Protocol Principal Investigator in the authoring and scientific development of the protocol. It contains the language required in protocols submitted to the NCI, Division of Cancer Prevention (DCP). Please modify all sections as necessary to meet the scientific aims of the study and development of the protocol.

1. Each protocol submission consists of four parts:

    a. DCP Consortia Protocol Submission Worksheet (PSW): This document contains prompts for required administrative information. The PSW is required for all protocol submissions including the original protocol, revisions and amendments. It is available at http://prevention.cancer.gov/files/clinical-trials/consortia_psw.doc

    b. Main Body and Appendices of the protocol: This document provides standard language plus instructions and prompts for information required in each DCP protocol. The current protocol template is attached to these instructions, and is available at http://prevention.cancer.gov/clinicaltrials/management/pio/instructions. Please ensure the current version of the template always is used for protocol development.

    c. Additional Study-Related Documents: These documents include the Recruitment and Retention Plan, the Pharmacokinetic and Biomarker Methods Development Report, the Case Report Forms (CRFs) and attachments, the Data Management Plan (DMP), the Multi-Institutional Monitoring Plan (MIMP), and the Data and Safety Monitoring Plan (DSMP).

    The Recruitment and Retention Plan, Pharmacokinetic and Biomarker Methods Development Report, CRFs and attachments, and protocol-specific addenda to the DMP, MIMP and DSMP are submitted with the initial protocol. These documents are not considered an integral part of the protocol. Unless required by local practices, these documents do not need to be submitted to the local Institutional Review Board (IRB) and should not be referenced in the protocol.

    The PSW includes a checklist for all study-related documents (protocol, informed consent, and additional study-related documents) that must accompany each protocol submission. The DMP, MIMP, and DSMP have been standardized and approved for each consortium. Please reference these approved plans on the PSW, and submit supplemental information or addenda to these plans (*e.g.*, a protocol-specific addendum to the DMP) only as required.

    d. Protocol budget

2. An "administratively complete" protocol submission must include the following components:

    a. First submission
        i. DCP Consortia Protocol Submission Worksheet
        ii. Protocol including the informed consent document
            1. A protocol document version number and date must be on the cover page.
            2. All pages of the protocol must include a header that identifies the protocol by DCP protocol number, protocol document version date and version number. Pagination must be complete.
            3. The table of contents sections and page numbers must match the protocol.
        iii. All appendices (correct header and pagination)
        iv. All Additional Study-Related Documents (Recruitment and Retention Plan, Pharmacokinetic and Biomarker Methods Development Report, CRFs and attachments, supplemental information or addenda to the standardized DCP-approved documents (DMP, MIMP, and DSMP).

        v.   Protocol budget

    b.   All subsequent submissions (protocol revisions and amendments) must include:
        i.   Cover letter with a point-by-point response to DCP reviewer required and recommended changes with references to the changed document section.
        ii.   An updated Protocol Submission Worksheet (PSW)
        iii.   Amended protocol budget, if applicable, or a statement indicating that the proposed revision or amendment will not result in a change to the budget.
        iv.   "Tracked changes" or highlighted version of the protocol with informed consent and study-related documents, as appropriate, indicating changes from previous version
        v.   Clean copy of all documents with highlights removed
        vi.   Any changes to the CRFs or other study-related documents resulting from a protocol revision or amendment must be included with the submission for review and approval.
        vii.   Standard font indicates suggested language that should be retained in the document.
        viii.   **Bold font** indicates language that must be retained in the document.
        ix.   Blank space or _____ indicates that you should fill in the appropriate information.

"Administratively Incomplete" submissions will be returned to the Consortium Lead PI for completion. The review process will begin following receipt of an administratively complete submission.

3.   All sections in the Protocol Template should be retained within the body of the document. If not appropriate for a given study, please insert "Not Applicable" after the section number and delete the corresponding text.

4.   *All Protocol Template instructions and prompts are in italics. Italicized information should be deleted prior to submitting the protocol to DCP.*

5.   DCP terminology for changes to protocol:

    a.   Changes made prior to the initial DCP study approval are "Revisions"

    b.   Changes made after DCP approval are "Amendments"

6.   Indicate changes using the 'tracked changes' function, highlighting, or underlining new or modified text in protocol revisions or amendments to facilitate the review process.

7.   All document submissions must be sent electronically to Head, DCP Protocol Information Office (NCI_DCP_PIO@mail.nih.gov). Documents submitted elsewhere will not be accepted for review.

8.   DCP Consortia forms are available at http://prevention.cancer.gov/clinicaltrials/management/pio/instructions. Additional information is available on the DCP website at http://prevention.cancer.gov/clinicaltrials/management/consortia.

Questions:
Contact the DCP Protocol Information Office at (301) 496-0090 or e-mail NCI_DCP_PIO@mail.nih.gov

COVER PAGE

DCP Protocol #: *This number will be assigned by DCP and may be the same as or different from the local protocol number. The DCP protocol number must appear on all protocol document versions and all communication to DCP.*

Local Protocol #: *Insert your local protocol # for this study. If a local protocol number has not been assigned, indicate 'pending'. DEFINITION: The local protocol number is assigned by the Lead Organization according to local institutional conventions or Consortium guidelines.*

<u>PROTOCOL TITLE</u>

Consortium Name:	*Insert name of Consortium*
Name of Consortium Principal Investigator:	*Name & Title of the Principal Investigator of Consortium Lead Organization*
	Address
	Address
	Telephone
	Fax
	E-mail address

Organization Name:	*Organization name*
Protocol Principal Investigator:	*Protocol Principal Investigator*
	Investigator's Specialty
	Address
	Address
	Telephone
	Fax
	E-mail address

Organization:	*Organization name*
Investigator:	*Investigator's Name*
	Investigator's Specialty
	Address
	Address
	Telephone
	Fax
	E-mail address

Organization:	*Organization name*
Investigator:	*Investigator's Name*
	Investigator's Specialty
	Address
	Address
	Telephone
	Fax
	E-mail address

Organization:	*Organization Name*
Statistician:	*Statistician Name*
	Address
	Address
	Telephone
	Fax
	E-mail address

NOTE: If this is a multi-institution study:
1. *The protocol title page(s) <u>must</u> include the name and address of <u>each participating institution</u> and any <u>affiliates participating in the study</u>.*
2. *The protocol title page(s) must include the names of <u>all investigators</u> at each institution; his/her telephone, Fax, and e-mail address.*
3. *Indicate the protocol lead investigator responsible for the study at each institution; his/her telephone, Fax, and e-mail address.*

IND Sponsor: *NCI/Division of Cancer Prevention (or other Sponsor)*
6130 Executive Blvd., Room 2117
Bethesda, MD 20892 (For FedEx, use Rockville, MD 20852)
(301) 496-8563

IND# _____

Agent(s)/Supplier: _Study Agent(s) /Supplier Name_

NCI Contract # _N01-CN-xxxxx_

Protocol Version Date: _(Date)_

Protocol Revision or Amendment # _Revision or Amendment #_

SCHEMA

Please provide a schema for the study.

Protocol Title

Study Population

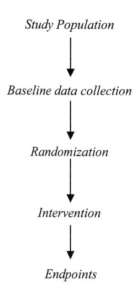

Baseline data collection

Randomization

Intervention

Endpoints

TABLE OF CONTENTS

1. **OBJECTIVES**

Study objectives are concise statements of the primary and secondary clinical and statistical questions that the study is designed to answer. Each objective should be stated as specifically and succinctly as possible. Both primary and secondary hypotheses must relate to the hypotheses presented in the rationale (section 2.3) and should be consistent with the objectives described in the statistical section (section 13.0). Clearly differentiate between primary and secondary objectives. Number the objectives in order of priority.

    1.1   **Primary Objectives** – *Insert primary protocol objective.*

    1.2   **Secondary Objectives** – *Insert secondary protocol objectives, if pertinent.*

2. **BACKGROUND**

    2.1   <u>***Study Disease***</u>

        Please provide background information on the study disease. (May not be applicable in phase 1 trials).

    2.2   <u>***Study Agent***</u>

        Please provide background information on the study agent, including information to support safety issues and the rationale for the study dose and duration of exposure.

    2.3   **Rationale**

        Please provide the background rationale for evaluating this agent in this cohort/target organ. Present possible mechanisms and/or theoretical framework for conducting the study. Include relevant literature review and pertinent preclinical, pilot, and preliminary and/or unpublished data to support conduct of the trial. Clearly state the hypotheses for the primary and secondary objectives. Justify selection of target population, agent, endpoints and choice of techniques for endpoint assessment, measurement of drugs, metabolites and drug effects. Describe the contributions that the proposed study will make to the current knowledge base.

3. **SUMMARY OF STUDY PLAN**

For the convenience of the reader, this section should provide a brief synopsis of the following points:
- *Study design*
- *Number of participants to be enrolled (total number and number per arm)*

        Example: A maximum of 25 participants will be accrued into each of four intervention arms. Three additional participants are anticipated to accrue per arm to account for an anticipated drop out rate of 10%. Assuming a screening rate of approximately 25 participants per month and an accrual rate of approximately 8–10 participants per month, we expect the study to be complete within 18–24 months.

- *Brief description of the study population*
- *Intervention plan, including doses, dose groups, and duration of exposure to the study agent.*

        Example: Participants will be given two 30 gram tubes of study agent at the baseline visit and at months 3, 6, 9, and 12. Participants will take study agent for 54 ± 2 weeks (minimum) to 102 ± 2 weeks (maximum). Duration of administration will depend on when a participant is randomized in relationship to when the final participant is randomized. The study will be terminated when all participants have...

- *Description of run-in period, if applicable*
- *Time points for performing study assessments*
- *Description of measurements taken to meet study objectives*
- *Description of clinical procedures, lab tests or other measurements taken to monitor effects of study agent on human safety and to minimize risks*
- *Duration of study*

4. PARTICIPANT SELECTION

4.1 Inclusion Criteria

4.1.1 *Please insert specific health risk or disease requirements. State methods for assessing risk or disease requirements, e.g., risk assessment tools, clinical evaluation, pathology review criteria, etc. For populations with cancer or precancer, include requirements for histological confirmation of diagnosis, time from diagnosis, and disease status at entry.*

4.1.2 *Please state allowable type and amount of prior therapy, if applicable. Include separate definitions for duration as needed. Include site/total dose for prior radiation exposure as needed.*

4.1.3 Age ≥18 years. *Please state reason for age restriction. If applicable, the following text can be used.*
Because no dosing or adverse event data are currently available on the use of *Study Agent* in participants <18 years of age, children are excluded from this study but will be eligible for future pediatric trials, if applicable.

4.1.4 *ECOG performance status ≤1 (Karnofsky ≥70%)*

4.1.5 Participants must have normal organ and marrow function as defined below:
Insert baseline lab parameters appropriate to agent and cohort, for example:

X	*Leukocytes*	*≥3,000/μL*
X	*Absolute neutrophil count*	*≥1,500/μL*
X	*Platelets*	*≥100,000/μL*
X	*Total bilirubin*	*within normal institutional limits*
X	*AST (SGOT)/ALT (SGPT)*	*≤1.5 X institutional ULN*
X	*Creatinine*	*within normal institutional limits*

4.1.6 *Insert other appropriate inclusion criteria relevant to the methodology of the study.*

4.1.7 *Please use or modify the following paragraph as appropriate:*

The effects of *Study Agent* on the developing human fetus at the recommended therapeutic dose are unknown. For this reason and because *Agent Class* are known to be teratogenic, women of child-bearing potential and men must agree to use adequate contraception (hormonal or barrier method of birth control; abstinence) prior to study entry and for the duration of study participation. Should a woman become pregnant or suspect she is pregnant while participating in this study, she should inform her study physician immediately.

4.1.8 Ability to understand and the willingness to sign a written informed consent document.

4.2 Exclusion Criteria

4.2.1 *List contraindications to participation based on agent pharmacology and metabolism, toxicology, clinical and methodology considerations.*

4.2.2   *Healthy volunteers may be required to demonstrate absence of chronic medical conditions or regular use of certain medications.*

4.2.3   Participants may not be receiving any other investigational agents.

4.2.4   History of allergic reactions attributed to compounds of similar chemical or biologic composition to *Study Agent.*

4.2.5   Uncontrolled intercurrent illness including, but not limited to, ongoing or active infection, symptomatic congestive heart failure, unstable angina pectoris, cardiac arrhythmia, or psychiatric illness/social situations that would limit compliance with study requirements.

4.2.6   *The investigator(s) must state a medical or scientific reason if pregnant or nursing participants or participants who are cancer survivors or those who are HIV-positive will be excluded from the study. Detailed information regarding these special populations is available in the DCP Clinical Trials Resource. Suggested text is provided below:*

Pregnant women are excluded from this study because *Study Agent is a/an Agent Class* agent with the potential for teratogenic or abortifacient effects. Because there is an unknown but potential risk for adverse events in nursing infants secondary to treatment of the mother with *Study Agent,* Breastfeeding should be discontinued if the mother is treated with *Study Agent.*

4.3   Inclusion of Women and Minorities

Both men and women (as applicable) and members of all races and ethnic groups are eligible for this trial.

Women and members of minority groups and their subpopulations must be included in the study population of research involving human subjects, unless a clear and compelling rationale and justification are provided indicating that inclusion is inappropriate with respect to the health of the participants or the purpose of the research. NIH requires accrual estimates by gender/race/ethnicity. This information should be recorded on the DCP Protocol Submission Worksheet (PSW). Additional information regarding the NIH policy is available in the Early Phase Prevention Trials Consortia section of the DCP website Resource.

4.4   Recruitment and Retention Plan

Please provide a short synopsis of strategies to be used for recruitment and retention for the target population. However, the detailed specifics of the plan (including gender and minority recruitment strategies, as per NIH guidelines) must be provided in the Recruitment and Retention Plan that is part of the Additional Study-Related Documents submitted with the protocol. Since the detailed Recruitment and Retention Plan is not part of the protocol, please do not reference it here.

Recruitment and retention efforts should be evaluated routinely by the study staff and modified as necessary to promote rapid accrual and to assure 100% retention of participants. Following initial review and approval by the DCP Protocol and Safety Review Committee (PSRC), revisions to the plan should be electronically submitted to the DCP Protocol Information Office.

A sample generic Recruitment and Retention Plan is provided in the Additional Study-Related Document guidelines. The plan should include three phases: Pre-Initiation phase, Active Recruitment phase, and Retention phase (which include adherence strategies). The sample generic plan may be used as a guideline or checklist and is not intended to be followed in entirety nor to preclude any additional strategies. Recruitment and Retention Plans should be tailored to the characteristics of the individual protocol, sample size, target population, clinical sites and resources.

5. **AGENT ADMINISTRATION**

Intervention will be administered on an *inpatient/outpatient* basis. Reported adverse events (AEs) and potential risks are described in Section 6.2.

5.1   Dose Regimen and Dose Groups

Please describe the regimen and dose groups. State any special precautions or warnings relevant for study agent administration. Each dose group should specify:
- *Agent(s)*
- *Daily dose(s) and regimen(s) for each agent (e.g., two capsules bid)*
- *Duration (days/weeks/months) for each agent.*

5.2   <u>Study Agent</u> Administration

- *Indicate who will administer the agent,*
- *How much agent (e.g., number of pills) should be administered at how many times/day (be specific; for example: 20 mg capsules, 100 capsules/bottle, 2 bottles distributed at the baseline visit and at months 3, 6, 9, etc.),*
- *Time of day dose is to be taken,*
- *Special instructions for taking the agent (e.g., with morning meal).*

5.3   Run-in Procedures

If the study includes a placebo run-in phase prior to randomization to assess compliance, please describe the procedure, including method of administering placebo, dose, duration, and methods for assessing compliance. Compliance should be clearly defined.

5.4   Contraindications

Indicate any restrictions that participants should follow when using the agent (e.g., limit sun exposure, dietary restrictions, etc.).

5.5   Concomitant Medications

Indicate any limitations on medications, herbs, and vitamin and mineral supplements (other than study agents) while participating in the study. Include time period for the limitation, if applicable.

All medications (prescription and over-the-counter), vitamin and mineral supplements, and/or herbs taken by the participant will be documented on the concomitant medication CRF and will include: start and stop date, dose and route of administration, and indication. Medications taken for a procedure (*e.g.*, biopsy) should also be included.

5.6   Dose Modification

Explicitly identify when dose modifications are appropriate. Modifications and the factors predicating dose modification should be explicit and clear. If dose modifications are anticipated, please provide a dose de-escalation schema with modifications expressed as a specific dose or amount rather than as a percentage of the starting or previous dose. Also indicate if the agent supply may be used for dose modifications or will an additional supply (smaller doses) be needed to achieve dose modification. If applicable, describe procedures for increasing dose following a toxicity-required dose reduction.

5.7   Adherence/Compliance

5.7.1   *Provide a definition of compliance that will be used to describe when participants are considered evaluable for statistical analysis.*

5.7.2   *Describe the method(s) used to monitor each participant's agent compliance. Methods may include diaries, pill counts, drug/metabolite plasma levels, and/or drug effect biomarkers.*

6.   PHARMACEUTICAL INFORMATION

6.1   <u>Study Agent (IND #, IND Sponsor)</u>

Confidential pharmaceutical information for investigational study agents supplied by NCI, DCP will be provided as an attachment to the LOI approval letter and should be inserted here.

Non-DCP supplied agents: insert appropriate agent information here. Specify:
- *Formulation to be used in this study*
- *Justification for this formulation if other formulations are available*
- *Physical description of agent*
- *List of excipients*

6.2   Reported Adverse Events and Potential Risks

The list of "Reported Adverse Events and Potential Risks" included in the LOI approval letter should be inserted here.

Non-DCP supplied agents: describe the toxicity profile and related data for the agent at the selected doses and schedule.

6.3   Availability

<u>Study Agent</u>   is an investigational agent supplied to investigators by the Division of Cancer Prevention (DCP), NCI.

Example: Agent A and Agent B are investigational agents for chemoprevention studies provided by NCI/DCP. Agent C will be supplied to NCI/DCP by XXX (20 mg capsules, 30 capsules/bottle). Agent D and matching placebo D will be supplied to NCI/DCP by XXX (50 mg capsules, 30 capsules/bottle).

Non-DCP supplied agents: delete the above statement and specify source and availability of supply.

Example: Agent XXX and matching placebo will be manufactured and supplied by XXX. Agent XXX and matching placebo will be packaged in bottles containing 100 capsules.

*If the study agent is provided by NCI under a Cooperative Research and Development Agreement (CRADA) or Clinical Trials Agreement (CTA) with the manufacturer, the appropriate text below must be included in the protocol **and the incorrect text deleted**. Information on the study agent's CRADA/CTA status will be provided in the LOI approval letter.*

<u>Study Agent</u>   is provided to the NCI under a Cooperative Research and Development Agreement (CRADA) between <u>*Agent Manufacturer*</u> and the DCP, NCI (see Section 12.7).

<u>Study Agent</u> is provided to the NCI under a Clinical Trials Agreement (CTA) between <u>*Agent Manufacturer*</u> and the DCP, NCI (see Section 12.7).

231

6.4 Agent Distribution

Agents will only be released by NCI, DCP after documentation of IRB approval of the DCP-approved protocol and consent is provided to DCP and the collection of all Essential Documents is complete (see DCP website for description of Essential Documents).

NCI, DCP-supplied agents may be requested by the Investigator (or their authorized designees) at each Organization. DCP guidelines require that the agent be shipped directly to the institution or site where the agent will be prepared and administered. DCP does not permit the transfer of agents between institutions (unless prior approval from DCP is obtained). <u>DCP does not automatically ship agents; the site must make a request.</u> Agents are requested by completing the DCP Clinical Drug Request form (NIH-986) (to include complete shipping contact information) and faxing or mailing the form to the DCP agent repository contractor:

Dr. Bruce Diel
MRIGlobal
DCP Repository
425 Volker Blvd.
Kansas City, MO 64110
Phone: (816) 360-5369
FAX: (816) 753-5359
Emergency Telephone: (816) 360-3800

For non-DCP supplied agents indicate the manufacturer, supplier and mechanism for distribution. DCP procedures for agent distribution and the required forms are available on the DCP website.

6.5 Agent Accountability

The Investigator, or a responsible party designated by the Investigator, must maintain a careful record of the inventory and disposition of all agents received from DCP using the NCI Drug Accountability Record Form (DARF). The Investigator is required to maintain adequate records of receipt, dispensing and final disposition of study agent. This responsibility has been delegated to ____ [*insert responsible party*] ___. Include on receipt record from whom the agent was received and to whom study agent was shipped, date, quantity and batch or lot number. On dispensing record, note quantities and dates study agent was dispensed to and returned by each participant.

DCP requirements for agent accountability and the required forms are available on the DCP website.

6.6 Packaging and Labeling

___[Agent]__ will be packaged by __[manufacturer or NCI, DCP]___.

DCP will package, label and distribute agent for all DCP-supplied agents. Occasionally, a pharmaceutical collaborator or the site performs one or more of these activities. DCP will send a draft label to the Principal Investigator and the DCP regulatory support contractor for review and approval. Final labels are printed and attached to the bottle prior to shipping to the site. DCP will provide information regarding packaging (container, amount of agent per container) and labeling in the LOI approval letter. The information provided by DCP should be inserted into this section of the protocol.

Example: Each bottle will be labeled with a one-part label identifying study specific information, such as Study title, DCP protocol number, dosing instructions, recommended storage conditions, the name and address of the distributor, randomization number, and a caution statement indicating that the agent is limited by United States law to investigational use only and the agent should be kept out of reach of children.

Protocols using non-DCP supplied agents: describe in detail how the agent will be packaged and distributed, including container, amount of agent per container, container label information, and if blinded, how the label will be constructed to maintain the blind. Label information should include dose, number of doses per day, time of day for dosing, with or without food, and any other specific instructions.

6.7 Storage

Provide instructions regarding proper storage of the agent at the study site(s). Storage temperatures should be expressed as a range, not a specific number. For example, room temperature should be specified (e.g., between 59°F and 86°F).

6.8 Registration/Randomization

Give specific details on how a participant will be registered in a trial. For randomized trials, describe the procedure for randomizing a participant to a dose group. (May refer to Section 13.3).

6.9 Blinding and Unblinding Methods

For blinded studies, describe blinding and unblinding methods. Address the following points:
- *Procedure for retaining the blind (including specific procedures for protecting the blind should data collected in the study offer evidence of a participant's assignment to a particular study arm)*
- *Individual authorized to break the blind*
- *Circumstances for breaking the blind*
- *Procedure for breaking the blind*

The NCI Medical Monitor and/or Scientific Monitor must be notified that the blind has been broken.

> *Provide DCP Medical Monitor Name and title (see LOI Decision Letter)*
> NCI/Division of Cancer Prevention
> *Insert the full contact information including address, telephone number, FAX number, and e-mail of the DCP Medical Monitor*

6.10 Agent Destruction/Disposal

DCP-supplied agents: at the completion of investigation, all unused study agent will be returned to NCI, DCP Repository according to the DCP "Guidelines for AGENT RETURNS" and using the DCP form "Return Drug List".

The Guidelines and form are available on the DCP website.

Non-DCP agents, provide the following procedure for handling the unused drug: method of disposal, documentation of disposal, and any other relevant standard operating procedures.

7. CLINICAL EVALUATIONS AND PROCEDURES

7.1 Schedule of Events

A table that lists baseline testing/pre-study evaluation, agent administration, study assessments, procedures and case report forms should be included. A sample schedule of events is provided on the following page. The protocol should state the expected duration of participation in the study and the sequence and duration of all trial periods, including follow-up, if any.

7.2 Baseline Testing/Prestudy Evaluation

Describe all procedures (including registration and randomization) that must be completed for a participant before the study intervention may begin. Note any time restrictions for testing (e.g., pre-study labs must be done within 14 days of registration).

Specify the amount of study agent that will be distributed to the participant at each visit. Also describe how the participant will return study agent for example: Day 0, participants will be randomized to receive either study agent or placebo and will be given a supply of study agent (3 bottles for a total of 90 capsules); day 60, participants will return any unused study agent and will be given a supply of study agent (3 bottles for a total of 90 capsules).

Refer to Section 5.3, Run-In Procedures, if applicable.

7.3 Evaluation During Study Intervention

Indicate the procedures to be performed during the study intervention phase.

7.4 Evaluation at Completion of Study Intervention

Specify the evaluations that must be performed at the discontinuation of study agent. Ensure that these evaluations are consistent with the endpoints described in the objectives and statistical analysis sections of the protocol.

7.5 Post-intervention Follow-up Period

If a defined post-intervention follow-up period is required, specify observations or tests to be performed. Define the length and purpose of the follow-up period.

7.6 Methods for Clinical Procedures

If applicable, document any special processes, instructions or methodology for clinical procedures required by the protocol, such as invasive procedures and imaging. Include special instructions for procedure prep (e.g., NPO after midnight) and scheduling instructions for tests that may be available only at certain locations or times.

SCHEDULE OF EVENTS

Evaluation/ Procedure	Registration	Baseline	Randomization	Months 1–3	Months 4–5	Month 6 or Early Termination	Follow-Up Visit
Informed Consent	X						
Assess Eligibility	X	X					
Medical History		X					
Physical Exam		X					
Vital Signs/ Height and Weight		X		X		X	
Laboratory Tests		X		X		X	
X-Rays		X				X	
EKG		X				X	
Biopsies		X				X	
Biomarkers		X				X	
Study Evaluations/ Assessments		X		X		X	
Concomitant Medications		X		X	X	X	X
Dispense Study Agent			X	X			
Collect Study Agent						X	
Review Agent Diary/Record			X	X		X	
Adverse Events				X	X	X	X
Telephone Contact					X		X

8. CRITERIA FOR EVALUATION AND ENDPOINT DEFINITION

Delineation of study endpoints, methods for measuring or evaluating, and timing of endpoint ascertainment should be described here.

8.1 Primary Endpoint

Depending on the study hypotheses and design, the primary endpoint may be an incidence of invasive or preinvasive disease (e.g., polyp incidence), clinical response (e.g., change in number and severity of leukoplakia by physical exam), histologic or cytologic response (e.g., change in severity of dysplasia in biopsy materials), and/or modulation of surrogate endpoint biomarkers (SEBs). Define endpoints clearly and briefly describe methods and intervals for assessment. A detailed description of methods should be included in the Pharmacokinetic and Biomarker Method Development Report document (part of the Additional Study-Related Documents that are submitted with the protocol) as appropriate. Do not reference the Pharmacokinetic and Biomarker Method Development Report here since it is not an actual part of the protocol.

8.2 Secondary Endpoints

As appropriate, secondary endpoints (serum/plasma/tissue agent/metabolite levels, other agent effect biomarkers) should be defined clearly. Methods for assessment should be referenced in this section with detailed descriptions of laboratory and computer modeling procedures provided in the required "Pharmacokinetic and Biomarker Method Development Report" document (part of the additional Study-Related Documents).

8.3 Off-Agent Criteria

Participants may stop taking study agent for the following reasons: completed the protocol-prescribed intervention, adverse event or serious adverse event, inadequate agent supply, noncompliance, concomitant medications, medical contraindication, or *specify other reasons, if applicable*. Participants will continue to be followed, if possible, for safety reasons and in order to collect endpoint data according to the schedule of events. *The protocol should state whether and how subjects are to be replaced, if applicable.*

8.4 Off-Study Criteria

Participants may go 'off-study' for the following reasons: the protocol intervention and any protocol-required follow-up period is completed, adverse event/serious adverse event, lost to follow-up, non-compliance, concomitant medication, medical contraindication, withdraw consent, death, determination of ineligibility (including screen failure), pregnancy, or *specify other reasons, if applicable.*

8.5 Study Termination

NCI, DCP as the study sponsor has the right to discontinue the study at any time.

9. CORRELATIVE/SPECIAL STUDIES

9.1 Rationale for Methodology Selection

Provide the rationale for selecting the assay methodology, particularly in cases where various assays are available that may assess different qualities of the marker (example: mutation analysis vs. *IHC for p53; gene expression* vs. *protein expression). Methodology should be included, as appropriate, in the Pharmacokinetic and Biomarker Methods Development Report.*

9.2 Comparable Methods

Discuss the comparability of the methods proposed to those previously used and the likelihood that the resulting data will be able to be compared to existing data.

10. SPECIMEN MANAGEMENT

10.1 Laboratories

Identify the laboratory(ies) that will perform each analysis for each specimen. Where appropriate, list individuals who will perform analysis and/or procedures for conducting consensus reviews of specimens.

10.2 Collection and Handling Procedures

For each type of specimen obtained, please describe the following
- *Amount to be collected*
- *When specimen should be obtained (e.g., fasting, prior to a.m. dose)*
- *Processing of specimen (e.g., details of tissue fixation, embedding, processing and sectioning)*
- *Labeling of specimen*
- *Tracking of specimens (e.g., logs or tracking sheets for participants)*
- *Temperature storage requirements*
- *Storage duration*

Note: If this section is too lengthy, please place this information in an appendix to the protocol.

10.3 Shipping Instructions

Include this section only if specimens will be shipped to an off-site laboratory for analysis. For each specimen, describe the following: packaging, carrier requirements, when specimens may be shipped, and name, address, and telephone number of the person to whom the specimens are being sent. Indicate compliance with the International Air Transport Association (IATA) Dangerous Goods Regulations.

10.4 Tissue Banking

Indicate methods and procedures for tissue banking here.

Biologic specimens collected during the conduct of each clinical trial that are not used during the course of the study will be considered deliverables under the contract and thus the property of the NCI. At study completion, NCI reserves the option to either retain or relinquish ownership of the unused biologic specimens. If NCI retains ownership of specimens, the Contractor shall collect, verify and transfer the requested biologic specimens from the site to a NCI-specified repository or laboratory at NCI's expense.

11. REPORTING ADVERSE EVENTS

DEFINITION: AE means any untoward medical occurrence associated with the use of a drug in humans, whether or not considered drug related. An AE can therefore be any unfavorable and unintended sign (including a clinically significant abnormal laboratory finding), symptom, or disease temporally associated with participation in a study, whether or not related to that participation. This includes all deaths that occur while a participant is on a study.

A list of AEs that have occurred or might occur (Reported Adverse Events and Potential Risks) can be found in Section 6.2, Pharmaceutical Information, as well as the Investigator Brochure or package insert.

11.1 Adverse Events

11.1.1 Reportable AEs

All AEs that occur after the informed consent is signed (including run-in) must be recorded on the AE CRF (paper and/or electronic) whether or not related to study agent.

11.1.2 AE Data Elements:
- AE reported date
- AE Verbatim Term
- Common Terminology Criteria for Adverse Events v4.0 (CTCAE) AE term
- Event onset date and event ended date
- Severity grade

- Attribution to study agent (relatedness)
- Whether or not the event was reported as a serious adverse event (SAE)
- Whether or not the subject dropped due to the event
- Action taken with the study agent
- Outcome of the event
- Comments

11.1.3   Severity of AEs

11.1.3.1 Identify the adverse event using the NCI Common Terminology Criteria for Adverse Events (CTCAE) version 4.0. The CTCAE provides descriptive terminology and a grading scale for each adverse event listed. A copy of the CTCAE can be found at http://ctep.cancer.gov/protocolDevelopment/electronic_applications/ctc.htm

AEs will be assessed according to the CTCAE grade associated with the AE term. AEs that do not have a corresponding CTCAE term will be assessed according to the general guidelines for grading used in the CTCAE v4.0. as stated below.

CTCAE v4.0 general severity guidelines:

Grade	Severity	Description
1	Mild	Mild; asymptomatic or mild symptoms; clinical or diagnostic observations only; intervention not indicated.
2	Moderate	Moderate; minimal, local or noninvasive intervention indicated; limiting age-appropriate instrumental activities of daily living (ADL)*.
3	Severe	Severe or medically significant but not immediately life-threatening; hospitalization or prolongation of hospitalization indicated; disabling; limiting self-care ADL**.
4	Life-threatening	Life-threatening consequences; urgent intervention indicated.
5	Fatal	Death related to AE.

ADL

*Instrumental ADL refers to preparing meals, shopping for groceries or clothes, using the telephone, managing money, *etc*.

**Self-care ADL refers to bathing, dressing and undressing, feeding self, using the toilet, taking medications, and not bedridden.

11.1.4   Assessment of relationship of AE to treatment

The possibility that the adverse event is related to study agent will be classified as one of the following: not related, unlikely, possible, probable, definite.

11.1.5   Follow-up of AEs

All AEs, including lab abnormalities that in the opinion of the investigator are clinically significant, will be followed according to good medical practices and documented as such.

11.2   Serious Adverse Events

11.2.1   DEFINITION: Fed. Reg. 75, Sept. 29, 2010 defines SAEs as those events, occurring at any dose, which meet any of the following criteria:
- Results in death

- Is life threatening (*Note: the term life-threatening refers to an event in which the patient was at risk of death at the time of the event; it does not refer to an event which hypothetically might have caused death if it were more severe*).
- Requires inpatient hospitalization or prolongation of existing hospitalization
- Results in persistent or significant incapacity or substantial disruption of the ability to conduct normal life functions
- Is a congenital abnormality/birth defect
- Important medical events that may not result in death, be life-threatening or require hospitalization may be considered serious when, based upon appropriate medical judgment, they may jeopardize the patient or subject and may require medical or surgical intervention to prevent one of the outcomes listed.

Based on FDA's Guidance for Industry and Investigators: Safety Reporting Requirements for INDs and BA/BE Studies, it is possible to list specific serious adverse events for routine reporting (not using the SAE Report Form) that are anticipated to occur in the study population at some frequency independent of drug exposure (e.g., characteristics of the study population, natural progression of the disease, background event rates, co-morbid conditions, and past experience with similar populations). For example, in a long-term osteoporosis trial in an elderly population, it would be reasonable to list myocardial infarction, but unreasonable to list acute narrow angle glaucoma, an event that can occur in this elderly population, but is relatively rare. A plan for monitoring the frequency of these events in the treatment group vs. the concomitant or historical control group should be provided in the protocol. If aggregate analysis indicates a higher frequency in the treatment group, this should be reported as a serious adverse event in a narrative format.

11.2.2   Reporting SAEs to DCP

11.2.2.1   The Lead Organization and all Participating Organizations will report SAEs on the DCP SAE form found at http://prevention.cancer.gov/files/clinical-trials/SAE_form.doc.

11.2.2.2   Contact the DCP Medical Monitor by phone within 24 hours of knowledge of the event.

Provide DCP Medical Monitor Name and title (see LOI Decision Letter)

NCI/Division of Cancer Prevention

Insert the full contact information including address, telephone number, FAX number, and e-mail of the DCP Medical Monitor

Include the following information when calling the Medical Monitor:
- Date and time of the SAE
- Date and time of the SAE report
- Name of reporter
- Call back phone number
- Affiliation/Institution conducting the study
- DCP protocol number
- Title of protocol
- Description of the SAE, including attribution to drug and expectedness

11.2.2.3   The Lead Organization and all Participating Organizations will FAX written SAE reports to the DCP Medical Monitor within 48 hours of learning of the event using the paper SAE form. The written SAE reports will also be FAX'ed [(650) 691-

4410) or e-mailed (safety@ccsainc.com)] to DCP's Regulatory Contractor, CCS Associates (phone: (650) 691-4400).

11.2.2.4   The DCP Medical Monitor and regulatory staff will determine which SAEs require FDA submission.

11.2.2.5   The Lead Organization and all Participating Organizations will comply with applicable regulatory requirements related to reporting SAEs to the IRB/IEC.

11.2.2.6   Follow-up of SAE

Site staff should send follow-up reports as requested when additional information is available. Additional information should be entered on the DCP SAE form in the appropriate format. Follow-up information should be sent to DCP as soon as available. *The protocol should state the length of time for follow-up of an SAE. Usually SAEs are followed until resolved, especially for those related to the study agent.*

12.   STUDY MONITORING

12.1   Data Management

This study will report clinical data using the DCP Oracle® Clinical Remote Data Capture (OC-RDC) web-based application managed by DCP's monitoring contractor. The OC-RDC will be the database of record for the protocol and subject to NCI and FDA audit. All OC-RDC users will be trained to use the RDC system and will comply with the instructions in the protocol-specific "RDC User Manual" provided to the Consortium Lead PI by the DCP Monitoring Contractor as well as applicable regulatory requirements such as 21 CFR; Part 11.

An approved Master Data Management Plan that is applicable to all studies within the Consortium will be on file at DCP. If there are any changes required to the Master DMP that are specific to this protocol only, then DMP Attachment #1 should be submitted with the protocol as part of the set of "Additional Study-Related Documents". Any changes or updates to the Master Data Management Plan following DCP approval should be submitted separately to the DCP Protocol Information Office for approval.

12.2   Case Report Forms

Participant data will be collected using protocol-specific case report forms (CRF) developed from the standard set of DCP Chemoprevention CRF Templates and utilizing NCI-approved Common Data Elements (CDEs). The approved CRFs will be used to create the electronic CRF (e-CRF) screens in the OC-RDC application. Site staff will enter data into the e-CRF for transmission to DCP according to pre-established DCP standards and procedures. Amended CRFs will be submitted to the DCP Protocol Information Office for review and approval. Approved changes will be programmed into the OC-RDC database by the DCP Monitoring Contractor.

The site will use DCP Chemoprevention CRF Templates from the DCP website to develop study-specific CRFs. The DCP templates contain NCI Common Data Elements (CDEs); use of these standardized terms facilitates data collection and analysis across studies. The standard template set may require modification to capture the unique data elements (i.e., biomarkers) of each protocol. NCI CDEs, where available, shall be used for all CRF modifications.

The CRFs and attachments will be submitted with the protocol for DCP PSRC review as part of the set of "Additional Study-Related Documents". The DCP Monitoring Contractor will work with the sites to finalize the CRFs. DCP must approve the final CRFs prior to study initiation. CRFs may require changes throughout the conduct of the clinical trial. The need for change may result from protocol amendments or other reasons. Amended CRFs and attachments should be submitted to the DCP Protocol Information Office for review and approval. Studies may be initiated using paper CRFs.

12.3   Source Documents

The protocol should state what constitutes a source document. Data recorded directly on the CRFs (i.e., no prior written or electronic record of data), which will be considered as source data should be identified.

12.4   Data and Safety Monitoring Plan

NIH and NCI policy requires a Data and Safety Monitoring Plan (DSMP) to document the institution's procedures to ensure safety of participants, validity of data, and the appropriate termination of studies for which significant benefits or risks have been uncovered or when it appears that the trials cannot be concluded successfully. Risks associated with participation in research must be minimized to the extent practical and the method and degree of monitoring should be commensurate with risk. The guidelines, essential elements and sample plans are available at: http://cancer.gov/clinicaltrials/conducting/dsm-guidelines. Please note that the requirements differ depending on whether a trial is conducted under an IND.

An approved Master DSMP applicable to all studies within a Consortium will be on file at DCP. If there are any changes required to the Master DSMP that are specific to this protocol only, then DSMP Attachment #1 should be submitted with the protocol as part of the set of "Additional Study-Related Documents".

Please provide a brief summary of the Master DSMP in this section.

12.5   Sponsor or FDA Monitoring

The NCI, DCP (or their designee), pharmaceutical collaborator (or their designee), or FDA may monitor/audit various aspects of the study. These monitors will be given access to facilities, databases, supplies and records to review and verify data pertinent to the study.

Please refer to the monitoring section (Step 3) of the Early Phase Prevention Trials area of the DCP website for information regarding DCP site visit procedures and requirements.

12.6   Record Retention

Clinical records for all participants, including CRFs, all source documentation (containing evidence to study eligibility, history and physical findings, laboratory data, results of consultations, *etc.*), as well as IRB records and other regulatory documentation will be retained by the Investigator in a secure storage facility in compliance with Health Insurance Portability and Accountability Act (HIPAA), Office of Human Research Protections (OHRP), Food and Drug Administration (FDA) regulations and guidances, and NCI/DCP requirements, unless the standard at the site is more stringent. The records for all studies performed under an IND will be maintained, at a minimum, for two years after the approval of a New Drug Application (NDA). For NCI/DCP, records will be retained for at least three years after the completion of the research. NCI will be notified prior to the planned destruction of any materials. The records should be accessible for inspection and copying by authorized persons of the Food and Drug Administration. If the study is done outside of the United States, applicable regulatory requirements for the specific country participating in the study also apply.

12.7   Cooperative Research and Development Agreement (CRADA)/Clinical Trials Agreement (CTA)

If the study agent is provided by DCP under a CRADA or CTA with the manufacturer, this section must be included in the protocol, but the inappropriate text (CTA or CRADA) should be deleted. Information on the study agent's CRADA/CTA status will be provided in the approved LOI response. If neither a CRADA nor CTA applies to the study agent, this section should be marked "N/A" and the text below deleted.

The agent(s) supplied by DCP, NCI, used in this protocol, is/are provided to the NCI under a Collaborative Agreement (CRADA, CTA) between the Pharmaceutical Company(ies) [hereinafter referred to as Collaborator(s)] and the NCI Division of Cancer Prevention. Therefore, the following obligations/guidelines, in addition to the provisions in the "Intellectual Property Option to Collaborator" contained within the terms of award, apply to the use of Agent(s) in this study:

12.7.1   Agent(s) may not be used for any purpose outside the scope of this protocol, nor can Agent(s) be transferred or licensed to any party not participating in the clinical study. Collaborator(s) data for Agent(s) are confidential and proprietary to Collaborator(s) and shall be maintained as such by the investigators. The protocol documents for studies utilizing investigational agents contain confidential information and should not be shared or distributed without the permission of the NCI. If a patient participating on the study or participant's family member requests a copy of this protocol, the individual should sign a confidentiality agreement. A suitable model agreement can be downloaded from the DCP website.

12.7.2   For a clinical protocol where there is an investigational Agent used in combination with (an) other investigational Agent(s), each the subject of different collaborative agreements, the access to and use of data by each Collaborator shall be as follows (data pertaining to such combination use shall hereinafter be referred to as "Multi-Party Data".):

12.7.3   NCI must provide all Collaborators with prior written notice regarding the existence and nature of any agreements governing their collaboration with NIH, the design of the proposed combination protocol, and the existence of any obligations that would tend to restrict NCI's participation in the proposed combination protocol.

12.7.4   Each Collaborator shall agree to permit use of the Multi-Party Data from the clinical trial by any other Collaborator solely to the extent necessary to allow said other Collaborator to develop, obtain regulatory approval, or commercialize its own investigational agent.

12.7.5   Any Collaborator having the right to use the Multi-Party Data from these trials must agree in writing prior to the commencement of the trials that it will use the Multi-Party Data solely for development, regulatory approval, and commercialization of its own investigational agent.

12.7.6   Clinical Trial Data and Results and Raw Data developed under a collaborative agreement will be made available exclusively to Collaborator(s), the NCI, and the FDA, as appropriate. All data made available will comply with HIPAA regulations.

12.7.7   When a Collaborator wishes to initiate a data request, the request should first be sent to the NCI, who will then notify the appropriate investigators of Collaborator's wish to contact them.

12.7.8   Any manuscripts reporting the results of this clinical trial must be provided to DCP for immediate delivery to Collaborator(s) for advisory review and comment prior to submission for publication. Collaborator(s) will have 30 days (or as specified in the CTA) from the date of receipt for review. Collaborator shall have the right to request that publication be delayed for up to an additional 30 days in order to ensure that Collaborator's confidential and proprietary data, in addition to Collaborator(s)'s intellectual property rights, are protected. Copies of abstracts must be provided to DCP for forwarding to Collaborator(s) for courtesy review as soon as possible and preferably at least three days prior to submission, but in any case, prior to presentation at the meeting or publication in the proceedings. Press releases and other media presentations must also be forwarded to DCP prior to release. Copies of any manuscript, abstract, and/or press release/media presentation should be sent to:

> Head, DCP Protocol Information Office
> 6130 Executive Boulevard, Room 2050
> Rockville, MD 20852
> E-mail: NCI_DCP_PIO@mail.nih.gov

The Protocol Information Office will forward manuscripts to the DCP Project Officer for distribution to the Collaborator(s). No publication, manuscript or other form of public disclosure shall contain any of Collaborator's confidential/proprietary information.

13. STATISTICAL CONSIDERATIONS

13.1 Study Design/Description

*The study design and provide a brief description. Indicate the type of study (e.g., phase I, phase II, observational) as applicable. Include justification for the selection of the particular study design. If a randomized study, indicate whether blinding is used and the methodology to ensure the blinding. Indicate whether or not the study employs intent to treat principles. If applicable indicate both the range of true values of the primary endpoint sufficiently promising to justify further testing of the agent (e.g., **true** response rate of at least 20%) and a range of values sufficiently discouraging to justify no further testing of the agent (e.g., **true** response rate no greater than 5%). Consider early testing for sufficiently discouraging results (e.g., interim analysis). Indicate the decision rule for declaring the agent promising based on the **observed value** of the primary endpoint. Provide the probability of a positive result, given that the true value falls within the promising range, and the probability of a negative result (along with the probability of early negative termination), given that the true value falls within the discouraging range.*

13.2 Randomization/Stratification

Methods for randomization and stratification are described and justified. Blocking and/or other techniques used to balance intervention assignments are described completely. Indicate whether interim analysis and efficacy determination will be done for each stratum individually.

13.3 Accrual and Feasibility

Specify the planned sample size and accrual rate (e.g., participants/month). Total sample size (including gender and minority considerations) and sampling strategy are described and justified for testing the primary and secondary hypotheses.

13.4 Primary Objective, Endpoint(s), Analysis Plan

Describe the primary objective of the study. Define the primary endpoints and indicate how the analysis plan will satisfy the primary objective of the study. Definition of the primary endpoint(s) should indicate time-points considered in computing the primary endpoint from the data observed. The analysis plan should consider the appropriateness for the particular type of endpoint (for example continuous, binary, time-dependent). Analysis plans should indicate the planned statistical test used to evaluate the objectives of the study along with power calculations and sample size requirements. When known, provide pilot or historical data to support power calculations. Clearly state all assumptions for the power calculations and indicate whether significance levels are one- or two-sided values. Consideration should be given to handling missing data if applicable.

13.5 Secondary Objectives, Endpoints, Analysis Plans

Describe the secondary objectives of the study. Define the secondary endpoints and indicate how the analysis plan will satisfy the secondary objectives of the study. Definition of the secondary endpoint(s) should indicate time-points considered in computing the secondary endpoint from the data observed. The analysis plan should consider the appropriateness for the particular type of endpoint (for example continuous, binary, time-dependent). Analysis plans should indicate the planned statistical test used to evaluate the secondary objectives of the study. Clearly indicate whether significance levels are one- or two-sided values. Consideration should be given to handling missing data if applicable.

13.6 Reporting and Exclusions

Definition of compliance is clearly stated. Non-compliance is sufficiently addressed. Particular consideration is given to dropouts, drop-ins, and lost-to-follow up. Handling of missing data or data from non-compliers is described. Any methods used to impute missing data should be described.

13.7 Evaluation of Toxicity

All participants will be evaluable for toxicity from the time of their first dose of *[Study Agent]* .

13.8 Evaluation of Response

All participants included in the study must be assessed for response to intervention, even if there are major protocol deviations or if they are ineligible.

All of the participants who met the eligibility criteria (with the possible exception of those who did not receive study agent) will be included in the main analysis. All conclusions regarding efficacy will be based on all eligible participants.

Subanalyses may be performed on the subsets of participants, excluding those for whom major protocol deviations have been identified (e.g., early death due to other reasons, early discontinuation of intervention, major protocol violations, etc.). However, subanalyses may not serve as the basis for drawing conclusions concerning efficacy, and the reasons for excluding participants from the analysis should be clearly reported. For all measurements of response, the 95% confidence intervals should also be provided.

13.9 Interim Analysis

If relevant to the study agent and study design, provide a plan for interim analysis and stopping rules. Include plans for monitoring the progress of the trial to implement early termination.

13.10 Ancillary Studies

Address the following, as appropriate:
- *If known, indicate the prevalence of the marker*
- *Specify how any cut points will be determined*
- *Specify the statistical power of the correlative study for the endpoint chosen*
- *If relevant, indicate what corrections will be made for multiple comparisons*
- *If appropriate, indicate relevant clinical endpoint, and a plan for how this endpoint will be correlated with the target(s) or marker(s).*

14. ETHICAL AND REGULATORY CONSIDERATIONS

14.1 Form FDA 1572

Prior to initiating this study, the Protocol Lead Investigator at the Lead or Participating Organization(s)will provide a signed Form FDA 1572 stating that the study will be conducted in compliance with regulations for clinical investigations and listing the investigators, at each site that will participate in the protocol. All personnel directly involved in the performance of procedures required by the protocol and the collection of data should be listed on Form FDA 1572.

14.2 Other Required Documents

14.2.1   Signed and dated current (within two years) CV or biosketch for all study personnel listed on the Form FDA 1572 and Delegation of Tasks form for the Lead Organization and all Participating Organizations.

14.2.2   Current medical licenses (where applicable) for all study personnel listed on Form FDA 1572 and Delegation of Tasks form for the Lead Organization and all Participating Organizations.

14.2.3   Lab certification (*e.g.*, CLIA, CAP) and lab normal ranges for all labs listed on Form FDA 1572 for the Lead Organization and all Participating Organizations.

14.2.4   Documentation of training in "Protection of Human Research Subjects" for all study personnel listed on the FDA Form 1572 and Delegation of Tasks form for the Lead Organization and all Participating Organizations.

14.2.5   Documentation of Federalwide Assurance (FWA) number for the Lead Organization and all Participating Organizations.

14.2.6   Signed Investigator's Brochure/Package Insert acknowledgement form.

14.2.7   Delegation of Tasks form for the Lead Organization and all Participating Organizations signed by the Principal Investigator for each site and initialed by all study personnel listed on the form.

14.2.8   Signed and dated NCI, DCP Financial Disclosure Form for all study personnel listed on Form FDA 1572 for the Lead Organization and all Participating Organizations.

14.3 Institutional Review Board Approval

Prior to initiating the study and receiving agent, the Investigators at the Lead Organization and the Participating Organization(s) must obtain written approval to conduct the study from the appropriate IRB. Should changes to the study become necessary, protocol amendments will be submitted to the DCP PIO according to DCP Amendment Guidelines. The DCP-approved amended protocol must be approved by the IRB prior to implementation.

14.4 Informed Consent

All potential study participants will be given a copy of the IRB-approved Informed Consent to review. The investigator will explain all aspects of the study in lay language and answer all questions regarding the study. If the participant decides to participate in the study, he/she will be asked to sign and date the Informed Consent document. The study agent(s) will not be released to a participant who has not signed the Informed Consent document. Subjects who refuse to participate or who withdraw from the study will be treated without prejudice.

Participants must be provided the option to allow the use of blood samples, other body fluids, and tissues obtained during testing, operative procedures, or other standard medical practices for further research purposes. *If applicable, statement of this option may be included within the informed consent document or may be provided as an addendum to the consent. A Model Consent Form for Use of Tissue for Research is available through a link in the DCP website.*

Prior to study initiation, the informed consent document must be reviewed and approved by NCI, DCP, the Consortium Lead Organization, and the IRB at each Organization at which the protocol will be implemented. Any subsequent changes to the informed consent must be approved by NCI, DCP, the Consortium Lead Organization's IRB, and then submitted to each organization's IRB for approval prior to initiation.

14.5 Submission of Regulatory Documents

All regulatory documents are collected by the Consortia Lead Organization and reviewed for completeness and accuracy. Once the Consortia Lead Organization has received complete and accurate documents from a participating organization, the Consortium Lead Organization will forward the regulatory documents to the DCP Regulatory Contractor:

> Paper Document/CD-ROM Submissions:
> Regulatory Affairs Department
> CCS Associates
> 1923 Landings Drive
> Mountain View, CA 94043
> Phone: 650-691-4400
> Fax: 650-691-4410
>
> E-mail Submissions:
> regulatory@ccsainc.com

Regulatory documents that do not require an original signature may be sent electronically to the Consortium Lead Organization for review, which will then be electronically forwarded to the DCP Regulatory Contractor.

14.6 Other

This trial will be conducted in compliance with the protocol, Good Clinical Practice (GCP), and the applicable regulatory requirements.

15. Financing, Expenses, and/or Insurance

Sample Informed Consent Form

RESEARCH SUBJECT INFORMED CONSENT FORM

Prospective Research Subject: Read this consent form carefully and ask as many questions as you like before you decide whether you want to participate in this research study. You are free to ask questions at any time before, during, or after your participation in this research.

This is a generic sample form to help you address most situations. Please adapt as appropriate for your research protocol and institution. *Pending rulemaking for classified human subject research will require additional elements of consent.*

Project Information

Project Title:	Project Number:
Site IRB Number:	Sponsor:
Principal Investigator:	Organization:
Location:	Phone:
Other Investigators:	Organization:
Location:	Phone:

---

1. PURPOSE OF THIS RESEARCH STUDY

- Include 3–5 sentences written in non-technical language (8th grade reading level): *"You are being asked to participate in a research study designed to …"*.

2. PROCEDURES

- Describe procedures: *"You will be asked to do …"*.
- Identify any procedures that are experimental/investigational/non-therapeutic.
- Define expected duration of subject's participation.
- Indicate type and frequency of monitoring during and after the study.

3. POSSIBLE RISKS OR DISCOMFORT

- Describe known or possible risks. If unknown, state so.
- Indicate if there are special risks to women of childbearing age; if relevant, state that study may involve risks that are currently unforeseeable, e.g. to developing fetus.
- If subject's participation will continue over time, state: *"any new information developed during the study that may affect your willingness to continue participation will be communicated to you"*.
- If applicable, state that a particular treatment or procedure may involve risks that are currently unforeseeable (to the subject, embryo or fetus, for example.)

4. OWNERSHIP AND DOCUMENTATION OF SPECIMENS

- Describe ownership, use, disposal, and documentation (identification) procedures for specimens or samples taken for study purposes.

5. POSSIBLE BENEFITS

- Describe any benefits to the subject that may be reasonably expected. If the research is not of direct benefit to the participant, explain possible benefits to others.

6. FINANCIAL CONSIDERATIONS

- Explain any financial compensation involved or state: *"There is no financial compensation for your participation in this research"*.
- Describe any additional costs to the subject that might result from participation in this study.

7. AVAILABLE TREATMENT ALTERNATIVES

- If the procedure involves an experimental treatment, indicate whether other non-experimental (conventional) treatments are available and compare the relative risks (if known) of each.

8. AVAILABLE MEDICAL TREATMENT FOR ADVERSE EXPERIENCES

- *"This study involves (minimal risk) (greater than minimal risk)"*. In the event that greater than minimal risk is involved, provide the subject with the following information.
  "If you are injured as a direct result of taking part in this research study, emergency medical care will be provided by [name] medical staff or by transporting you to your personal doctor or medical center. Neither the [your site name] nor the Federal government will be able to provide you with long-term medical treatment or financial compensation except as may be provided through your employer's insurance programs or through whatever remedies are normally available at law".

9. CONFIDENTIALITY

- Describe the extent to which confidentiality of records identifying the subject will be maintained.
  "Your identity in this study will be treated as confidential. The results of the study, including laboratory or any other data, may be published for scientific purposes but will not give your name or include any identifiable references to you".
  "However, any records or data obtained as a result of your participation in this study may be inspected by the sponsor, by any relevant governmental agency (e.g. U.S. Department of Energy), by the [your site name] Institutional Review Board, or by the persons conducting this study, provided that such inspectors are legally obligated to protect any identifiable information from public

disclosure, except where disclosure is otherwise required by law or a court of competent jurisdiction. These records will be kept private in so far as permitted by law".

In addition, list steps to protect confidentiality such as codes for identifying data.

10. TERMINATION OF RESEARCH STUDY

You are free to choose whether or not to participate in this study. There will be no penalty or loss of benefits to which you are otherwise entitled if you choose not to participate. You will be provided with any significant new findings developed during the course of this study that may relate to or influence your willingness to continue participation. In the event you decide to discontinue your participation in the study,

- *These are the potential consequences that may result: (list)*
- *Please notify (name, telephone no., etc.) of your decision or follow this procedure (describe), so that your participation can be orderly terminated.*

In addition, your participation in the study may be terminated by the investigator without your consent under the following circumstances. (Describe) It may be necessary for the sponsor of the study to terminate the study without prior notice to, or consent of, the participants in the event that (Describe circumstances, such as loss of funding.)

11. AVAILABLE SOURCES OF INFORMATION

- Any further questions you have about this study will be answered by the Principal Investigator:
  Name:
  Phone Number:
- Any questions you may have about your rights as a research subject will be answered by:
  Name:
  Phone Number:
- In case of a research-related emergency, call:
  Day Emergency Number:
  Night Emergency Number:

12. AUTHORIZATION

I have read and understand this consent form, and I volunteer to participate in this research study. I understand that I will receive a copy of this form. I voluntarily choose to participate, but I understand that my consent does not take away any legal rights in the case of negligence or other legal fault of anyone who is involved in this study. I further understand that nothing in this consent form is intended to replace any applicable Federal, state, or local laws.

Participant Name (Printed or Typed):
Date:
Participant Signature:
Date:
Principal Investigator Signature:
Date:
Signature of Person Obtaining Consent:
Date:

10. TERMINATION OF RESEARCH STUDY

11. AVAILABLE SOURCES OF INFORMATION

12. AUTHORIZATION

Sample Case Report Form

From National Cancer Institute http://prevention.cancer.gov/clinicaltrials/management/pio/instructions

SCREENING

INSTITUTION CODE	PARTICIPANT ID	VISIT TYPE	VISIT DATE (MM/DD/YYYY)
_____	_____	_____	__ __ / __ __ / __ __ __ __

Date Screening Informed
Consent Signed: __ __ / __ __ / __ __ __ __
(MM/DD/YYYY)

☐ Not Applicable

Screening Date: __ __ / __ __ / __ __ __ __
(MM/DD/YYYY)

☐ Not Applicable

Is this participant a screen failure?　☐ Yes　☐ No　**(If Yes, complete Off Study form)**

If yes, specify primary reason for screen failure: ☐ Investigator decision

☐ Participant decision

☐ Did not meet eligibility criteria

☐ Other, specify: _____

Comments: _____

_____

_____

Who referred participant?

☐ Physician

☐ Health Care Provider

☐ Family/friend

☐ Self

☐ Other, specify:

_____

How did participant find out about the study?

☐ Physician

☐ Nurse

☐ Family/friend

☐ NCI web site

☐ Written material

☐ Unknown

☐ Other, specify:

_____

252

INCLUSION CRITERIA

INSTITUTION CODE	PARTICIPANT ID	VISIT TYPE	VISIT DATE (MM/DD/YYYY)
_____	_____	_____	__ __ / __ __ / __ __ __ __

List each inclusion criteria question here exactly as stated in the protocol. Modify the question numbers as appropriate. Gray out any boxes within the N/A column that do not allow N/A as a valid response.

	Criteria	Yes	No	N/A
1				
2				
3				
4				
5				
6				
7				
8				
9				
10				
11				
12				

253

EXCLUSION CRITERIA

INSTITUTION CODE	PARTICIPANT ID	VISIT TYPE	VISIT DATE (MM/DD/YYYY) __ __ / __ __ / __ __ __ __
_____	_____	_____	

List each exclusion criteria question here exactly as stated in the protocol. Modify the question numbers as appropriate. Gray out any boxes within the N/A column that do not allow N/A as a valid response.

	Criteria	Yes	No	N/A
1				
2				
3				
4				
5				
6				
7				
8				
9				
10				
11				
12				

REGISTRATION

INSTITUTION CODE	PARTICIPANT ID	VISIT TYPE	VISIT DATE *(MM/DD/YYYY)*
_____	_____	_____	__ __ / __ __ / __ __ __ __

Registering Consortium: _____

Gender: ☐ Male ☐ Female ☐ Unknown ☐ Unspecified   Date of Birth *(MM/DD/YYYY)*: __ __ / __ __ / __ __ __ __

Race:
(Check all that apply)
☐ White
☐ Black or African American
☐ Native Hawaiian or Other Pacific Islander
☐ Asian
☐ American Indian or Alaska Native
☐ Unknown
☐ Not Reported

Ethnicity: ☐ Hispanic or Latino
☐ Not Hispanic or Latino
☐ Unknown
☐ Not Reported

Date Study Informed
Consent Signed: __ __ / __ __ / __ __ __ __
(MM/DD/YYYY)

Date of Registration: __ __ / __ __ / __ __ __ __
(MM/DD/YYYY)

Does the participant satisfy all of the eligibility criteria?   ☐ Yes   ☐ No   **(If No, complete Off Study form)**

RANDOMIZATION

INSTITUTION CODE	PARTICIPANT ID	VISIT TYPE	VISIT DATE (MM/DD/YYYY)
_____	_____	_____	__ __ / __ __ / __ __ __ __

RANDOMIZATION ☐ Not Applicable

Date Participant Randomized: __ __ / __ __ / __ __ __ __ (MM/DD/YYYY)	Randomization Number: _____

RUN-IN ☐ Not Applicable

Date Run-In Started: __ __ / __ __ / __ __ __ __ (MM/DD/YYYY)	Date Run-In Ended: __ __ / __ __ / __ __ __ __ (MM/DD/YYYY)

WASHOUT ☐ Not Applicable

Date Washout Started: __ __ / __ __ / __ __ __ __ (MM/DD/YYYY)	Date Washout Ended: __ __ / __ __ / __ __ __ __ (MM/DD/YYYY)

256

INTERVENTION ADMINISTRATION
(BLINDED STUDY)

INSTITUTION CODE	PARTICIPANT ID	VISIT TYPE	VISIT DATE _(MM/DD/YYYY)_
_____	_____	_____	__ __ / __ __ / __ __ __ __

Agent #	Agent/Placebo	Dose	Dose Units	Frequency	Date Agent Provided (to Participant) _(MM/DD/YYYY)_	Date Agent Started _(MM/DD/YYYY)_
1					__ __ / __ __ / __ __ __ __	__ __ / __ __ / __ __ __ __
2					__ __ / __ __ / __ __ __ __	__ __ / __ __ / __ __ __ __
3					__ __ / __ __ / __ __ __ __	__ __ / __ __ / __ __ __ __

257

INTERVENTION ADMINISTRATION
(NON-BLINDED STUDY - Agent is known)

INSTITUTION CODE	PARTICIPANT ID	VISIT TYPE	VISIT DATE (MM/DD/YYYY)
_____	_____	_____	__ __ / __ __ / __ __ __ __

Agent #	Agent/Placebo	Dose	Dose Units	Frequency	Date Agent Provided (to Participant) (MM/DD/YYYY)	Date Agent Started (MM/DD/YYYY)
1					__ __ / __ __ / __ __ __ __	__ __ / __ __ / __ __ __ __
2					__ __ / __ __ / __ __ __ __	__ __ / __ __ / __ __ __ __
3					__ __ / __ __ / __ __ __ __	__ __ / __ __ / __ __ __ __

INTERVENTION ADMINISTRATION
(OTHER MODALITIES)

INSTITUTION CODE	PARTICIPANT ID	VISIT TYPE	VISIT DATE *(MM/DD/YYYY)*
____	____	____	__/__/__

Intervention #	Intervention Type (surgery, radiation, active surveillance, etc.)	Intervention Name	Intervention Dose (if applicable)	Dose Units (if applicable)	Start Date (MM/DD/YYYY)	End Date (MM/DD/YYYY)	Duration	Duration Units
1					__/__/____	__/__/____		
2					__/__/____	__/__/____		
3					__/__/____	__/__/____		

259

BASELINE MEDICAL/SURGICAL HISTORY

INSTITUTION CODE	PARTICIPANT ID	VISIT TYPE	VISIT DATE (MM/DD/YYYY)
_____	_____	_____	___ ___ / ___ ___ / ___ ___ ___ ___

Check here if <u>all</u> body systems are normal: ☐

Body System	Normal	Abnormal	Not Assessed	Comments (Required if Abnormal; provide condition/diagnosis)
H/E/E/N/T	☐	☐	☐	
Neck	☐	☐	☐	
Respiratory	☐	☐	☐	
Cardiovascular	☐	☐	☐	
Gastrointestinal	☐	☐	☐	
Musculoskeletal	☐	☐	☐	
Dermatologic	☐	☐	☐	
Hematopoietic/Lymph	☐	☐	☐	
Endocrine/Metabolic	☐	☐	☐	
Genitourinary	☐	☐	☐	
Breasts	☐	☐	☐	
Neurologic	☐	☐	☐	

Does the participant have any allergies?　　☐ Yes　　☐ No

If Yes, specify: _____

BASELINE MEDICAL/SURGICAL HISTORY (continued)

INSTITUTION CODE	PARTICIPANT ID	VISIT TYPE	VISIT DATE (MM/DD/YYYY)
_____	_____	_____	__ __ / __ __ / __ __ __ __

Specify Other Body System/Site	Normal	Abnormal	Comments (Required if Abnormal; provide condition/diagnosis)
	☐	☐	
	☐	☐	
	☐	☐	
	☐	☐	
	☐	☐	
	☐	☐	
	☐	☐	
	☐	☐	
	☐	☐	
	☐	☐	
	☐	☐	
	☐	☐	

BASELINE SYMPTOMS

INSTITUTION CODE	PARTICIPANT ID	VISIT TYPE	VISIT DATE (MM/DD/YYYY)
_____	_____	_____	__ __ / __ __ / __ __ __ __

Check here if none reported (no baseline symptoms): ☐

Symptom Description	Onset Date (MM/DD/YYYY)	Grade*	Comments
	__ __ / __ __ / __ __ __ __		
	__ __ / __ __ / __ __ __ __		
	__ __ / __ __ / __ __ __ __		
	__ __ / __ __ / __ __ __ __		
	__ __ / __ __ / __ __ __ __		
	__ __ / __ __ / __ __ __ __		
	__ __ / __ __ / __ __ __ __		
	__ __ / __ __ / __ __ __ __		
	__ __ / __ __ / __ __ __ __		
	__ __ / __ __ / __ __ __ __		
	__ __ / __ __ / __ __ __ __		
	__ __ / __ __ / __ __ __ __		

*Grade
1 = Mild; 2 = Moderate; 3 = Severe; 4 = Life Threatening

BASELINE SYMPTOMS (continued)

INSTITUTION CODE	PARTICIPANT ID	VISIT TYPE	VISIT DATE (MM/DD/YYYY)
_____	_____	_____	__ __ / __ __ / __ __ __ __

Symptom Description	Onset Date (MM/DD/YYYY)	Grade*	Comments
	__ __ / __ __ / __ __ __ __		
	__ __ / __ __ / __ __ __ __		
	__ __ / __ __ / __ __ __ __		
	__ __ / __ __ / __ __ __ __		
	__ __ / __ __ / __ __ __ __		
	__ __ / __ __ / __ __ __ __		
	__ __ / __ __ / __ __ __ __		
	__ __ / __ __ / __ __ __ __		
	__ __ / __ __ / __ __ __ __		
	__ __ / __ __ / __ __ __ __		
	__ __ / __ __ / __ __ __ __		
	__ __ / __ __ / __ __ __ __		

*Grade
1 = Mild; 2 = Moderate; 3 = Severe; 4 = Life Threatening

PHYSICAL EXAM

INSTITUTION CODE	PARTICIPANT ID	VISIT TYPE	VISIT DATE (MM/DD/YYYY)
_____	_____	_____	__ __ / __ __ / __ __ __ __

Examination Date *(MM/DD/YYYY)*: __ __ / __ __ / __ __ __ __ ☐ Not Done

Height: __ __ __ . __ __ ☐ cm ☐ Not Obtained ☐ in	Weight: __ __ __ . __ __ ☐ kg ☐ Not Obtained ☐ lb	Temperature: __ __ __ . __ __ ☐ °C ☐ Not Obtained ☐ °F
Pulse Rate: __ __ __ ☐ Not Obtained	Respiration Rate: __ __ __ ☐ Not Obtained	Blood Pressure: __ __ __ / __ __ __ ☐ Not Obtained Systolic (mm Hg) Diastolic (mm Hg)

ECOG Performance Status: ☐ 0 ☐ 1 ☐ 2 ☐ 3 ☐ 4

Check here if NO body systems were examined: ☐

Body System/Site	Normal	Abnormal	Not Examined	Comments (Required if Abnormal; provide condition/diagnosis)
Appearance	☐	☐	☐	
Skin	☐	☐	☐	
H/E/E/N/T	☐	☐	☐	
Thyroid	☐	☐	☐	
Chest	☐	☐	☐	
Lungs	☐	☐	☐	
Breasts	☐	☐	☐	
Heart	☐	☐	☐	
Abdomen	☐	☐	☐	
Musculoskeletal	☐	☐	☐	
Genitalia	☐	☐	☐	
Pelvis	☐	☐	☐	
Rectal	☐	☐	☐	
Prostate	☐	☐	☐	
Vascular	☐	☐	☐	
Neurological	☐	☐	☐	
Lymph Nodes	☐	☐	☐	

PHYSICAL EXAM (continued)

INSTITUTION CODE	PARTICIPANT ID	VISIT TYPE	VISIT DATE (MM/DD/YYYY)
_____	_____	_____	__ __ / __ __ / __ __ __ __

Specify Other Body System/Site	Normal	Abnormal	Comments (Required if Abnormal; provide condition/diagnosis)
	☐	☐	
	☐	☐	
	☐	☐	
	☐	☐	
	☐	☐	
	☐	☐	
	☐	☐	
	☐	☐	
	☐	☐	
	☐	☐	
	☐	☐	
	☐	☐	

TOBACCO USE ASSESSMENT

INSTITUTION CODE	PARTICIPANT ID	VISIT TYPE	VISIT DATE (MM/DD/YYYY)
_____	_____	_____	__ __ / __ __ / __ __ __ __

Have you smoked 100 cigarettes or more during your lifetime?	☐ Yes	*(If yes, please complete Sections 1& 2 below)*
	☐ No	*(If no, complete section 2 only)*

Section 1

At what age did you begin smoking regularly?	_____ (Age in years)	☐ Don't know ☐ Never regular
Do you currently smoke cigarettes regularly?	☐ Yes ☐ No	
At what age did you stop smoking cigarettes on a regular basis?	_____ (Age in years)	☐ Don't know ☐ Still smoking
How many years have you been smoking (or did smoke) regularly?	_____ (Years)	☐ Don't know
On the average, about how many cigarettes a day do (or did) you smoke? (1 pack = 20 cigarettes)	_____ (Number of Cigarettes per day)	

Section 2

Have you ever smoked this type of tobacco on a regular basis?	Response	If yes, how many years did you smoke this type of tobacco?	If yes, how many did you usually smoke?	
Non-filtered (plain) cigarettes	☐ Yes ☐ No	_____	_____ per	☐ Day ☐ Week ☐ Month
Filtered cigarettes	☐ Yes ☐ No	_____	_____ per	☐ Day ☐ Week ☐ Month
Low tar cigarettes	☐ Yes ☐ No	_____	_____ per	☐ Day ☐ Week ☐ Month
Pipe	☐ Yes ☐ No	_____	_____ per	☐ Day ☐ Week ☐ Month
Cigar	☐ Yes ☐ No	_____	_____ per	☐ Day ☐ Week ☐ Month

AE AND CONMED EVALUATION FORM

INSTITUTION CODE	PARTICIPANT ID
_____	_____

Visit Type	Visit Date (MM/DD/YYYY)	Were any new or changes in Adverse Events reported? [1] (either the first report of a new AE or changes to previously reported AEs?)		Were any new or changes in Concomitant Medications reported? [2] (either the first report of a new Conmed or changes to previously reported Conmed?)	
Registration /Randomization	___/___/_____ ☐ N/A (visit did not occur)	☐ Yes	☐ No ☐ N/A	☐ Yes ☐ Not Evaluated	☐ No ☐ N/A
Month 1	___/___/_____ ☐ N/A (visit did not occur)	☐ Yes	☐ No ☐ N/A	☐ Yes ☐ Not Evaluated	☐ No ☐ N/A
Month 2	___/___/_____ ☐ N/A (visit did not occur)	☐ Yes	☐ No ☐ N/A	☐ Yes ☐ Not Evaluated	☐ No ☐ N/A
Month 3	___/___/_____ ☐ N/A (visit did not occur)	☐ Yes	☐ No ☐ N/A	☐ Yes ☐ Not Evaluated	☐ No ☐ N/A
Month 4	___/___/_____ ☐ N/A (visit did not occur)	☐ Yes	☐ No ☐ N/A	☐ Yes ☐ Not Evaluated	☐ No ☐ N/A
Month 5	___/___/_____ ☐ N/A (visit did not occur)	☐ Yes	☐ No ☐ N/A	☐ Yes ☐ Not Evaluated	☐ No ☐ N/A
Month 6	___/___/_____ ☐ N/A (visit did not occur)	☐ Yes	☐ No ☐ N/A	☐ Yes ☐ Not Evaluated	☐ No ☐ N/A
Follow up	___/___/_____ ☐ N/A (visit did not occur)	☐ Yes	☐ No ☐ N/A	☐ Yes ☐ Not Evaluated	☐ No ☐ N/A

[1] If Yes is selected; the Adverse Event form must be completed. If No and/or N/A is selected for ALL visits, NONE must be checked on the AE form

[2] If Yes is selected; the Concomitant Medication form must be completed. If No and/or N/A is selected for ALL visits, NONE must be checked on the Concomitant Medications form

CONCOMITANT MEDICATIONS

INSTITUTION CODE	PARTICIPANT ID
_____	_____

At end of study only: check this box if participant did not take any concomitant medications ☐ None

Medication Reported Date (MM/DD/YYYY)	Medication	Dose	Units	Frequency	Reason	Start Date (MM/DD/YYYY)	Stop Date (MM/DD/YYYY)	Continuing
__/__/__						__/__/__	__/__/__	☐
__/__/__						__/__/__	__/__/__	☐
__/__/__						__/__/__	__/__/__	☐
__/__/__						__/__/__	__/__/__	☐
__/__/__						__/__/__	__/__/__	☐
__/__/__						__/__/__	__/__/__	☐
__/__/__						__/__/__	__/__/__	☐
__/__/__						__/__/__	__/__/__	☐
__/__/__						__/__/__	__/__/__	☐
__/__/__						__/__/__	__/__/__	☐

CLINICAL LABORATORY DATA
HEMATOLOGY

INSTITUTION CODE	PARTICIPANT ID	VISIT TYPE	VISIT DATE *(MM/DD/YYYY)*
_____	_____	_____	__ __ / __ __ / __ __ __ __

Date Specimen Collected: __ __ / __ __ / __ __ __ __
(MM/DD/YYYY)

Please indicate results for all completed tests or check the Not Obtained box if a test was not performed. Indicate if test is out of range (as defined by the lab where the specimen was analyzed) and provide the physician's assessment of clinical significance for completed tests only.

Lab Test	Not Obtained	Result	Units	Out of Range Yes	Out of Range No	Clinically Significant Yes	Clinically Significant No	Clinically Significant Unknown	Comments
RBC	☐			☐	☐	☐	☐	☐	
Hemoglobin	☐			☐	☐	☐	☐	☐	
Hematocrit	☐			☐	☐	☐	☐	☐	
Platelets	☐			☐	☐	☐	☐	☐	
WBC	☐			☐	☐	☐	☐	☐	
DIFFERENTIAL									
Neutrophils, %	☐		%	☐	☐	☐	☐	☐	
Bands, %	☐		%	☐	☐	☐	☐	☐	
Lymphocytes, %	☐		%	☐	☐	☐	☐	☐	
Monocytes, %	☐		%	☐	☐	☐	☐	☐	
Eosinophils, %	☐		%	☐	☐	☐	☐	☐	
Basophils, %	☐		%	☐	☐	☐	☐	☐	

269

CLINICAL LABORATORY DATA
BLOOD CHEMISTRY

INSTITUTION CODE	PARTICIPANT ID	VISIT TYPE	VISIT DATE (MM/DD/YYYY)
_____	_____	_____	__ __ / __ __ / __ __ __ __

Date Specimen Collected: __ __ / __ __ / __ __ __ __   Fasting: ☐ Yes   ☐ No   ☐ Unknown
(MM/DD/YYYY)

Please indicate results for all completed tests or check the Not Obtained box if a test was not performed. Indicate if test is out of range (as defined by the lab where the specimen was analyzed) and provide the physician's assessment of clinical significance for completed tests only.

Lab Test	Not Obtained	Result	Units	Out of Range		Clinically Significant			Comments
				Yes	No	Yes	No	Unknown	
Sodium	☐			☐	☐	☐	☐	☐	
Potassium	☐			☐	☐	☐	☐	☐	
Chloride	☐			☐	☐	☐	☐	☐	
Bicarbonate	☐			☐	☐	☐	☐	☐	
Creatinine	☐			☐	☐	☐	☐	☐	
Glucose, Serum	☐			☐	☐	☐	☐	☐	
BUN	☐			☐	☐	☐	☐	☐	
Alkaline Phosphatase	☐			☐	☐	☐	☐	☐	
LDH	☐			☐	☐	☐	☐	☐	
SGOT/AST	☐			☐	☐	☐	☐	☐	
SGPT/ALT	☐			☐	☐	☐	☐	☐	
Bilirubin, Total	☐			☐	☐	☐	☐	☐	
Total Protein	☐			☐	☐	☐	☐	☐	
Albumin	☐			☐	☐	☐	☐	☐	
Calcium	☐			☐	☐	☐	☐	☐	
Phosphorus	☐			☐	☐	☐	☐	☐	
Uric Acid	☐			☐	☐	☐	☐	☐	
Cholesterol	☐			☐	☐	☐	☐	☐	
Triglycerides	☐			☐	☐	☐	☐	☐	

CLINICAL LABORATORY DATA
URINE

INSTITUTION CODE	PARTICIPANT ID	VISIT TYPE	VISIT DATE *(MM/DD/YYYY)*
_____	_____	_____	__ __ / __ __ / __ __ __ __

Date Specimen Collected: __ __ / __ __ / __ __ __ __
(MM/DD/YYYY)

Please indicate results for all completed tests or check the Not Obtained box if a test was not performed. Indicate if test is out of range (as defined by the lab where the specimen was analyzed) and provide the physician's assessment of clinical significance for completed tests only.

Lab Test	Not Obtained	Result	Out of Range Yes	Out of Range No	Clinically Significant Yes	Clinically Significant No	Clinically Significant Unknown	Comments
Appearance (include color & transparency)	☐		☐	☐	☐	☐	☐	
pH	☐		☐	☐	☐	☐	☐	
Specific Gravity	☐		☐	☐	☐	☐	☐	
Protein	☐		☐	☐	☐	☐	☐	
Glucose	☐		☐	☐	☐	☐	☐	
Ketones	☐		☐	☐	☐	☐	☐	
Blood	☐		☐	☐	☐	☐	☐	

PREGNANCY SPECIMEN DATA

INSTITUTION CODE	PARTICIPANT ID	VISIT TYPE	VISIT DATE (MM/DD/YYYY)
_____	_____	_____	__ __ / __ __ / __ __ __ __

If "participant is male" or "participant is female and not of childbearing potential" and pregnancy specimen data was NOT COLLECTED please select the corresponding check-box below.

Otherwise, if participant is female and is of childbearing potential, please complete the form by indicating results for all completed tests or check the "Not Obtained box" if a test was not performed.

Reason pregnancy data was not collected:
- ☐ Participant is male
- ☐ Participant is female and not of childbearing potential

Lab Test	Pregnancy Test Type	Result	Date Specimen Collected (MM/DD/YYYY)
Pregnancy	☐ Urine ☐ Serum	☐ Not Obtained ☐ Positive ☐ Negative	__ __ / __ __ / __ __ __ __

OUTCOME OF PREGNANCY

INSTITUTION CODE	PARTICIPANT ID	VISIT TYPE	VISIT DATE
			_ _ / _ _ / _ _ _ _
			(MM/DD/YYYY)

Pregnancy Test Date: _ _ / _ _ / _ _ _ _   Delivery Date: _ _ / _ _ / _ _ _ _
  (MM/DD/YYYY)   *(MM/DD/YYYY)*

Delivery Type: ☐ Vaginal   Reason for Cesarean: _____
  ☐ Cesarean

Neonate(s)

Gender	Weight (kg)	Length (cm)	One minute Apgar Score	Five minute Apgar Score	Was an abnormality discovered when neonate was assessed?	Specify abnormality	Contributing Factors	Pregnancy Outcome
☐ Male ☐ Female ☐ Unknown	_ _ . _ _	_ _ . _			☐ Yes* ☐ No			☐ Full Term Live Birth ☐ Induced/Elective Abortion ☐ Miscarriage/Spontaneous Abortion* ☐ Neonatal Death* ☐ Preterm Live Birth ☐ Weeks Gestation ___ ☐ Stillbirth*
☐ Male ☐ Female ☐ Unknown	_ _ . _ _	_ _ . _			☐ Yes* ☐ No			☐ Full Term Live Birth ☐ Induced/Elective Abortion ☐ Miscarriage/Spontaneous Abortion* ☐ Neonatal Death* ☐ Preterm Live Birth ☐ Weeks Gestation ___ ☐ Stillbirth*

* Complete SAE Report Form

Obstetric History (check all that apply)	
☐ Gravida	Total number of pregnancies including current: ___
☐ Para	Total number of pregnancies resulting in live births: ___ Total number of stillbirths ___
☐ Abortus	Total number of miscarriages: ___ Total number of therapeutic abortions: ___

CLINICAL LABORATORY DATA
OTHER LAB TESTS

INSTITUTION CODE	PARTICIPANT ID	VISIT TYPE	VISIT DATE (MM/DD/YYYY)
_____	_____	_____	__ __ / __ __ / __ __ __ __

Date Specimen Collected: __ __ / __ __ / __ __ __ __   Fasting: ☐ Yes ☐ No ☐ Unknown
(MM/DD/YYYY)

Please indicate the test name and results for all other completed tests. Indicate if test is out of range (as defined by the lab where specimen was analyzed) and provide the physician's assessment of clinical significance.

Lab Test	Result	Units	Out of Range Yes	Out of Range No	Clinically Significant Yes	Clinically Significant No	Clinically Significant Unknown	Comments
			☐	☐	☐	☐	☐	
			☐	☐	☐	☐	☐	
			☐	☐	☐	☐	☐	
			☐	☐	☐	☐	☐	
			☐	☐	☐	☐	☐	
			☐	☐	☐	☐	☐	
			☐	☐	☐	☐	☐	
			☐	☐	☐	☐	☐	
			☐	☐	☐	☐	☐	
			☐	☐	☐	☐	☐	
			☐	☐	☐	☐	☐	
			☐	☐	☐	☐	☐	

PARTICIPANT CONTACT FORM

INSTITUTION CODE	PARTICIPANT ID	VISIT TYPE	DATE OF CONTACT
			(MM/DD/YYYY)
_____	_____	_____	___ / ___ / ___

Contact Type:
- ☐ Home Phone
- ☐ Work Phone
- ☐ Home Cell
- ☐ Work Cell
- ☐ Email
- ☐ Work Email
- ☐ Regular Mail

Contact Time _____ : _____
(hr:mm per 24 hour clock)
☐ Unknown

Contact Result:
- ☐ Spoke to Patient/Participant
- ☐ Spoke to family member
- ☐ Spoke to friend
- ☐ Left voicemail message
- ☐ Email contact with Patient/Participant
- ☐ Mail contact with Patient/Participant
- ☐ No contact made   (End this form; do not complete remaining questions)

Did the participant report any symptoms or adverse events?
- ☐ Yes   (Complete AE CRF)
- ☐ No
- ☐ Too early to evaluate

Were any changes in concomitant medications reported?
[Either new medications started or previous medications stopped]?
- ☐ Yes   (Complete Con Med CRF)
- ☐ No
- ☐ N/A

Is the participant compliant with protocol intervention per telephone conversation or email?
- ☐ Yes
- ☐ No
- ☐ Unknown

275

COMPLIANCE

INSTITUTION CODE	PARTICIPANT ID	VISIT TYPE	VISIT DATE *(MM/DD/YYYY)*
_____	_____	_____	___ / ___ / _____

First Dose taken this period *(MM/DD/YYYY)*: ___ / ___ / _____

Last Dose taken this period *(MM/DD/YYYY)*: ___ / ___ / _____

Was agent interrupted during this period? ☐ Yes ☐ No ☐ N/A

If Yes, indicate number of interruptions this period: _____

Was agent regimen modified during this period? ☐ Yes ☐ No ☐ N/A

(If Yes is selected for either question, complete Agent Interruption/Modification form)

Amount of agent provided at last visit: _____ ☐ N/A

Amount of agent returned this visit: _____

Amount of agent taken during this period: _____

Amount of agent missing/not accounted for this period: _____

Is the participant compliant with protocol intervention? ☐ Yes ☐ No ☐ Unknown

If No, specify reason for noncompliance: _____

_____

Was agent provided at this visit? ☐ Yes ☐ No ☐ N/A

Amount of agent provided at this visit: _____

AGENT INTERRUPTION / MODIFICATION FORM

INSTITUTION CODE	PARTICIPANT ID	VISIT TYPE	VISIT DATE *(MM/DD/YYYY)*
			__/__/__

Agent Interruptions:

Interruption Number	Specify Date Stopped *(MM/DD/YYYY)*	Reason Stopped	Specify Reason Stopped	Was Agent Restarted?	If Yes, specify date restarted *(MM/DD/YYYY)*	Specify Reason Restarted
1	__/__/__	☐ Investigator decision, specify ☐ Participant decision, specify ☐ AE/SAE, specify ☐ Other, specify		☐ Yes ☐ No ☐ N/A	__/__/__	☐ Investigator decision ☐ Participant decision
2	__/__/__	☐ Investigator decision, specify ☐ Participant decision, specify ☐ AE/SAE, specify ☐ Other, specify		☐ Yes ☐ No ☐ N/A	__/__/__	☐ Investigator decision ☐ Participant decision
3	__/__/__	☐ Investigator decision, specify ☐ Participant decision, specify ☐ AE/SAE, specify ☐ Other, specify		☐ Yes ☐ No ☐ N/A	__/__/__	☐ Investigator decision ☐ Participant decision
4	__/__/__	☐ Investigator decision, specify ☐ Participant decision, specify ☐ AE/SAE, specify ☐ Other, specify		☐ Yes ☐ No ☐ N/A	__/__/__	☐ Investigator decision ☐ Participant decision

Agent Modifications:

Modification Number	Specify Date Modified *(MM/DD/YYYY)*	Specify new regimen:		
		Dose	Units	Frequency
1	__/__/__			
2	__/__/__			
3	__/__/__			
4	__/__/__			

ADVERSE EVENTS

INSTITUTION CODE	PARTICIPANT ID
_____	_____

At end of study only: check this box if participant experienced no adverse events ☐ **None**

Adverse Event Reported Date *(MM/DD/YYYY)*	Adverse Event Verbatim Term	CTCAE Term (v4.0)	Event Onset Date *(MM/DD/YYYY)*	Event End Date *(MM/DD/YYYY)*	Grade	Attribution	Reported as SAE?	Action	Outcome	Dropped due to this AE?	Comments
__/__/____			__/__/____	__/__/____							
__/__/____			__/__/____	__/__/____							
__/__/____			__/__/____	__/__/____							

Grade	Attribution: Relation to Study Agent	Reported as SAE?	Action	Outcome	Dropped due to this AE?
1 = Mild	1 = Unrelated	1 = Yes	1 = Agent Withdrawn 5 = Unknown	1 = Resolved 5 = Fatal	1 = Yes
2 = Moderate	2 = Unlikely	2 = No	2 = Agent Dose Reduced 6 = Not Applicable	2 = Resolving 6 = Unknown	2 = No
3 = Severe	3 = Possible		3 = Agent Dose Increased	3 = Not Resolved	
4 = Life Threatening	4 = Probable		4 = Agent Dose Not Changed	4 = Resolved with sequelae	
5 = Death	5 = Definite				

OFF STUDY*

INSTITUTION CODE	PARTICIPANT ID	FORM DATE (MM/DD/YYYY)
_____	_____	__ __ / __ __ / __ __ __ __

Date On Follow-up: __ __ / __ __ / __ __ __ __
(MM/DD/YYYY)
☐ Not Applicable

Date Off Follow-up: __ __ / __ __ / __ __ __ __
(MM/DD/YYYY)
☐ Not Applicable

Date Off Study: __ __ / __ __ / __ __ __ __
(MM/DD/YYYY)

Date of Last Contact: __ __ / __ __ / __ __ __ __
(MM/DD/YYYY)

Date Last Study Agent Taken: __ __ / __ __ / __ __ __ __
(MM/DD/YYYY)
☐ Not Applicable

Reason Off Study   (Please mark only the primary reason. Reasons **other than Completed Study** require explanation below)

☐ Completed study

☐ Ineligible

☐ AE/SAE **(complete AE CRF & SAE form, if applicable)**

☐ Lost to follow-up

☐ Non-compliant participant

☐ Concomitant medication

☐ Medical contraindication

☐ Pregnancy

☐ Withdraw consent

☐ Death **(complete Death Report CRF & SAE form)**

☐ Other

Reason Explanation: _____

_____

*This form must be completed for all participants that have signed an informed consent, including screen failures.

279

DEATH REPORT

INSTITUTION CODE	PARTICIPANT ID	FORM DATE *(MM/DD/YYYY)*
_____	_____	___ ___ / ___ ___ / ___ ___ ___ ___

Date of Death *(MM/DD/YYYY)*: ___ ___ / ___ ___ / ___ ___ ___ ___

Place of Death:

☐ Hospital (Submit discharge summary to NCI, DCP)

☐ Other, specify: _____

☐ Unknown

Cause of Death:

☐ AE/SAE

☐ Other, specify: _____

☐ Unknown

Autopsy performed?　　☐ Yes (Submit autopsy report to NCI, DCP when available)

☐ No

☐ Unknown

SPECIMEN ACQUISITION
BLOOD

INSTITUTION CODE	PARTICIPANT ID	VISIT TYPE	VISIT DATE (MM/DD/YYYY)
_____	_____	_____	__ / __ / __

Pre-agent Administration

Specimen #	Not Obtained	Date Specimen Collected (MM/DD/YYYY)	Time Specimen Collected (hr:mm per 24 hour clock)	Storage Temperature (Centigrade)	Date Specimen Shipped (MM/DD/YYYY)
	☐	__ / __ / __	__ : __		__ / __ / __
	☐	__ / __ / __	__ : __		__ / __ / __

Post-agent Administration

Specimen #	Not Obtained	Date Specimen Collected (MM/DD/YYYY)	Time Specimen Collected (hr:mm per 24 hour clock)	Date Last Study Agent Taken (MM/DD/YYYY)	Time Last Study Agent Taken (hr:mm per 24 hour clock)	Storage Temperature (Centigrade)	Date Specimen Shipped (MM/DD/YYYY)
	☐	__ / __ / __	__ : __	__ / __ / __	__ : __		__ / __ / __
	☐	__ / __ / __	__ : __	__ / __ / __	__ : __		__ / __ / __
	☐	__ / __ / __	__ : __	__ / __ / __	__ : __		__ / __ / __
	☐	__ / __ / __	__ : __	__ / __ / __	__ : __		__ / __ / __
	☐	__ / __ / __	__ : __	__ / __ / __	__ : __		__ / __ / __
	☐	__ / __ / __	__ : __	__ / __ / __	__ : __		__ / __ / __
	☐	__ / __ / __	__ : __	__ / __ / __	__ : __		__ / __ / __

SPECIMEN ACQUISITION
URINE

INSTITUTION CODE	PARTICIPANT ID	VISIT TYPE	VISIT DATE (MM/DD/YYYY)
_____	_____	_____	__/__/____

Pre-agent Administration

Specimen #	Not Obtained	Date Specimen Collected (MM/DD/YYYY)	Time Specimen were Collected (hr:mm per 24 hour clock)	Date Last Urine Void (MM/DD/YYYY)	Time Last Urine Void (hr:mm per 24 hour clock)	Urine Volume ml	Storage Temperature (Centigrade)	Date Specimen Shipped (MM/DD/YYYY)
	☐	__/__/____	__:__	__/__/____	__:__			__/__/____
	☐	__/__/____	__:__	__/__/____	__:__			__/__/____

Post-agent Administration

Specimen #	Not Obtained	Date Specimen Collected (MM/DD/YYYY)	Time Specimen were Collected (hr:mm per 24 hour clock)	Date Last Study Agent Taken (MM/DD/YYYY)	Time Last Study Agent Taken (hr:mm per 24 hour clock)	Date Last Urine Void (MM/DD/YYYY)	Time Last Urine Void (hr:mm per 24 hour clock)	Urine Volume ml	Storage Temperature (Centigrade)	Date Specimen Shipped (MM/DD/YYYY)
	☐	__/__/____	__:__	__/__/____	__:__	__/__/____	__:__			__/__/____
	☐	__/__/____	__:__	__/__/____	__:__	__/__/____	__:__			__/__/____
	☐	__/__/____	__:__	__/__/____	__:__	__/__/____	__:__			__/__/____
	☐	__/__/____	__:__	__/__/____	__:__	__/__/____	__:__			__/__/____
	☐	__/__/____	__:__	__/__/____	__:__	__/__/____	__:__			__/__/____
	☐	__/__/____	__:__	__/__/____	__:__	__/__/____	__:__			__/__/____

SPECIMEN ACQUISITION TISSUE

INSTITUTION CODE	PARTICIPANT ID	VISIT TYPE	VISIT DATE (MM/DD/YYYY)
_____	_____	_____	___ / ___ / ___

Pre-agent Administration

Specimen #	Not Obtained	Tissue Type	Location	Date Specimen Collected (MM/DD/YYYY)	Time Specimen Collected (hr:mm per 24 hour clock) (if unknown report UNK)	Storage Temperature (Centigrade)	Date Specimen Shipped (MM/DD/YYYY)
	☐			___ / ___ / ___	___ : ___		___ / ___ / ___
	☐			___ / ___ / ___	___ : ___		___ / ___ / ___

Post-agent Administration

Specimen #	Not Obtained	Date Specimen Collected (MM/DD/YYYY)	Tissue Type	Location	Time Specimen Collected (hr:mm per 24 hour clock) (if unknown report UNK)	Date Last Study Agent Taken (MM/DD/YYYY)	Time Last Study Agent Taken (hr:mm per 24 hour clock) (if unknown report UNK)	Storage Temperature (Centigrade)	Date Specimen Shipped (MM/DD/YYYY)
	☐	___ / ___ / ___			___ : ___	___ / ___ / ___	___ : ___		___ / ___ / ___
	☐	___ / ___ / ___			___ : ___	___ / ___ / ___	___ : ___		___ / ___ / ___
	☐	___ / ___ / ___			___ : ___	___ / ___ / ___	___ : ___		___ / ___ / ___
	☐	___ / ___ / ___			___ : ___	___ / ___ / ___	___ : ___		___ / ___ / ___
	☐	___ / ___ / ___			___ : ___	___ / ___ / ___	___ : ___		___ / ___ / ___
	☐	___ / ___ / ___			___ : ___	___ / ___ / ___	___ : ___		___ / ___ / ___

PHARMACOKINETICS RESULTS
BLOOD

INSTITUTION CODE	PARTICIPANT ID	VISIT TYPE	VISIT DATE *(MM/DD/YYYY)*
_____	_____	_____	___/___/___

Specimen #	Not Obtained	Date Specimen Collected *(MM/DD/YYYY)*	Time Specimen Collected *(hr:mm per 24 hour clock) (if unknown report UNK)*	Result	Units	Other Result	Date Specimen Analyzed *(MM/DD/YYYY)*
	☐	___/___/___	___:___			☐ Not assayed ☐ Below limit of detection	___/___/___
	☐	___/___/___	___:___			☐ Not assayed ☐ Below limit of detection	___/___/___
	☐	___/___/___	___:___			☐ Not assayed ☐ Below limit of detection	___/___/___
	☐	___/___/___	___:___			☐ Not assayed ☐ Below limit of detection	___/___/___
	☐	___/___/___	___:___			☐ Not assayed ☐ Below limit of detection	___/___/___
	☐	___/___/___	___:___			☐ Not assayed ☐ Below limit of detection	___/___/___
	☐	___/___/___	___:___			☐ Not assayed ☐ Below limit of detection	___/___/___

PHARMACOKINETICS RESULTS
URINE

INSTITUTION CODE	PARTICIPANT ID	VISIT TYPE	VISIT DATE *(MM/DD/YYYY)*
___	___	___	__/__/__

Specimen #	Not Obtained	Date Specimen Collected *(MM/DD/YYYY)*	Time Specimen Collected *(hr:mm per 24 hour clock) (if unknown report UNK)*	Result	Units	Other Result	Date Specimen Analyzed *(MM/DD/YYYY)*
	☐	__/__/__	__:__			☐ Not assayed ☐ Below limit of detection	__/__/__
	☐	__/__/__	__:__			☐ Not assayed ☐ Below limit of detection	__/__/__
	☐	__/__/__	__:__			☐ Not assayed ☐ Below limit of detection	__/__/__
	☐	__/__/__	__:__			☐ Not assayed ☐ Below limit of detection	__/__/__
	☐	__/__/__	__:__			☐ Not assayed ☐ Below limit of detection	__/__/__
	☐	__/__/__	__:__			☐ Not assayed ☐ Below limit of detection	__/__/__
	☐	__/__/__	__:__			☐ Not assayed ☐ Below limit of detection	__/__/__

PHARMACOKINETICS RESULTS
TISSUE

INSTITUTION CODE	PARTICIPANT ID	VISIT TYPE	VISIT DATE
_____	_____	_____	__/__/____ (MM/DD/YYYY)

Specimen #	Not Obtained	Tissue Type	Location	Date Specimen Collected (MM/DD/YYYY)	Time Specimen Collected (hr:mm per 24 hour clock) (if unknown report UNK)	Result	Units	Other Result	Date Specimen Analyzed (MM/DD/YYYY)
	☐			__/__/____	__:__			☐ Not assayed ☐ Below limit of detection	__/__/____
	☐			__/__/____	__:__			☐ Not assayed ☐ Below limit of detection	__/__/____
	☐			__/__/____	__:__			☐ Not assayed ☐ Below limit of detection	__/__/____
	☐			__/__/____	__:__			☐ Not assayed ☐ Below limit of detection	__/__/____
	☐			__/__/____	__:__			☐ Not assayed ☐ Below limit of detection	__/__/____
	☐			__/__/____	__:__			☐ Not assayed ☐ Below limit of detection	__/__/____
	☐			__/__/____	__:__			☐ Not assayed ☐ Below limit of detection	__/__/____

COMMENTS

INSTITUTION CODE	PARTICIPANT ID	VISIT TYPE	VISIT/FORM DATE (MM/DD/YYYY)
_____	_____	_____	___ ___ / ___ ___ / ___ ___ ___ ___

Form Code	Field Name	Comments

FORM CODES:

AE (ADVERSE EVENTS)	EXCL (EXCLUSION CRITERIA)	OFFST (OFF STUDY)	REG (REGISTRATION)
AECMD (AE & CON MED EVALUATION)	INCL (INCLUSION CRITERIA)	OUTPG (OUTCOME OF PREGNANCY)	SCRN (SCREENING)
AGINT (AGENT INTERRUPTION MODIF)	INTAD (INTERVENTION ADMIN)	PE1 (PHYSICAL EXAM PAGE 1)	SPCBL (SPECIMEN ACQUISITION BLOOD)
CNTCT (PARTICIPANT CONTACT FORM)	LABBC (BLOOD CHEMISTRY)	PE2 (PHYSICAL EXAM PAGE 2)	SPCUR (SPECIMEN ACQUISITION URINE)
COMM1 (COMMENTS PAGE 1)	LABHM (HEMATOLOGY)	PKBL (PK BLOOD)	SPCTS (SPECIMEN ACQUISITION TISSUE)
COMM2 (COMMENTS PAGE 2)	LABOT (OTHER LABS)	PKTS (PK TISSUE)	SYMP1 (BASELINE SYMPTOMS PAGE 1)
COMP (COMPLIANCE)	LABUR (URINE)	PKURN (PK URINE)	SYMP2 (BASELINE SYMPTOMS PAGE 2)
CONMD (CONCOMITANT MEDS)	MEDHX1 (MEDICAL HISTORY PAGE 1)	PREG (PREGNANCY SPECIMEN DATA)	TOBAC (TOBACCO USE ASSESSMENT)
DEATH (DEATH REPORT)	MEDHX2 (MEDICAL HISTORY PAGE 2)	RAND (RANDOMIZATION)	VERIF (VERIFICATION)

287

COMMENTS (continued)

INSTITUTION CODE	PARTICIPANT ID	VISIT TYPE	VISIT/FORM DATE (MM/DD/YYYY)
_____	_____	_____	__ __ / __ __ / __ __ __ __

Form Code	Field Name	Comments

FORM CODES:

AE (ADVERSE EVENTS)	EXCL (EXCLUSION CRITERIA)	OFFST (OFF STUDY)	REG (REGISTRATION)
AECMD (AE & CON MED EVALUATION)	INCL (INCLUSION CRITERIA)	OUTPG (OUTCOME OF PREGNANCY)	SCRN (SCREENING)
AGINT (AGENT INTERRUPTION MODIF)	INTAD (INTERVENTION ADMIN)	PE1 (PHYSICAL EXAM PAGE 1)	SPCBL (SPECIMEN ACQUISITION BLOOD)
CNTCT (PARTICIPANT CONTACT FORM)	LABBC (BLOOD CHEMISTRY)	PE2 (PHYSICAL EXAM PAGE 2)	SPCUR (SPECIMEN ACQUISITION URINE)
COMM1 (COMMENTS PAGE 1)	LABHM (HEMATOLOGY)	PKBL (PK BLOOD)	SPCTS (SPECIMEN ACQUISITION TISSUE)
COMM2 (COMMENTS PAGE 2)	LABOT (OTHER LABS)	PKTS (PK TISSUE)	SYMP1 (BASELINE SYMPTOMS PAGE 1)
COMP (COMPLIANCE)	LABUR (URINE)	PKURN (PK URINE)	SYMP2 (BASELINE SYMPTOMS PAGE 2)
CONMD (CONCOMITANT MEDS)	MEDHX1 (MEDICAL HISTORY PAGE 1)	PREG (PREGNANCY SPECIMEN DATA)	TOBAC (TOBACCO USE ASSESSMENT)
DEATH (DEATH REPORT)	MEDHX2 (MEDICAL HISTORY PAGE 2)	RAND (RANDOMIZATION)	VERIF (VERIFICATION)

VERIFICATION

INSTITUTION CODE	PARTICIPANT ID	FORM DATE *(MM/DD/YYYY)*
_____	_____	__ __ / __ __ / __ __ __ __

The Investigator signature on this form should be obtained after ALL the Case Report Forms for this participant have been completed.

"I have reviewed all the Case Report Forms for the above participant and agree that they are accurate and complete."

_____

Investigator's Signature

__ __ / __ __ / __ __ __ __

Date of Investigator's Signature
(MM/DD/YYYY)

_____

Investigator Name (PLEASE PRINT)

Sample Statistical Analysis Plan

APPROVAL SIGN-OFF

<<Protocol Title>>

AUTHOR SIGNATURE

Prepared by: _____   Date:_____

    <<Name>>

    <<Title>>, Biostatistics

APPROVAL SIGNATURES

Approved by: _____   Date:_____

    <<Name>>

    <<Title>>, Biometrics

Approved by: _____   Date:_____

    <<Name>>

    <<Title>>, Clinical Affairs

Approved by: _____   Date:_____

    <<Name>>

    <<Title>>, Regulatory Affairs

Approved by: _____   Date:_____

    <<Name>>

    <<Title>>, Global Pharmacovigilance and Risk Management

STATISTICAL ANALYSIS PLAN

Protocol Title:

Protocol Number:

Sponsor:

Date of SAP:

Version:

TABLE OF CONTENTS

1. INTRODUCTION

Provide general background of study referring to version of specific protocol associated with systems analysis plan (SAP).

2. OBJECTIVES

2.1. Primary Objectives and Endpoints

Copy directly from associated protocol.

2.2. Secondary Objectives and Endpoints

Copy directly from associated protocol.

3. STUDY DESIGN

Copy directly from associated protocol.

4. ABBREVIATIONS AND DEFINITIONS
4.1. Abbreviations

Include in table list of abbreviations used in SAP.

Abbreviation	Description

4.2. Definitions

Provide specific definitions as required.

5. STATISTICAL METHODS
5.1. General Considerations

Describe summary measures, significance level, etc.

5.2. Statistical Tests: Primary and Secondary Endpoints

The null and alternative hypotheses for the primary and secondary endpoints should be specified in this section.

5.3. Sample Size

If appropriate, present sample size calculations including power, treatment effect, significance level, and associated test used for derivation. Include as much detail for future reproducibility.

If calculation of sample size is unconventional, reference(s) or the algorithm should be provided.

5.4. Interim Analysis

Provide details of interim analyses.

5.5. Randomization and Stratification

Provide general randomization procedure.

5.6. Early Termination and Unscheduled Visits

Provide details on how to account for data from unscheduled visits and data from early termination visits.

5.7. Analysis Datasets

Describe analysis datasets to be used.

5.8. Subject Disposition

Describe approach of presenting subject disposition.

5.9. Demographic and Baseline Characteristics

Describe approach for summarizing demographic and baseline characteristics.

5.10. Missing Data

Describe how missing data will be handled.

5.11. Efficacy Analyses

Follow exact same sequence in protocol and describe how each of the endpoints will be analyzed. Describe here or separately handling of multiplicity.

5.11.1. PRIMARY ENDPOINT

5.11.2. SECONDARY ENDPOINTS

5.11.3. EXPLORATORY ENDPOINTS

5.12. Subgroup Analyses

For completeness, describe subgroups that are planned to be analyzed.

5.13. Safety Monitoring Committee

Describe plans for a safety monitoring committee and provide reference, as appropriate, to the charter of the committee.

5.14. Safety and Tolerability Analyses

Some items to include are plans for analyzing: adverse events, laboratory evaluations, and vital signs.

5.14.1. TOLERABILITY

Include this section as needed.

5.14.2. ADVERSE EVENTS

Present approach to presenting adverse events.

5.14.3. DEATHS

State how deaths will be described.

5.14.4. LABORATORY EVALUATIONS

Present plans for how laboratory measurements will be described.

5.14.5. VITAL SIGNS

Present plans for how vital signs will be described.

5.14.6. 12-LEAD ELECTROCARDIOGRAM

Present plans for how 12-lead electrocardiogram will be described.

5.14.7. PHYSICAL EXAMINATION

Present plans for how physical exams will be described.

5.14.8. OTHER (ADD OTHER SECTIONS AS NEEDED)

5.15. Pharmacokinetic and Pharmacodynamic Analyses

Present plans for PK/PD.

6. PLANNED TABLES, LISTINGS AND GRAPHS

Describe all tables, listings, and figures (TLF) that will be included in the clinical study report. Include TLF numbers and titles.

7. REFERENCES

Include all literature references used within the SAP.

8. APPENDICES

Make liberal use of appendices to improve readability of SAP.

Case Report Form Versioning Policy

DIVISION OF CANCER PREVENTION (DCP) POLICY FOR DCP CONSORTIA STUDIES: CASE REPORT FORM VERSIONING POLICY

Policy Statement: Case report forms (CRFs) will be versioned according to the DCP standard for CRF submission used at the time of protocol development. DCP standards are based on the CRF submission format.

PURPOSE:

The purpose of this document is to describe the proper method for updating the version number and/or version date for CRFs developed for DCP Consortia studies and to describe the relation of CRF versioning to protocol versioning.

BACKGROUND:

When the DCP Consortia study development began in 2003–2004, the required protocol template consisted of the protocol, informed consent and several appendices. In October 2005, DCP authored a new protocol template to better support the process of protocol development and submission. This update separated several of the appendices into individual "Additional Study-Related Documents" that include the following:

A. Recruitment and Retention Plan

B. Pharmacokinetic and Biomarker Methods Development Report

C. Case Report Form (CRF) Package

D. Data Management Plan (DMP)

E. Multi-Institutional Monitoring Plan (MIMP)

F. Data and Safety Monitoring Plan (DSMP)

The Consortia protocol template on the DCP website provides a description of the requirements for a complete submission of protocol documents to DCP:
(http://prevention.cancer.gov/clinicaltrials/management/pio/instructions).

A complete CRF package includes the documents listed below. The DCP website should be consulted at the time of CRF submission to ensure compliance with the current requirements for a CRF package.

Attachment #1 – Schedule of Forms*

Attachment #2 – Case Report Forms*

Attachment #3 – Coding Conventions

*Templates for the "Schedule of Forms" (Appendix A of the "CRF Instructions") and "CRFs" are included within the DCP Consortia Additional Study Related Documents Template, Item C. Refer to the URL provided above.

Since the versioning of the CRFs impacts the DCP Oracle Clinical Remote Data Capture (DCP OC-RDC) database, it is important to adhere to the CRF versioning standards specified in the protocol template.

IMPORTANT NOTE:

Regardless of the CRF submission standard utilized, if the study database is activated or is being developed, it is **_imperative_** that the site work closely with the DCP Monitoring Contractor, Westat, to coordinate CRF changes.

Westat uses the version number on the paper CRFs (pCRFs) as the version number for the electronic CRFs (eCRFs). Therefore, when the pCRFs are versioned, Westat will also version the eCRFs in the DCP OC-RDC database as the pCRFs must be keyed to the corresponding eCRF version.

For example, version 1 pCRFs must be keyed to version 1 of the eCRFs. If a new version of the pCRFs has been approved (version 2), coordination with Westat is essential so that the version 2 eCRFs are available for data entry as soon as possible after approval of the version 2 pCRFs. Version 2 pCRFs would, under normal circumstances, never be keyed to version 1 eCRFs.

PROCEDURE:

1. CURRENT STANDARD (DCP Consortia Chemoprevention Protocol Template): CRFs ARE SUBMITTED AS AN ATTACHMENT TO THE <u>CRF PACKAGE</u>:

NOTE: The CRF version number and date are not required to match the protocol version number and date, since this format (initiated in October 2005) does not require the protocol and CRFs to be submitted as a combined document.

a. During the CRF concurrence review process (prior to CRF approval), the consortium developing the CRFs must change the <u>version date</u> to differentiate each CRF submission. The version number and version date must be the same across all <u>CRF pages</u> within the CRF set.

b. If protocol revisions are requested as a result of the concurrence review, but no corresponding revisions to the CRFs are needed, then the CRF version number and date **should not** be changed.

<u>Any change to the CRF version number and date will affect DCP OC-RDC</u>. If the study is active in DCP OC-RDC, database downtime will be required to change the version number on all eCRFs in the database. Therefore, the practice of updating the CRF version number and date, in order to match the protocol version number and date, is strongly discouraged when there are no CRF content changes.

However, if the CRF version number and date are updated, a memo to file must be created to document the version of the eCRFs that will be used with the corresponding version of the pCRFs.

c. If revisions to the CRFs are requested during the concurrence review period (prior to CRF approval) but additional revisions to the protocol are NOT required, then only the <u>version date</u> of the CRF set needs to be updated for the revised CRF submission. This will allow the CRF version number to remain consistent with the protocol version number for easier tracking, although this is not a DCP requirement.

d. If both the protocol <u>AND</u> CRFs require changes as a result of the concurrence review, then BOTH the version number and the version date must be updated within the CRF set.

e. In some rare cases, changes may be implemented within the CRF set that will not affect the DCP OC-RDC database. Regardless of the DCP OC-RDC impact, a new version date should be assigned to any revised CRF submission. After review by the RDC team, if it is confirmed that the CRF changes do not need to be implemented within DCP OC-RDC, the CLO will be asked to draft and submit a memo to file to the DCP Monitoring Contractor, documenting which version of the eCRFs will be used to correspond with the new version of the pCRFs.

2. SUBMISSION STANDARD PRIOR TO OCTOBER 2005 (DCP Consortia Chemoprevention Protocol Template, version 1.0): CRFs INCLUDED AS AN APPENDIX WITHIN THE PROTOCOL:

NOTE: In this previous standard, the CRF version number and date match the protocol version number and date because they were considered one document. Any studies following this previous standard must follow the guidelines provided below.

a. The consortium developing the pCRFs must change the version date for pCRFs that are modified for a study. If the study is active in DCP OC-RDC, changes to the pCRF version information will require database downtime in order to change the version number on all eCRFs. The eCRF version information must match the version information for the pCRF and protocol.

b. The new version of the eCRFs can be developed while there is ongoing data entry to the old eCRF version. The database downtime includes time to test and activate the new version of the eCRFs and retire the old version.

Checklist for Study Close-out

CHECKLIST FOR STUDY CLOSE-OUT

Study Close-out Tasks *	Key Staff Point of Contact	Target Completion Timeline	Status			Comments
1. Draft manuscript submission to the PIO and Medical Monitor	Lead PI		☐ Yes	☐ No	☐ N/A	
2. Last participant off study at all PO sites (and CLO, if applicable)	CLO Site Coordinator		☐ Yes	☐ No	☐ N/A	
3. Submit Study Status Update Form to the PIO	CLO Site Coordinator		☐ Yes	☐ No	☐ N/A	
4. Notify the DCP Help Desk with a projected date for locking the database and sending the data sets to the Study Statistician	CLO Site Coordinator		☐ Yes	☐ No	☐ N/A	Early communication will ensure the target timeline is met.
5. PO data entry complete	PO Site Coordinator		☐ Yes	☐ No	☐ N/A	
6. PO data QA review(s) complete	PO Site Coordinator		☐ Yes	☐ No	☐ N/A	
7. Close-out visits complete at POs	CLO Monitor		☐ Yes	☐ No	☐ N/A	
8. Close-out visit at CLO complete (if applicable)	CLO Site Coordinator		☐ Yes	☐ No	☐ N/A	
9. Study agent returned to DCP drug repository	Site Pharmacist		☐ Yes	☐ No	☐ N/A	
10. Reconciled drug accountability records	Site Pharmacist		☐ Yes	☐ No	☐ N/A	
11. Research lab(s) analyses completed; results forwarded to data management staff	Research Lab Investigator(s)		☐ Yes	☐ No	☐ N/A	
12. Endpoint data from research labs uploaded to DCP OC-RDC	CLO Site Coordinator		☐ Yes	☐ No	☐ N/A	

Study Close-out Tasks *	Key Staff Point of Contact	Target Completion Timeline	Status			Comments
13. DCP OC-RDC database cleaned and locked for analysis	CLO Site Coordinator		☐ Yes	☐ No	☐ N/A	
14. DCP OC-RDC data sets delivered to Study Statisticians	CLO Site Coordinator		☐ Yes	☐ No	☐ N/A	
15. Final statistical analyses complete	Statistician		☐ Yes	☐ No	☐ N/A	
16. Medical Monitor agrees to unblind	Medical Monitor		☐ Yes	☐ No	☐ N/A	
17. Study unblinding (if applicable)	Statistician		☐ Yes	☐ No	☐ N/A	
18. Other required data not collected in DCP OC-RDC (biomarker data; individual surveys; etc.) available to DCP	Lead PI		☐ Yes	☐ No	☐ N/A	
19. Final manuscript submission to the PIO & Medical Monitor	Lead PI		☐ Yes	☐ No	☐ N/A	

* The tasks within this checklist are arranged in a logical sequence, though variations among protocols may require rearrangement or an overlap of tasks.

303

CLO: Consortium Lead Organization

DCP: Division of Cancer Prevention

DCP OC-RDC: Division of Cancer Prevention Oracle Clinical – Remote Data Capture

PI: Principal Investigator

PIO: Protocol Information Office

PO: Participating Organization

QA: Quality Assurance

Financial Disclosure Form

| National Cancer Institute, Division of Cancer Prevention (NCI, DCP) |
| FINANCIAL DISCLOSURE FORM |

TO BE COMPLETED BY INVESTIGATOR

The following information concerning _____, who is participating as a clinical investigator in the study:

_____

is submitted in accordance with 21 CFR part 54. Indicate by marking YES or NO if any of the financial interests or arrangements as described below apply to you, your spouse, or dependent children cumulatively. If the information changes during the course of the study or within one year after completion of the study, please notify NCI, DCP.

YES   NO

☐   ☐   Any financial arrangement entered into between the sponsor of the covered study and the clinical investigator involved in the conduct of the covered study, whereby the value of the compensation to the clinical investigator for conducting the study could be influenced by the outcome of the study (For example, compensation that is explicitly greater for a favorable outcome, or compensation to the investigator in the form of an equity interest in the sponsor or in the form of compensation tied to sales of the product, such as a royalty interest.) If yes, please attach details on a separate sheet.

☐   ☐   Any significant payments of other sorts made on or after February 2, 1999, from the sponsor of the covered study, excluding the costs of conducting this or any other clinical studies. This could include payments made to the investigator or institution to support activities that have a cumulative monetary value greater than $25,000 (*i.e.*, a grant to fund ongoing research, compensation in the form of equipment, retainer for ongoing consultation, or honoraria). If yes, please attach details on a separate sheet.

☐   ☐   Any proprietary or financial interest in the product tested in the covered study such as a patent, trademark, copyright, or licensing agreement. If yes, please attach details on a separate sheet.

☐   ☐   Any significant equity interest in the sponsor, defined in 21 CFR 54.2(b), as any ownership interest, stock options, or other financial interest whose value cannot be readily determined through reference to public prices (generally, interests in a nonpublicly traded corporation), or any equity interest in a publicly traded corporation that exceeds $50,000 during the time the clinical investigator is carrying out the study and for one year following completion of the study.

OR ☐   I hereby certify that none of the financial interests or arrangements listed above exist for myself, my spouse, or my dependent children.

Details of the individual's disclosable financial arrangements and interests are attached, along with a description of steps taken to minimize the potential bias of clinical study results by any of the disclosed arrangements or interests.

NAME	TITLE
FIRM/ORGANIZATION	
SIGNATURE	Date *(mm/dd/yyyy)*

Note: Page numbers followed by *f* indicate figures, *t* indicate tables and *b* indicate boxes.

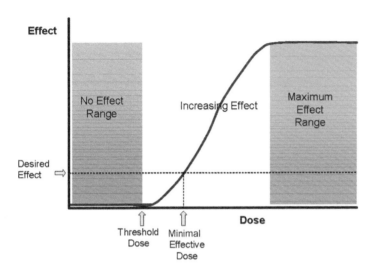

FIGURE 2.1
Dose—response curve.

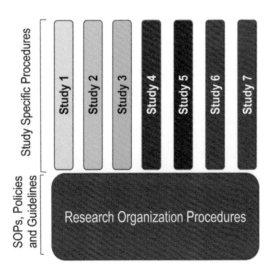

FIGURE 4.1
Standard operating procedures (SOPs), policies, and guidelines are applicable throughout an organization, whereas study-specific procedures provide additional detail to support the implementation of a specific protocol to standardize procedures throughout all the organizations involved in implementing the study.

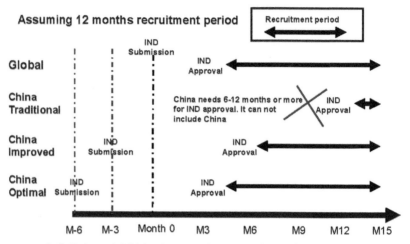

Bradley Marchant, Head of Clinical Development Asia, Pfizer Emerging Markets, IBC Shanghai meeting, April 7. 2010

FIGURE 8.2

How to include China in a global study, by planning early: a practical strategy for investigational new drug (IND) study in China.

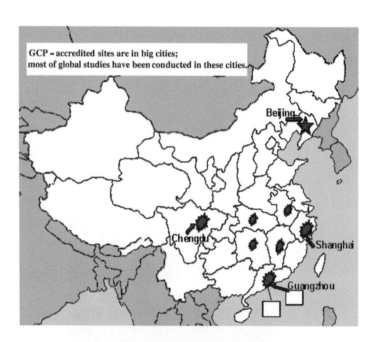

FIGURE 8.3

Main good clinical practice (GCP) sites in China. Most GCP-accredited sites are in big cities; most global studies have been conducted in these cities.

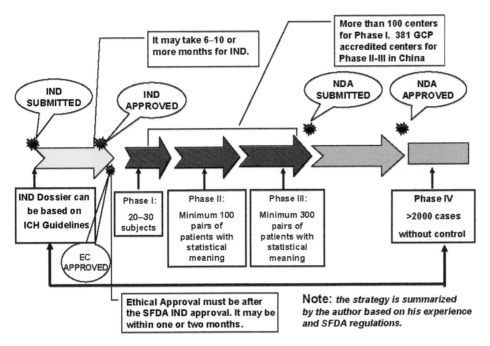

FIGURE 8.6
Investigational new drug strategy (IND) in China (manufacturing drug in China).

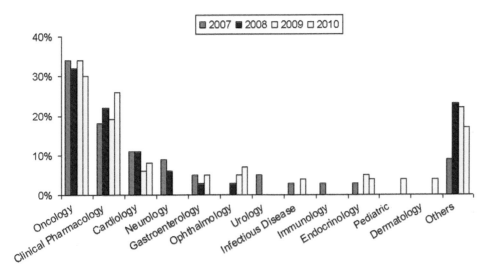

FIGURE 10.1
Percentage of clinical trials by therapeutic area in Singapore, from 2007 to 2010.[7]

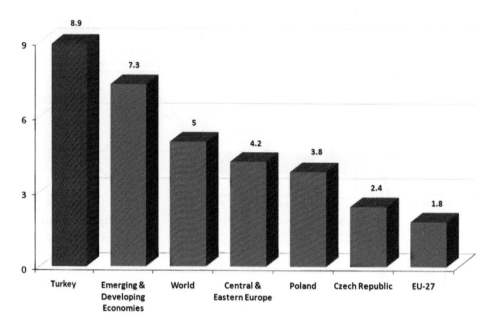

FIGURE 11.1
Real gross domestic product growth (%), 2010.

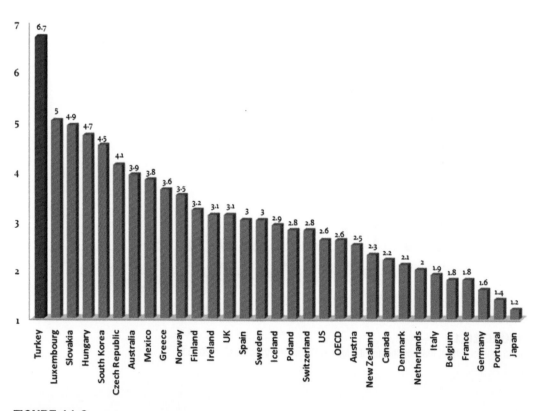

FIGURE 11.2
Annual average real gross domestic product growth (%) forecast in Organisation for Economic Co-operation and Development (OECD) countries, 2011–2017.

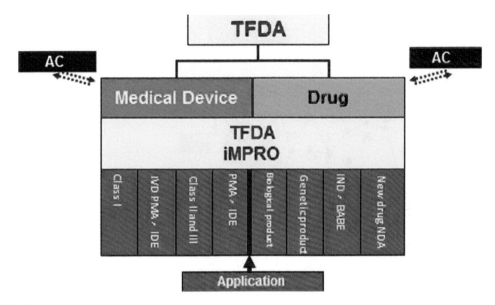

FIGURE 12.1

Excellence in regulatory science: in-house review capacity of the Center for Drug Evaluation/ Taiwan Food and Drug Administration (CDE/TFDA). The Integrated Medicinal Product Review Office (iMPRO) has integrated reviewers and project managers from TFDA and CDE since June 1, 2001. AC: ??; IVD: in vitro diagnostics; PMA: premarket approval; IDE: investigational device exemption; IND: investigational new drug; BABE: bioavailability and bioequivalence; NDA: new drug application.

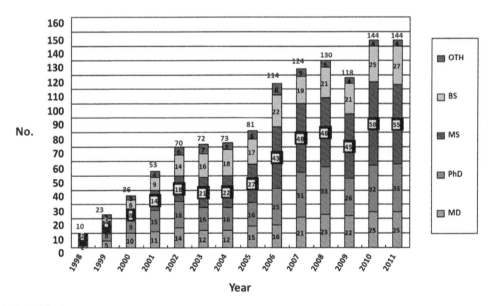

FIGURE 12.2

Full-time employees in the Center for Drug Evaluation (CDE), March 2011.

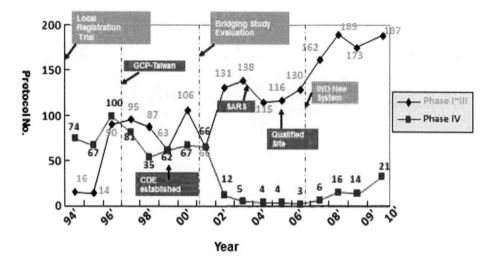

FIGURE 12.3

Built-up regulatory infrastructure: investigational new drugs (INDs) from 1994 to 2010 in Taiwan. GCP: good clinical practice; CDE: Center for Drug Evaluation.

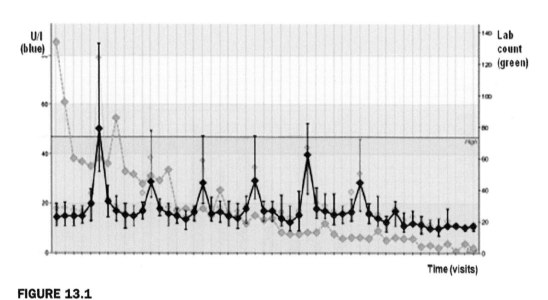

FIGURE 13.1

Ongoing surveillance and trend analysis of liver function tests showing potentially liver-toxic effects in a cyclic dosing scheme. *Source: IMRA—ICON Medical Review Application.*

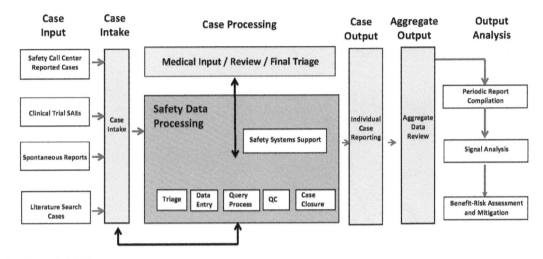

FIGURE 13.2
Summary of the major activities associated with pharmacovigilance. SAE: serious adverse event; QC: quality control.

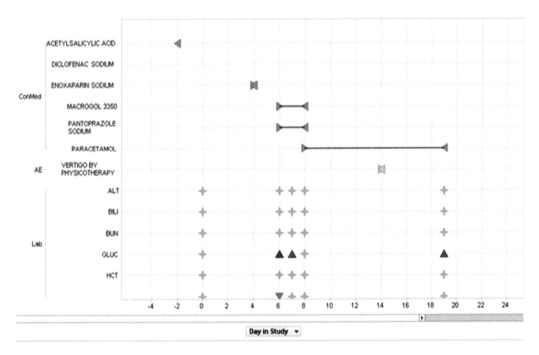

FIGURE 13.7
Subject profile. *Source: TIBCO Spotfire.*

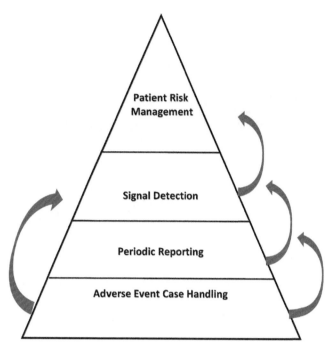

FIGURE 13.9
Pharmacovigilance activity pyramid.

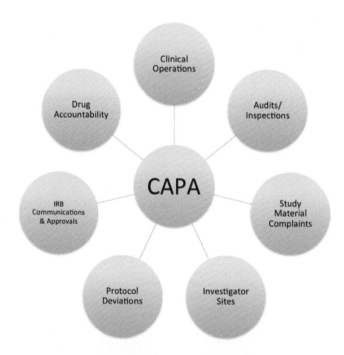

FIGURE 16.1
Sources for deficiencies that could lead to the need for corrective or preventive actions. CAPA: Corrective Action and Preventive Action; IRB: Institutional Review Board.

Printed and bound by CPI Group (UK) Ltd, Croydon, CR0 4YY

08/05/2025

01865026-0002